Drugs in Sport

Dr   vith
me   t to
gai   host
cor   into
acc   the
ha   ical
an

•

•   ncy

•   ting

•

•   ent

•

•

W   *ort*
pro   ers,
ath   and
pol

Da   ohn
M

Drugs in Sport

Fourth Edition

Edited by David R. Mottram

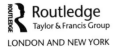

Routledge
Taylor & Francis Group

LONDON AND NEW YORK

First published 1988
Second edition 1996
Third edition 2003
Fourth edition 2005
by Routledge
2 Park Square, Milton Park, Abingdon, Oxon OX14 4RN

Simultaneously published in the USA and Canada
by Routledge
270 Madison Ave, New York, NY10016

Routledge is an imprint of the Taylor & Francis Group

Typeset in 10/12pt Times NR by Graphicraft Limited, Hong Kong
Printed and bound in Great Britain by TJ International Ltd, Padstow, Cornwall

British Library Cataloguing in Publication Data
A catalogue record for this book is available from the British Library

Library of Congress Cataloging in Publication Data
A catalog record has been requested

ISBN 0-415-37563-0 (hbk)
ISBN 0-415-37564-9 (pbk)

Coventry University

This edition of *Drugs in Sport* is dedicated to Alan George, our friend and colleague, who sadly died of cancer in 2004. Alan's contribution to the development of this book has been immeasurable.

Contents

Contributors

David Armstrong
Peter Elliott
Alan George
David Mottram
School of Pharmacy and Chemistry
Liverpool John Moores University
Byrom Street
Liverpool
L3 3AF
UK

Neil Chester
Don MacLaren
Tom Reilly
Centre for Sport and Exercise Sciences
School of Health and Human Sciences
15–21 Webster Street
Liverpool
L3 2ET
UK

Michele Verroken
UK Sport
40 Bernard Street
London
WC1N 1ST
UK

Chapter 1

An introduction to drugs and their use in sport

David R. Mottram

1.1 Definition of a drug

Drugs are chemical substances which, by interaction with biological targets, can alter the biochemical systems of the body. The branch of science investigating drug action is known as pharmacology. These interactions may be mediated through a variety of target tissues within the body. For example, effects on cardiac muscle by drugs such as ephedrine can lead to an increase in the force and rate of beating of the heart; stimulation of nerve endings in the central nervous system by drugs such as amphetamine can produce changes in mood and behaviour; interaction with metabolic processes, with drugs such as insulin, can be used in the treatment of disorders such as diabetes.

In this chapter, frequent reference is made to drugs on the World Anti-Doping Agency (WADA) list of doping classes and methods. The January 2005 version of this list is presented in Table 1.1.

1.2 Classification and description of drug names

Drugs are variously classified and described by their:

* generic name (international non-proprietary name: INN)
* proprietary name (manufacturer's name)
* mechanism of action

The generic name (INN) is the internationally recognized name of the drug and should normally be used when describing the drug.

When a pharmaceutical company first develops a new drug, it patents the drug under a proprietary name. When the patent expires, other pharmaceutical companies may produce the same drug but they give the drug their own proprietary name to distinguish their version of the drug from that of other companies. Examples of the classification and names of drugs subject to restrictions in sport are presented in Table 1.2.

Table 1.1 WADA prohibited classes of substances and prohibited methods – January 2005

| I | Substances and methods prohibited at all times (in- and out-of-competition) |

- S1 Anabolic agents
  1. Anabolic Androgenic Steroids (AAS)
  2. Other Anabolic Agents
- S2 Hormones and related substances
  1. Erythropoietin (EPO)
  2. Growth Hormone (hGH), Insulin-like Growth Factor (IGF-1), Mechano Growth Factors (MGFs)
  3. Gonadotrophins (LH, hCG)
  4. Insulin
  5. Corticotrophins
- S3 β_2-agonists
- S4 Agents with anti-estrogenic activity
- S5 Diuretics and other Masking Agents

- M1 Enhancement of oxygen transfer
- M2 Chemical and physical manipulation
- M3 Gene doping

II Substances and methods prohibited in-competition

- S6 Stimulants
- S7 Narcotics
- S8 Cannabinoids
- S9 Glucocorticosteroids

III Substances prohibited in particular sports
- P1 Alcohol
- P2 Beta Blockers

IV Specified substances

Source: www.wada-ama.org (January 2005).

Table 1.2 Examples of the classification and description of drugs by their names

Class of drug	Generic name	Proprietary names
Androgenic anabolic steroids	Stanozolol Nandrolone	Stromba Deca-Durabolin
Diuretics	Furosamide	Lasix
β_2-Agonists (bronchodilators)	Salbutamol	Ventolin; Aerolin
Narcotic analgesics	Morphine	Oramorph; Sevredol
Beta blockers	Atenolol Propranolol	Tenormin Inderal
Human growth hormone	Somatropin	Genotropin; Humatrope

Table 1.3 Examples of the classification of drugs by their mechanism of action and use

Class of drug	Pharmacological action	Therapeutic use in:
Diuretics	Prevention of reabsorption of water from the kidneys	Heart failure Hypertension
β_2-Agonists	Bronchodilation through stimulation of β_2-adrenoreceptors	Asthma Chronic obstructive pulmonary disease
Aspirin	Inhibition of prostaglandin synthesis	Mild pain Inflammation
	Reduction in platelet adhesion	Thrombotic diseases
Morphine	Agonist on opioid μ receptors	Severe pain
Beta blockers	Antagonists on β-adrenoreceptors	Angina Hypertension Cardiac arrhythmias Anxiety

The mechanism of action describes the pharmacology of the drug and the therapeutic use for which the drug is designed. For example, Table 1.3 lists the mechanism of action of some commonly used drugs in terms of their pharmacological action and the therapeutic uses for which they are prescribed.

1.3   Development of new drugs

Over the centuries, herbalists and apothecaries have experimented with potions derived from plant and animal sources. Indeed, some drugs are still derived from natural sources. For example, the morphine group of drugs is extracted from the fruiting head of the opium poppy (*Papaver somniferum*) and digoxin is derived from the foxglove plant (*Digitalis purpurea*). However, the majority of drugs are produced through chemical synthesis. The pharmaceutical industry is one of the largest and most successful international organizations. Companies are continually striving, through research and development, to produce new drugs. Current research into gene technology is likely to revolutionize the development of new drugs in the future.

The development of new drugs is monitored by government agencies who evaluate data on the activity and safety of new drugs before the company is awarded a product licence. In the USA the agency is the Food and Drug Administration (FDA), in the UK it is the Medicines Control Agency (MCA). Agencies do not always agree, therefore a drug may have a product licence in one country but not in another. The product licence states the therapeutic purpose(s) for which the drug may be used. This, again, may vary from one country to another. The development of new drugs can take between 10 and 12 years and cost several hundred million dollars.

Table 1.4 Examples of dosage forms for drugs used in sport

Generic drug name	Dosage forms
Testosterone (androgenic anabolic steroid)	Oral capsules Intramuscular injection Transdermal patches
Terbutaline (bronchodilator)	Aerosol inhaler Oral tablets Syrup Injection
Hydrocortisone (corticosteroid)	Oral tablets Injection Ear/eye drops Cream/ointment
Pethidine (narcotic analgesic)	Oral tablets Injection
Chorionic gonadotrophin (peptide hormone)	Injection

1.4   Dosage forms for drug delivery to the body

There are many different dosage forms through which drugs can be delivered to particular sites in the body. Examples of dosage forms for drugs subject to restrictions in sport are presented in Table 1.4. The selection of the most appropriate dosage form depends on a number of factors:

1. Speed of action

   - Oral preparations are slow to be absorbed from the gastrointestinal tract. Modified release tablets can slow this process even more, to give a longer duration of action.
   - Injections, particularly intravenous, are very rapid.
   - Aerosol inhalers provide rapid effects on the airways.
   - Transdermal patches provide a slow sustained delivery by absorption through the skin.

2. Site of action

   - Oral and most injection preparations lead to extensive distribution of the drug around the body.
   - Creams/ointments/ear drops/eye drops/aerosol inhalers are each delivered to the site where they are specifically needed.

3. Reduction of side-effects

   - Generally, the more widely distributed the drug is in the body, the greater the chance of side-effects. Therefore, topical administration has advantages over systemic delivery by mouth or by injection.

Table 1.5 Major routes of administration for drugs

Route	Examples of dosage forms
Oral	Tablets, capsules, syrups
Buccal	Lozenges, sublingual (dissolved under the tongue) tablets, buccal sprays
Injections	Intravenous, intramuscular, subcutaneous, intra-articular (into a joint such as the knee)
Topical	Dermatological (creams, ointments, lotions, sprays) Drops (ear, eye, nose)
Inhalation	Aerosols, dry powders
Rectal	Suppositories
Vaginal	Pessaries

1.5 The absorption, distribution, metabolism and elimination of drugs

For a drug to exert its effect it must reach its site of action. This will involve its passage from the site of administration to the cells of the target tissue or organ. The principal factors which can influence this process are absorption, distribution, metabolism and elimination. Consideration of these factors is known as the **pharmacokinetics** of drug action.

Absorption

The absorption of a drug is, in part, dependent upon its route of administration (Table 1.5). Most drugs must enter the bloodstream in order to reach their site of action and the most common route of administration for this purpose is orally, in either liquid or tablet form. Absorption from the gut can be affected by:

- lipid solubility of the drug (strong acids or bases are generally poorly absorbed)
- gastrointestinal motility
- gastrointestinal pH (acidity)
- physicochemical interaction with the contents of the gut (enzymes, food, other drugs)

Where a drug is required to act more rapidly, or is susceptible to breakdown in the gastrointestinal tract, the preferred route of administration is by injection. There are a number of routes through which drugs are injected and the main ones are subcutaneous (under the skin), intramuscular (into a muscle) and intravenous (directly into the bloodstream via a vein).

Many drugs can be applied topically for a localized response. This may take the form of applying a cream, ointment or lotion to an area of skin for treatment of abrasions, lesions, infections or other such dermatological conditions. Topical applications may also involve applying drops to the eye, the ear or the nose. Drugs administered by a topical route are not normally absorbed into the body to the same extent as drugs administered orally. Consequently, the WADA regulations regarding glucocorticosteroids specify that: 'All glucocorticosteroids are prohibited when administered orally, rectally, intravenously or intramuscularly. Their use requires a Therapeutic Use Exemption certificate. Dermatological preparations are not prohibited.'

Distribution

Apart from topical administration, a significant proportion of a drug will reach the bloodstream. Most drugs are then dissolved in the water phase of the blood plasma. Within this phase some of the drug molecules may be bound to proteins and thus may not be freely diffusible out of the plasma. This will affect the amount of drug reaching its target receptors. Plasma protein binding is but one factor in the complicated equation of drug distribution. As a general rule the amount of drug reaching its target tissue is a small proportion of the total drug in the body. Most of the drug remains in solution within the various fluid compartments of the body.

The principal fluid compartments are: the plasma, the interstitial spaces between the cells and the fluid within the cells of the body (intracellular). These compartments are separated by capillary walls and cell membranes, respectively. Therefore, drugs which can pass through the capillary wall but are unable to cross cell membranes are distributed in the extracellular space and those drugs which permeate all membranes are found within the total body water.

Very few molecules, with the exception of proteins, are unable to cross capillary walls; hence, most drugs, except those which extensively bind to plasma protein, can be found outside the plasma. For a drug to be able to penetrate cell membranes it must be lipid soluble as well as water soluble. The majority of drugs are lipid soluble and are therefore widely distributed throughout the total body water. Drugs which are not lipid soluble are unable to penetrate the cells of the gastrointestinal tract and are therefore poorly absorbed orally. Such drugs must be administered by injection.

An additional obstruction to the passage of drugs occurs at the 'blood–brain barrier' which comprises a layer of cells which covers the capillary walls of the vessels supplying the brain. This barrier effectively excludes molecules which are poorly lipid soluble. The blood–brain barrier is an important factor to be considered in drug design since a drug's ability to cross this barrier can influence its potential for centrally mediated side-effects.

Metabolism

The body has a very efficient system for transforming chemicals into safer molecules which can then be excreted by the various routes of elimination. This process is known as metabolism and many drugs which enter the body undergo metabolic change.

There are several enzyme systems which are responsible for producing metabolic transformations. These enzymes are principally located in the cells of the liver but may also be found in other cells. They produce simple chemical alteration of the drug molecules by processes such as oxidation, reduction, hydrolysis, acetylation and alkylation.

The consequences of drug metabolism may be seen in a number of ways:

1. An active drug is changed into an inactive compound. This is a common metabolic process and is largely responsible for the termination of the activity of a drug.
2. An active drug can be metabolized into another active compound. The metabolite may have the same pharmacological action as the parent drug or it may differ in terms of higher or lower potency or a different pharmacological effect.
3. An active drug can be changed into a toxic metabolite.
4. An inactive drug can be converted into pharmacologically active metabolites. This mechanism can occasionally be used for beneficial purposes where a drug is susceptible to rapid breakdown before it reaches its site of action. In this case a 'prodrug' can be synthesized which is resistant to breakdown, but which will be metabolized to the active drug on arrival at its target tissue.

Generally speaking, the metabolism of drugs results in the conversion of lipid-soluble drugs into more water-soluble metabolites. This change affects distribution, in that less lipid-soluble compounds are unable to penetrate cell membranes. The kidneys are able to excrete water-soluble compounds more readily than lipid-soluble molecules since the latter can be reabsorbed in the kidney tubules and therefore re-enter the plasma.

Metabolism is a very important factor in determining a drug's activity since it can alter the drug's intrinsic activity, its ability to reach its site of action, and its rate of elimination from the body. Many drugs are completely metabolized before being excreted in the urine. **The WADA testing procedures in doping control detect both the parent drug and its metabolite(s), where appropriate.**

Elimination

There are many routes through which drugs can be eliminated from the body:

- kidneys (urine)
- salivary glands (saliva)
- sweat glands (sweat)
- pulmonary epithelium (exhaled gases)
- mammary glands (mammary milk)
- rectum (faeces)

Excretion via the rectum in the faeces may take place either by passage from the blood into the colon or through secretion with the bile.

The most important route for drug excretion, however, is through the kidneys into the urine. Most drugs and their metabolites are small molecules which are water soluble and as such can be easily filtered through the capillaries within the glomeruli of the kidneys. Having been filtered out from the plasma, the molecules may be reabsorbed, to a greater or lesser extent, from the renal tubules. This will depend on their lipid/water partition coefficients, and on whether there is a specific membrane carrier transport system for the particular molecule. The net effect, in all cases, is that a constant fraction of the drug is eliminated at each passage of the blood through the kidney filtration system. The drug and/or its metabolites are then voided with the urine. It is for this reason that **urine sampling is the principal method used in dope testing**. The methods available for detecting drugs and their metabolites are extremely sensitive and capable of determining both the nature and the concentration of the drug/metabolite present.

Peptide hormones, which are synthesized in the body, have produced difficulties with regard to dope testing. At the time of writing, a suitable test for human growth hormone, acceptable to the WADA, had not been implemented, despite significant resources having been invested in developmental research. On the other hand, an accredited testing system for erythropoietin (EPO) was introduced for the first time at the Sydney 2000 Olympic Games. The test comprised both a urine-based and a blood-based test and relied on the fact that EPO, used by athletes, is derived from recombinant DNA technology. This instils subtle differences in the properties of recombinant EPO (rEPO) compared with endogenous EPO, produced by the body. The urine test used electrophoretic techniques to distinguish between rEPO and EPO (Lasne and de Ceaurriz, 2000). The blood test identified characteristic changes in blood cell morphology, induced by rEPO (Parisotto et al., 2001). From 2004, the urine test alone was considered robust enough as a test for EPO.

Pharmacological means have been used in an attempt to mask drug-taking activities. These have included the concomitant use of drugs such as probenecid, whose therapeutic use is in the treatment of gout. Probenecid has also been used for many years in combination with certain antibiotics, as it will delay the excretion of these antibiotics and therefore prolong their antibacterial effect within the body. This property of probenecid has been used by competitors to try to delay the excretion of banned drugs such as anabolic steroids and thereby avoid detection. However, this effect is not absolute and the testing procedures are sophisticated enough to detect minute quantities of drugs in the urine. Probenecid itself has been on the IOC/WADA list of banned substances since 1987.

1.6   Effect of exercise on pharmacokinetics

Under most circumstances exercise does not affect the pharmacokinetics of drug action. During severe or prolonged exercise, blood flow within the body will be altered, with a decrease in blood supply to the gastrointestinal tract and to the kidneys. However, there is little documentary evidence to suggest that such changes significantly affect the pharmacokinetics of the majority of drugs.

1.7   Drugs and their targets

Ideally, a drug should interact with a single target to produce the desired effect within the body. However, all drugs possess varying degrees of side-effects, largely dependent on the extent to which they interact with sites other than their primary target. During their development, drugs undergo a rigorous evaluation in an endeavour to achieve maximum selectivity. The aim of selectivity is to increase the drug's ability to interact with those sites responsible for inducing the desired therapeutic effect whilst reducing the drug's tendency to interact with secondary target sites which are responsible for producing its side-effects.

Drugs can interact with enzymes, carrier molecules and ion channels in cell walls to produce their pharmacological effect. However, the sites through which most drug molecules interact are known as receptors. These receptors are normally specific areas within the structure of cells. They may be located intracellularly but most receptor sites are found on cell membranes. Receptors are present within cells to enable naturally occurring substances, such as neurotransmitters, to induce their biochemical and physiological functions within the body. We exploit the fact that receptors exist, by designing drugs to stimulate (agonists) or block (antagonists) (see section 1.8, below) these receptors and thereby intensify or reduce biochemical processes within the body.

The interaction between a drug (ligand) and a receptor is the first step in a series of events which eventually leads to a biological effect. This process is illustrated in Figure 1.1. The drug-receptor interaction can therefore be thought of as a trigger mechanism. There are many different receptor sites

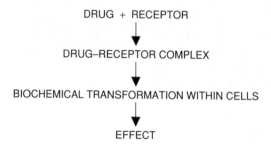

DRUG + RECEPTOR

↓

DRUG–RECEPTOR COMPLEX

↓

BIOCHEMICAL TRANSFORMATION WITHIN CELLS

↓

EFFECT

Figure 1.1 The drug–receptor process.

within the body, each of which possesses its own specific arrangement of recognition sites. Drugs are designed to interact with the recognition sites of particular receptors thereby inducing an effect in the tissue within which the receptors lie. The more closely a drug can fit into its recognition site the greater the triggering response and therefore the greater the potency of the drug on that tissue. In designing drugs it is sometimes necessary to sacrifice some degree of potency on the target receptor site in order to decrease the drug's ability to interact on other receptors. A tendency towards the therapeutic effect and away from side-effects is thereby achieved, thus producing a greater degree of selectivity.

1.8   Agonists and antagonists

A drug which mimics the action of an endogenous biochemical substance (i.e. one which occurs naturally in the body) is said to be an **agonist**. The potency of agonists depends on two parameters:

- **affinity** – the ability to bind to receptors
- **efficacy** – the ability, once bound to the receptor, to initiate changes which lead to effects

Another group of drugs used in therapeutics is known as **antagonists**. They also have the ability to interact with receptor sites but, unlike agonists, do not trigger the series of events leading to a response. Their pharmacological effect is produced by preventing the body's own biochemical agents from interacting with the receptors and therefore inhibiting particular physiological processes.

A typical example of this can be seen with the group of drugs known as the beta blockers. They exert their pharmacological and therapeutic effects by occupying beta receptors without stimulating a response but, by so doing, prevent the neurotransmitter noradrenaline (norepinephrine) and

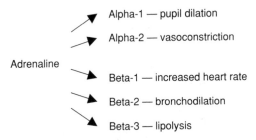

Alpha-1 — pupil dilation

Alpha-2 — vasoconstriction

Adrenaline

Beta-1 — increased heart rate

Beta-2 — bronchodilation

Beta-3 — lipolysis

Figure 1.2 Some physiological effects of adrenaline mediated through the five principal classes of adrenergic receptors.

the hormone adrenaline (epinephrine) from interacting with these receptors. One of the physiological functions mediated by noradrenaline and adrenaline through beta receptors is to increase heart rate in response to exercise or stress, therefore the administration of a beta blocker antagonizes this effect thereby maintaining a lower heart rate under stress conditions.

The principle of drug selectivity applies equally to agonists and antagonists. Research into drug–receptor interactions has led to a greater understanding of receptor structure and function, consequently, the original concepts of receptors have had to be modified. There are now many examples of receptor subclassification allowing for a greater degree of selectivity in drug design.

This can be illustrated by looking at the effect of adrenaline (epinephrine) on adrenergic receptors. We know that there are at least five subclasses of adrenergic receptors, known as alpha-1 (α_1) alpha-2 (α_2) beta-1 (β_1) beta-2 (β_2) and beta-3 (β_3). Adrenaline can interact with all of these receptors producing a variety of physiological effects, some of which are shown in Figure 1.2. The drug called salbutamol was developed to have a selective effect on β_2-receptors. It therefore produces bronchodilation, without the other effects associated with adrenaline. As such it is a first-line drug in the treatment of asthma. The selective nature of salbutamol is recognized by WADA who permit its use in sport (subject to Therapeutic Use Exemption approval) whilst other less selective sympathomimetics are banned.

1.9 Side-effects of drugs

It is important to remember that all drugs, even the most selective, produce side-effects. For patients taking drugs for therapeutic purposes, these side-effects may be deemed acceptable when weighed against the beneficial therapeutic effects of the drug (the risk:benefit ratio). However, no such counterbalance exists for individuals, such as athletes, taking drugs for non-therapeutic purposes. In this case, side-effects can only be perceived as detrimental to health.

Table 1.6 Side-effects associated with some drugs that are commonly misused in sport

Class of drugs	Side-effects
Amphetamines	Restlessness; irritability; tremor; insomnia; cardiac arrhythmias; aggression; addiction (Knopp *et al.*, 1997)
β_2-Agonists	Tremor; tachycardia; cardiac arrhythmias; insomnia; headache (Prather *et al.*, 1995)
Narcotic analgesics	Constipation; respiratory depression; addiction
Anabolic androgenic steroids	Acne; hypertension; mania; depression; aggression; liver and kidney tumours In females: masculinization; cliteromegaly In males: testicular atrophy; gynaecomastasia (Tucker, 1997)
Diuretics	Dehydration; muscular cramp (Caldwell, 1987)
Human growth hormone	In children: gigantism In adults: acromegaly (hypertension; diabetes; muscular weakness; thickening of the skin) (Healy and Russell-Jones, 1997)
Erythropoietin	Flu-like symptoms; hypertension; thromboses (Anon, 1992)

Some side-effects to drugs occur at normal, therapeutic dose levels whilst other side-effects are experienced only at higher dose levels. It should be remembered that, in many instances, athletes are taking drugs in doses far in excess of those required for therapeutic purposes and in so doing increase the risk of experiencing side-effects. Side-effects associated with some of the drugs that are commonly misused in sport are shown in Table 1.6.

Drug toxicity can to a large extent be predictable. The side-effects of drugs are usually well documented as a result of extensive toxicity studies during the development of the drug and from adverse reaction reporting once the drug is on the market. These predictable toxic effects are more pronounced when the drug is taken in overdose. This could occur intentionally (suicide, murder) or accidentally. Accidental overdose may result from children mistaking drugs for sweets; iatrogenic (physician produced) toxicity, resulting from incorrect dosing of patients; patient-induced toxicity when the patient does not comply with the prescribed method of treatment. Accidental toxicity can easily occur with athletes who self-medicate themselves without appreciating the full implications of their actions. The naive philosophy that if one tablet produces a particular desired effect then three tablets must be three times as good frequently prevails in these circumstances.

In addition to predictable toxicity, there are numerous ways in which non-predictable toxicity can occur following the administration of therapeutic or even sub-therapeutic doses of drugs. An example of this is **idiosyncrasy**

where a drug produces an unusual reaction within a
effect is normally genetically determined and is often d
deficiency, resulting in the patient's over-reaction to th
due to their inability to metabolize the drug.

A second type of non-predictable toxicity is **drug aller**
qualitatively altered reaction of the body to a drug. It differs
toxicity to drugs in that the patient will only exhibit the reaction if they have
been previously exposed to the drug or a closely related chemical. This
initial exposure to the drug, or its metabolite, sensitizes the patient by inducing an allergic response. The drug combines with a protein within the body
to produce an antigen, which, in turn, leads to the formation of other proteins called antibodies. This reaction in itself does not induce toxic effects.
However, subsequent exposure to the drug will initiate an antigen–antibody
reaction. This allergic reaction can manifest itself in a variety of ways. An
acute reaction is known as anaphylaxis and normally occurs within one
hour of taking the drug. This response frequently involves the respiratory
and cardiovascular systems and is often fatal. Subacute allergic reactions
usually occur between 1 and 24 hours after the drug is taken and the most
common manifestations involve skin reactions, blood dyscrasias, fever and
dysfunctions of the respiratory, kidney, liver and cardiovascular systems.
Examples of drugs known to produce such allergic responses are aspirin and
some antibiotics including penicillins and cephalosporins.

1.10 Complex drug reactions

Complex reactions may occur during long-term usage of a drug or where
more than one drug is being taken simultaneously.

The dose regime for a drug is chosen with the objective of maintaining a
therapeutic dose level within the body. This regime is determined by two
factors: the potency of the drug, which indicates the concentration required
at each administration and the rate of metabolism and excretion of the
drug, which dictates how frequently the dose has to be taken. If the frequency of administration exceeds the elimination rate of a drug, then **drug
cumulation** occurs, thereby increasing the likelihood of toxicity reactions.
The reason for a slow elimination may be related to a slow metabolism, a
strong tendency to plasma protein binding or an inhibition of excretion such
as occurs in patients with kidney disease.

The opposite response to cumulation is seen in patients with **drug
resistance**. This drug resistance may be genetically inherited or acquired.
The former type of resistance is not common in humans, though it is an
increasing problem in antibacterial therapy where pathogenic microbes can
develop genetic changes in their structure or biochemistry which renders
them resistant to antibiotic drugs. Acquired resistance to drugs, also known
as **tolerance**, can develop with repeated administration of a drug. Where

erance occurs, more drug is needed to produce the same pharmacological response.

A very rapidly developing tolerance is known as **tachyphylaxis** and is seen when a drug is repeatedly administered with a decreasing response to each administration. This is usually caused by a slow rate of detachment of the drug from its receptor sites, so that subsequent doses of the drug are unable to form the drug–receptor complexes which are required to produce an effect. Alternatively the drug may exert its response through the release of an endogenous mediator whose stores become rapidly depleted with consecutive doses of the drug.

There are several instances where the apparent tolerance to drugs cannot be explained in such simple terms and where other factors are evidently involved. A number of drugs acting on the central nervous system, particularly the group known as the narcotic analgesics, produce tolerance which is accompanied by **physical dependence**. This is a state in which an abrupt termination of the administration of the drug produces a series of unpleasant symptoms known as the abstinence syndrome. These symptoms are rapidly reversed after the readministration of the drug. A further manifestation of this problem involves psychogenic dependence in which the drug taker experiences an irreversible craving, or compulsion, to take the drug for pleasure or for relief of discomfort.

Where more than one drug is being taken there is a possibility for a **drug interaction** to occur. Less commonly, drugs may interact with certain foodstuffs, particularly milk products in which the calcium can bind to certain drugs and limit their absorption. The interactions are in the main, well documented (BNF, 2005). Their effects can range from minor toxicity to potential fatality. Such interactions may occur at the site of absorption where one agent may increase or decrease the rate or extent of absorption of the other. Alternatively drug interactions may affect the distribution metabolism or excretion of the interacting drugs. These types of interaction are known as pharmacokinetic drug interactions. A second type is the pharmacodynamic drug interaction where one drug can affect the response of another drug at its site of action. Interactions involving more than one drug that may be misused in sport are shown in Table 1.7.

1.11 Drugs and the law

The manufacture and supply of drugs is subject to legal control. This legislation may vary from country to country but the principles are the same.

The definition of a medicinal product

Medicinal product means any substance which is manufactured, sold, supplied, imported or exported for use in either or both of the following ways:

Table 1.7 Drug interactions between drugs which may be misused in sport

Interacting drugs	Nature of the interaction
Corticosteroids – human growth hormone	The growth promoting effect may be inhibited by corticosteroids
Corticosteroids – diuretics	Corticosteroids antagonize the diuretic effect. Plasma potassium levels may be decreased (hypokalaemia)
Corticosteroids – β_2-stimulants	High doses of these drugs increase the risk of hypokalaemia
Diuretics – beta blockers	Enhanced reduction in blood pressure (hypotension)
Diuretics – NSAIDs*	Diuretics increase the risk of kidney disease (nephrotoxicity) due to NSAIDs
Diuretics – β_2-stimulants	There is an increased risk of hypokalaemia if certain diuretics are taken with β_2-stimulants
NSAIDs* – beta blockers	NSAIDs antagonize the hypotensive effect of beta blockers

* NSAIDs (non-steroidal anti-inflammatory drugs) are not prohibited in sport by WADA, but are used commonly for the treatment of sporting injuries.

- administered to human beings or animals for medicinal purposes
- as an ingredient in the preparation of substances administered to human beings or animals for medicinal purposes

'Medicinal purpose' means any one or more of the following:

- treating or preventing disease
- diagnosing of disease or physiological condition
- contraception
- inducing anaesthesia
- otherwise preventing or interfering with the normal operation of physiological function

Classes of medicinal products

In the UK, as in many countries, there are three classes of medicinal products:

1. General sale list medicines (GSL).
2. Pharmacy medicines (P).
3. Prescription-only medicines (POM).

The law of the country dictates which medicines may be purchased and which can only be obtained through a prescription. In general these laws are similar from country to country, but exceptions do occur. This may tempt

Table 1.8 Drugs present in OTC medicines which are subject to WADA regulations

Drug	Present in certain medicines for:
Ephedrine	Coughs and colds
Methylephedrine	Hay fever
L-Methylamphetamine	
Cathine	
Morphine	Diarrhoea

athletes to travel to abroad, specifically to purchase a drug which is more readily available in another country. Alternatively, some drugs may be, illegally, obtained through internet sources.

Doctors may normally only prescribe drugs or medicines to patients for their licensed therapeutic use. Patients can obtain these **prescription-only medicines** (POMs) from medical practitioners in a hospital, clinic or community practice. Prescriptions are then dispensed by a pharmacist or, in some cases, by a dispensing doctor. Once the prescription has been dispensed, the medicine becomes the property of the patient.

Over-the-counter (OTC) medicines are available for purchase by the general public, without a prescription. These medicines are normally only available from a pharmacy (P medicines) although some medicines, such as aspirin and other analgesics, may be obtained in small pack sizes from other retail outlets (GSL medicines). OTC drugs pose particular problems for athletes, since a number of drugs subject to WADA regulations are available in OTC preparations. Some examples are given in Table 1.8. It is the responsibility of the athlete to ensure that they are not taking a banned substance, therefore advice from a pharmacist should be sought when an OTC medicine is purchased. Some OTC drugs, such as phenylephrine, phenylpropanolamine and pseudoephedrine, were removed from the WADA prohibited list in January 2004. However, they continue to be monitored by WADA in order to detect patterns of misuse in sport (see Chapter 2).

Controlled drugs (CDs), normally those drugs with addictive properties, are subject to further legal restrictions. In most countries CDs include:

*   hallucinogenic drugs (e.g. LSD and marijuana)
*   opiates (narcotic analgesics, e.g. morphine, heroin)
*   amphetamines
*   cocaine

For these drugs, the law states that it is illegal to possess such drugs, except where the user is a registered addict and has obtained their drug legally on prescription.

In some countries anabolic steroids, clenbuterol and some polypeptide hormones are classed as CDs as a further deterrent to their misuse in sport and in body building.

1.12 Nutritional supplements

In an attempt to enhance performance through ergogenic aids, without contravening WADA doping control regulations, many athletes have turned to 'natural' products and nutritional supplements. Unlike therapeutic drugs, nutritional supplements are not required to have strong scientific and clinical evidence that they are effective before being allowed to be sold to the public (Clarkson, 1996). They are not subject to the same independent, scientific scrutiny as that for regulated medicines (Herbert, 1999). Manufacturers may therefore make exaggerated claims regarding the ergogenic properties of their products (Beltz and Doering, 1993). It is a widely held view by athletes that by using such supplements, performance will be enhanced through replacement of the body's biochemical stores or by modification of the processes involved in weight control and energy function.

Nutritional supplements include vitamins, minerals, carbohydrate, protein and various extracts from plant sources. There is a commonly held view that 'natural' products are, by definition, free of toxic side-effects. This is clearly a misconception, particularly when it is remembered that in the early days of pharmacological science all drugs were derived from plant and animal sources and that many of these derivatives are amongst the most toxic chemicals known to man. Indeed, some nutritional supplements have the potential for harm (Beltz and Doering, 1993).

Many of these products are promoted as having ergogenic properties. Such claims are rarely substantiated by sound scientific data in peer-reviewed journals (Nieman and Pedersen, 1999). In recent times, there have been a number of high profile cases involving athletes who have tested positive for the anabolic steroid, nandrolone, where the athlete had claimed that they had ingested the steroid in a 'contaminated' nutritional supplement, an assertion which may be based on truth (Ayotte, 1999).

Whether WADA should revise its doping control regulations, to include nutritional supplements, is debatable (Williams, 1994; Mottram, 1999).

Vitamins

Vitamins are frequently taken by athletes on the supposition that they are experiencing a vitamin deficiency due to exercise and training regimes. However, Cotter (1988) has suggested that there is little evidence to suggest that exercise would necessitate vitamin supplementation.

In terms of using vitamin supplements as ergogenic aids, the B-complex vitamins have been taken because they are co-enzymes in the processes of red blood cell production and in the metabolism of fats and carbohydrates. Vitamin C is reputed to aid in the wound healing process and vitamin E has been claimed to increase aerobic capacity. All these claims for ergogenic properties of vitamins have been discussed by Barone (1988) but, in general, there is little evidence available to substantiate these claims.

Vitamins, taken in excess, are toxic. This applies particularly to the fat-soluble vitamins (A, D, E and K) which are stored in the body and which can therefore accumulate. Even the water-soluble vitamins (B and C) can produce toxic effects when taken in excess (Hecker, 1987).

In general, a balanced diet will provide the necessary nutritional requirements of vitamins. Vitamin supplements are only of benefit where there is a clear deficiency, such as occurs with an exceptional nutritional intake (Wadler and Hainlain, 1989).

Proteins and amino acids

Protein and amino acid supplements are frequently used by athletes, particularly where muscle development is of prime importance. Protein is obviously an essential component of a balanced diet but there is no experimental evidence to show that protein supplementation enhances metabolic activity or leads to increased muscle mass (Wilmore and Freund, 1986; Hecker, 1987).

Excessive intake of protein can produce toxic effects, due to overproduction of urea with a concomitant loss of water, leading to dehydration with a risk to the competitor of muscle cramp and an impairment of body temperature regulation. Manipulation of diet, to induce metabolic acidosis by reducing carbohydrate intake or increasing fat and protein intake, has shown impaired performance (MacLaren, 1997).

The amino acids, arginine and ornithine have been shown to stimulate the release of growth hormone (Bucci, 1989). Such an effect requires intravenous infusion of the amino acids. A similar effect following oral administration of arginine or ornithine has not been established. Furthermore, the literature does not support the idea that growth hormone releasers have an ergogenic effect (Beltz and Doering, 1993).

In general, it is considered that amino acids do not improve endurance performance (Wagenmakers, 1999) and that physically active individuals are advised to obtain necessary amino acids through consumption of natural, high quality protein foods, rather than through supplements (Williams, 1999).

Carbohydrate

Sports drinks, used to replace fluid, carbohydrate and electrolytes are widely used by athletes. During endurance exercise, suitable intake of such products has been shown to be beneficial for glycogen-depleted muscles and to enhance performance (Burke and Read, 1993).

Ginseng

Ginseng is a herbal preparation comprising a complex mixture of glycosides, known as ginsenosides. There are many varieties of plant from which ginsenosides are extracted and multiple preparations within which they are presented. No two preparations will therefore contain the same combination and dose of ginsenosides.

Ginseng has been used for thousands of years, particularly by the Chinese, and many claims have been made as to its therapeutic value. Few scientific experiments have been reported with regard to its performance-enhancing properties. Teves *et al.* (1983) failed to find any statistically significant difference in maximum aerobic capacity, heart rate or time to exhaustion during a comparative controlled trial on a small group of marathon runners.

Several disparate side-effects have been described (Siegel, 1979) as being common with long-term use of ginseng.

Creatine

Creatine is an amino acid present in skeletal muscle. Taking dietary supplements of creatine will add to the whole body creatine pool but the saturation point is soon achieved. Thereafter dietary creatine is simply excreted. Approximately half of the endogenous creatine is in the form of phosphocreatine. The development of muscle fatigue during exercise is associated with the depletion of muscle phosphocreatine stores. This results in an inability to resynthesize ATP at the normal rate, therefore the force of muscle contraction is reduced. Creatine ingestion will not increase the maximal force or power that an individual can produce, but will improve the ability to maintain performance close to maximum as exercise continues. Parallels to the use of creatine have been drawn with carbohydrate loading (Greenhaff, 1993).

Creatine has been the subject of many studies, but results are equivocal as to whether it produces ergogenic effects (Clarkson, 1996; Balsom, 1997; Demant and Rhodes, 1999). There are few reliable scientific data on possible adverse effects of creatine but its potential effect on renal dysfunction and electrolyte imbalance, leading to a predisposition to dehydration and heat-related illness, suggests caution in its use (Kayne, 1999).

Creatine is one of the most widely used legal supplements available to athletes, with an estimated 30 to 50 per cent of professional athletes using it on a regular basis (Puerini and Gorey, 2000).

L-Carnitine

L-Carnitine is synthesized in the kidneys and liver. It can be obtained through the diet from animal sources. L-Carnitine deficiency is extremely rare. It is required for the transport and oxidation of long-chain fatty acids into mitochondria for the production of energy. It is therefore postulated that ingesting more L-carnitine will lead to more fat being burned to supply energy. Athletes have used its supplementation in the diet to promote fat loss and to enhance aerobic and anaerobic capacity (Beltz and Doering, 1993). However, most placebo-controlled trials have failed to demonstrate any improvement in maximal oxygen uptake or in endurance performance in response to oral L-carnitine (Brown, 1993). A review by Cerretelli and Marconi (1990) was unable to show any beneficial effects on performance as a result of L-carnitine supplementation. At the dose ranges used, no reports of toxicity due to L-carnitine were described.

1.13   Why drugs are used in sport

Although there may be many reasons why sportsmen and women use drugs, four main reasons can be identified:

- Legitimate therapeutic use (prescription drug or self-medication).
- Performance continuation (treatment of sports injuries).
- Recreational/social use (legal and illegal).
- Performance enhancement.

In each of the above categories there are drugs which appear in the WADA list of banned substances.

Inevitably, clear distinctions cannot always be made between these uses. It would be easy to say that athletes should avoid taking drugs, for any reason, particularly at the time of a competition. However, there are many circumstances when drug taking is advisable, if not imperative for the general health and well being of the athlete. Therefore it would be prudent for athletes to consider the specific need for taking drugs and the full implications of their action.

There is a heavy reliance upon sophisticated dietary and training programmes to obtain the winning edge. Some so-called vitamin preparations and nutritional supplements may contain banned substances. There is no legal requirement for manufacturers to list all the contents of food supplements. To avoid any potential conflict with the doping regulations, these supplements are best avoided.

Legitimate therapeutic use of drugs

Like any other person, an athlete is liable to suffer from a major or minor illness that requires treatment with drugs. A typical example might involve a bacterial or fungal infection necessitating the use of an antibiotic or antifungal agent. How many sportsmen or women have experienced athlete's foot? Apart from the slight risk of side-effects due to the drug's action, it is difficult to perceive how such a treatment would affect an athlete's performance. A less common but more serious medical condition would be epilepsy or diabetes. Under these circumstances it would be inconceivable for an athlete to consider participating in sport without regular treatment with drugs.

For many minor illnesses, from which we all suffer from time to time, such as coughs, colds, gastrointestinal upsets and hay fever, it is possible to obtain medications without visiting the doctor. There is a wide range of preparations available for the treatment of minor illnesses which can be purchased from a pharmacy without the need for a doctor's prescription. The drugs contained in these over-the-counter (OTC) medications are relatively less potent than those available on prescription. Athletes should carefully scrutinize the label on any medication or substance which is being taken to ensure that a banned substance is not included in the medicine. Examples of such substances include the sympathomimetic amines, ephedrine, methylephedrine, cathine and L-methylamphetamine. Though dose levels are low in OTC medications, the sophisticated methods used for the analysis of urine are perfectly capable of detecting these drugs or their metabolites. The IOC introduced urinary cut-off levels for these OTC drugs in the late 1990s. If these drugs are detected in urine samples, at concentrations below the cut-off levels, the athlete will not be sanctioned.

It is also in the athlete's interest, in the event of visiting a medical practitioner, to discuss the nature of any drug treatment, to avoid the prescribing of prohibited substances wherever possible. As with any medical condition requiring treatment, a decision needs to be taken as to whether the athlete is fit to compete at all.

Performance continuation

Permitted drug treatments to alleviate the symptoms of minor ailments such as sore throats, colds and stomach upsets can be seen as simply allowing the athlete to continue performing during a temporary period of minor ill-health.

Athletes frequently experience injuries involving muscles, ligaments and tendons. Provided that the injury is not too serious, it is common for the athlete to take palliative treatment in the form of analgesic and anti-inflammatory drugs. This enables the athlete to continue to train and even compete during the period of recovery from the injury. The wisdom of such action is perhaps open to question but the use of analgesics under these circumstances is unlikely to confer an unfair advantage.

The doping regulations restrict the type of analgesics which can be used and control the methods of administration for drugs such as corticosteriods. In weighing up the consequences of giving a pain-killing injection, a doctor would probably take into account: the time available before the athlete is in competition and the extent of the injury. In contrast an athlete is more likely

Table 1.9 Drugs used socially or recreationally that are subject to WADA regulations

Drug	WADA regulation
Amphetamines	Prohibited class S6 (stimulants)
Cocaine	Prohibited class S6 (stimulants)
Narcotic analgesics	Prohibited class S7 (narcotics)
Alcohol	Prohibited in particular sports, class P1
Marijuana	Prohibited in particular sports, class S8

to be thinking about the effort which has been expended in reaching this stage, the remaining opportunities, the rewards from sponsors, the acclaim from family and friends, and often the risks of treatment are inadequately reviewed. Certainly, the inappropriate injection of corticosteroids could have deleterious effects on joints (Fredberg, 1997) and systemic complications are not uncommon (Leadbetter, 1990). Even non-steroidal anti-inflammatory drugs (NSAIDs), such as aspirin, though widely used, are liable to produce adverse effects such as gastrointestinal bleeding and ulceration (Weiler, 1992; Leadbetter, 1995). Hertel (1997) has suggested that NSAIDs may not hasten the return of injured athletes back to competition.

Recreational/social use

Many cultures, throughout the ages, have used the drugs listed in Table 1.9 for social and recreational purposes. These substances range from caffeine, a constituent of beverages frequently consumed in many societies, through the generally socially tolerated drugs, such as alcohol and marijuana, to the hard, addictive drugs such as the narcotic analgesics related to heroin and morphine and the psychomotor stimulants such as cocaine. The use of these drugs, particularly in Western cultures, has grown in recent years. This has been reflected in the increasing numbers of positive test results, particularly for marijuana, from WADA accredited laboratories.

Although these drugs may be taken in a social or recreational setting, they are all potential performance-enhancing drugs, hence their subjection to WADA regulations. Amphetamines, cocaine and narcotic analgesics are banned completely. Marijuana is banned in all sports whilst alcohol is prohibited only in certain sports such as archery, modern pentathlon and skiing.

Amphetamines

In the UK, it has been estimated that 10 per cent of 16- to 59-year-olds, rising to 20 per cent of 16- to 29-year-olds have tried amphetamines (Anon, 2000). Amphetamines are used socially to produce alertness and energy. However, they also impair judgement and concentration and heavy use leads to depression and anxiety. There is a risk of addiction with regular use of amphetamine (Knopp *et al.*, 1997).

Cocaine

Cocaine is a powerful stimulant. It is usually inhaled as a powder but a crystalline ('crack') form of cocaine is smoked as a vapour. The complex pharmacology of cocaine leads to a wide spectrum of adverse effects, including a negative effect on glycogenolysis, paranoid psychosis, seizures, hypertension and myocardial toxicity, which could lead to ischaemia, arrhythmias and sudden death, especially following intense exercise (Conlee, 1991; Eichner, 1993). Smoked 'crack' cocaine is more dangerous as the rate of absorption is greater, leading to a more intense effect on the cardiovascular system (Ghaphery, 1995). After regular use, addictive cravings for cocaine can persist for a period of months.

Some bizarre fatalities have been linked to concomitant use of cocaine with alcohol and anabolic steroids, which may have resulted from the production of a novel, cardiotoxic metabolite, norcocaine (Welder and Melchert, 1993).

Caffeine

Perhaps the most widely used social drug is caffeine, which is present in many of the beverages that we consume daily. These include tea, coffee and many soft drinks. At the levels at which caffeine is normally consumed its pharmacological effects are minimal. However, attempts have been made to use caffeine as a doping agent by taking supplements in the form of tablets or injections. Caffeine was on the IOC banned list but was removed by WADA in January 2004. However, it was placed still on the WADA Monitoring List in order to defect patterns of misuse in sport.

Narcotic analgesics

The narcotic analgesics are readily absorbed when taken orally, by injection or by inhalation. They are potent drugs whose effects are primarily on the central nervous system. The discovery of opiate receptors within the brain has helped in the understanding of the mode of action of morphine, heroin and other related narcotic analgesics. They appear to be mimicking the effect of certain endogenous opiates, known as endorphins and enkephalin. They depress certain centres of the brain resulting in reduced powers of concentration, fear and anxiety. Prolonged pain, more so than acute pain, is reduced. Some centres of the brain, such as the vomiting centre and those associated with salivation, sweating and bronchial secretion, are initially stimulated, though they become depressed on continued use of the drugs.

The respiratory and cough centres are depressed. Respiration becomes slow, it deepens and may be periodic in nature. Death as a result of overdose of narcotic analgesics normally occurs through respiratory depression. Characteristic side-effects of narcotic analgesics include constricted pupil size, dry mouth, heaviness of the limbs, skin itchiness, suppression of hunger and constipation. Athletes are in danger of addiction to analgesics as they attempt to mask injury to train or to compete (WHO, 1993).

Narcotic analgesics are renowned for their ability to cause tolerance and dependence in the regular user. Tolerance to the drugs occurs over a period of time and increasing dose levels are needed to produce the same pharmacological effect. Dependence on narcotic analgesics leads to physical withdrawal symptoms. Symptoms normally begin with sweating, yawning and running of the eyes and nose. These are followed by a period of restlessness which leads to insomnia, nausea, vomiting and diarrhoea. This is accompanied by dilation of the pupils, muscular cramp and a 'goose flesh' feeling of the skin commonly referred to as 'cold turkey'. Relief from the physical withdrawal symptoms of narcotic analgesics can be achieved by the readministration of these drugs, hence the difficulty that addicts experience in trying to terminate their dependence on narcotic analgesics. Methadone, a synthetic opiate, is used to treat heroin addiction. Methadone itself has addictive properties and accounts for many deaths through overdose.

Alcohol

Alcohol is the most commonly used drug in Britain, with only 7 per cent of males and 13 per cent of females describing themselves as non-drinkers (Anon, 2000). Though taken for recreational purposes, the effects of alcohol may well be manifested in the field of sport. Some sporting events even take place in an environment where alcohol is freely available both to the spectator and the performer. Alcohol suppresses inhibitions but also impairs judgement and reflexes. Alcoholics risk premature death through cirrhosis of the liver, accidents and suicide.

Marijuana

Marijuana (cannabis) is a drug derived from the hemp plant and which is normally taken by inhalation in the form of a cigarette ('joint') but can be taken orally. The precise mode of action of cannabis is not fully understood but the effects produced are principally euphoria and elation accompanied by a loss of perception of time and space. A single 'joint' can slow reactions for up to 24 hours.

Conflicting opinions exist on the dangers associated with prolonged use of cannabis. There is evidence that short-term recall memory can be impaired and that permanent brain damage may be induced. Marijuana can adversely affect psychomotor functions; these effects may last up to 24 hours following its use (Haupt, 1989).

Although unlikely to be used as a performance-enhancing substance in sport, events in recent years have shown that marijuana is used as part of the lifestyle of many athletes. This was illustrated in the landmark case of the Canadian snowboarder, Ross Rebagliati, who tested positive for marijuana and was stripped of his gold medal at the 1998 Winter Olympic Games in Nagano, only to be re-instated when the IOC and the International Ski Federation realized that they were each operating different rules regarding the banning of marijuana. Apart from the validity of the test result, Ross Rebagliati claimed that the marijuana was present in his body through secondary, passive smoking, not as an attempt at performance enhancement.

Over the years, controls have been introduced in motorized sports and a number of professional sports such as association football and rugby league. Since January 2004, marijuana has been prohibited by WADA in all sports.

Performance enhancement

This particular area of drug use is potentially the most serious threat to the credibility of competitive sport and has become subject to doping control regulations. It concerns the deliberate, illegitimate use of drugs in an attempt to gain an unfair advantage over fellow competitors.

It would be appropriate, at this point, to provide a definition of a performance-enhancing drug. Unfortunately a precise definition is extremely difficult to formulate for a number of reasons.

1. A particular drug which may be considered performance enhancing in one sport may well be deleterious to performance in another sport. Drugs with a sedative action, such as alcohol and beta blockers, would be considered useful in events such as rifle shooting where a reduced heart rate and steady stance are important. However, these drugs would be counterproductive, if not dangerous, in most other sports.
2. Should performance-enhancing drugs be defined by the fact that they are 'synthetic' or 'unnatural' substances to the body? This type of definition would exclude testosterone and other naturally occurring peptide hormones which are used for illicit purposes. 'Blood doping', the method by which competitors store quantities of their own or other blood in a frozen state and re-infuse it prior to competing in an attempt to increase oxygen carrying capacity, would also be excluded by such a definition.
3. Should substances used in special diets, such as vitamin supplements, be classed as performance-enhancing drugs? Certainly other naturally occurring substances, such as creatine and L-carnitine, have been widely used in the expectation that they would enhance performance.

4. Perhaps the greatest difficulty in precisely defining performance-enhancing drugs concerns the prescribing and use of drugs which can be perceived as possessing performance-enhancing properties but which are used for legitimate therapeutic purposes. This problem is readily illustrated when considering athletes who suffer from asthma. One of the most important classes of drugs used for their treatment is the group of bronchodilators, many of which are sympathomimetics and therefore the subject of doping control. Since asthmatic attacks are frequently associated with stress, of which competitive exercise is an extreme case, then this obviously produces severe problems for the asthmatic if they are to avoid transgressing the doping control regulations. Selected bronchodilator sympathomimetics are allowed under doping control regulations.

WADA requires athletes to apply for Therapeutic Use Exemption in cases where a banned substance is required for a legitimate therapeutic purpose.

The issue of performance enhancement is one which will retain media attention at major sporting events. Definitions may actually obscure the fundamental principle as explained by Sir Arthur Porritt, first Chairman of the IOC Medical Commission: 'to define doping is, if not impossible, at best extremely difficult, and yet everyone who takes part in competitive sport or who administers it knows exactly what it means. The definition lies not in words but in integrity of character' (Porritt, 1965). In essence, it encompasses the principle of cheating, defined in the antidoping regulations of individual sports.

The remaining chapters of this book provide a detailed analysis of the substances used for performance enhancement in sport.

1.14 References

Anon (1992) Epoetin. An important advance. *Drug Ther. Bull.*, **30**, 29–32.
Anon (2000) *Drugs: dilemmas, choices and the law*. Joseph Rowntree Foundation, York, England.
Ayotte, C. (1999) Nutritional supplements and doping controls. *New Studies Athlet.*, **14**, 37–42.
Balsom, P.D. (1997) Creatine supplementation in humans. Esteve Foundation Symposium, Vol. 7. *The clinical pharmacology of sport and exercise*. Amsterdam, Excerpta Medica, 167–177.
Barone, S. (1988) Vitamins and athletes. In: *Drugs, athletes and physical performance*. J.A. Thomas (ed.), Plenum, New York, 1–9.
Beltz, S.D. and Doering, P.L. (1993) Efficacy of nutritional supplements used by athletes. *Clin. Pharm.*, **12**, 900–908.
BNF (2005) *British National Formulary. Appendix 1. Drug Interactions*. British Medical Association and Royal Pharmaceutical Society of Great Britain, London.
Brown, M. (1993) Performance enhancement. *Coaching Focus*, **23**, 5–6.

Bucci, L.R. (1989) Nutritional ergogenic aids. In: *Nutrition in exercise and sport.* I. Wolinsky and J.F. Hickson (eds), Boca Raton, Florida, 107–184.

Burke, L.M. and Read, R.S.D. (1993) Dietary supplements in sport. *Sports Med.,* **15**, 43–65.

Caldwell, J.E. (1987) Diuretic therapy and exercise performance. *Sports Med.,* **4**, 290–304.

Cerretelli, P. and Marconi, C. (1990) L-Carnitine supplementation in humans: the effects on physical performance. *Int. J. Sports Med.,* **11**, 1–14.

Clarkson, P.M. (1996) Nutrition for improved sport performance: current issues on ergogenic aids. *Sports Medicine,* **21**, 393–401.

Conlee, R.K. (1991) Amphetamine, caffeine and cocaine. *Perspectives in exercise science and sports medicine.* Brown and Benchmark, New York, 285–328.

Cotter, R. (1988) Nutrition, fluid balance and physical performance. In: *Drugs, athletes and physical performance.* J.A. Thomas (ed.), Plenum, New York, 31–40.

Demant, T.W. and Rhodes, E.C. (1999) Effects of creatine supplementation on exercise performance. *Sports Med.,* **28**, 49–60.

Eichner, E.R. (1993) Ergolytic drugs in medicine and sports. *Amer. J. Med.,* **94**, 205–211.

Fredberg, U. (1997) Local corticosteroid injection in sport: review of literature and guidelines for treatment. *Scand. J. Med. Sci. Sports,* **7**, 131–139.

Ghaphery, N.A. (1995) Performance-enhancing drugs. *Orthop. Clin. North Amer.,* **26**, 433–442.

Greenhaff, P. (1993) Update-creatine ingestion and exercise performance, *Coaching Focus,* **23**, 3–4.

Haupt, H. (1989) Drugs in athletics. *Clin. Sports Med.,* **18 (3)**.

Healy, M.-L. and Russell-Jones, D. (1997) Growth hormone and sport: abuse, potential benefits, and difficulties in detection. *Br. J. Sports Med.,* **31**, 267–268.

Hecker, A.L. (1987) Nutrition and physical performance. In: *Drugs and performance in sports.* R.H. Strauss (ed.), Saunders, Philadelphia, 23–52.

Herbert, D.L. (1999) Recommending or selling nutritional supplements enhances potential legal liability for sports medicine practitioners. *Sports Med. Alert,* **5 (11)**, 91–92.

Hertel, J. (1997) The role of nonsteroidal anti-inflammatory drugs in the treatment of acute soft tissue injury. *J. Athletic Train.,* **32**, 350–358.

Kayne, S. (1999) Creatine: The athlete's wonder supplement? *Pharmaceut. J.,* **263**, 906–908.

Knopp, W.D., Wang, T.W. and Bacch, B.R. Jr. (1997) Ergogenic drugs in sports. *Clin. Sports Med.,* **16**, 375–392.

Lasne, F. and de Ceaurriz, J. (2000) Recombinant erythropoietin in urine. *Nature,* **405**, 635.

Leadbetter, W.B. (1990) Corticosteroid injection therapy in sports injuries. In: *Sports-induced inflammation.* American Academy of Orthopaedic Surgeons, Park Ridge, Illinois, 527–545.

Leadbetter, W.B. (1995) Anti-inflammatory therapy in sports injury. The role of nonsteroidal drugs and corticosteroid injection. *Clin. Sports Med.,* **14**, 353–410.

MacLaren, D.P.M. (1997) Alkalinizers: influence of blood acid–base status on performance. In: *Esteve Foundation Symposium. Vol. 7. The clinical pharmacology of sport and exercise.* Amsterdam, Excerpta Medica, 157–165.

Mottram, D.R. (1999) Banned drugs in sport. Does the IOC list need updating? *Sports Med.*, **27**, 1–10.

Nieman, D.C. and Pedersen, B.K. (1999) Exercise and immune function: recent developments. *Sports Med.*, **27**, 73–80.

Parisotto, R., Wu, M., Ashenden, M.J. *et al.* (2001) Detection of recombinant human erythropoietin abuse in athletes utilizing markers of altered erythropoiesis. *Haematologica*, **86**, 128–137.

Porritt, A. (1965) Doping. *J. Sports Med. Phys. Fitness*, **5**.

Prather, I.D., Brown, D.E., North, P. *et al.* (1995) Clenbuterol: a substitute of anabolic steroids? *Med. Sci. Sports Exerc.*, **27**, 1118–1121.

Puerini, A.J. and Gorey, K. (2000) Sports and drugs in primary care. *Med. Health*, **83**, 169–172.

Siegel, R.K. (1979) Ginseng abuse syndrome: problems with the panacea. *JAMA*, **241**, 1614–1615.

Teves, J.E., Wright, J.E. and Welch, M.J. (1983) Effects of ginseng on repeated bouts of exhaustive exercise. *Med. Sci. Sports Exerc.*, **15**, 162.

Tucker, R. (1997) Abuse of anabolic-androgenic steroids by athletes and bodybuilders: a review. *Pharmaceut. J.*, **259**, 171–179.

Wadler, G.I. and Hainlain, B. (1989) *Drugs and the athlete*. Davis, Philadelphia.

Wagenmakers, A.J.M. (1999) Amino acid supplements to improve athletic performance. *Curr. Opin. Clin. Nutr. Metab. Care*, **2**, 539–544.

Weiler, J.M. (1992) Medical modifiers of sports injury. The use of nonsteroidal anti-inflammatory drugs (NSAIDs) in sports soft-tissue injury. *Clin. Sports Med.*, **11**, 625–644.

Welder, A.A. and Melchert, R.B. (1993) Cardiotoxic effects of cocaine and anabolic-androgenic steroids in the athlete. *J. Pharmacol. Toxicol. Methods*, **29**, 61–68.

Williams, M.H. (1994) The use of nutritional ergogenic aids in sports: is it an ethical issue? *Int. J. Sports Nutr.*, **4**, 120–131.

Williams, M.H. (1999) Facts and fallacies of purported ergogenic amino acid supplements. *Clin. Sports Med.*, **18**, 633–649.

Wilmore, J.H. and Freund, B.J. (1986) Nutritional enhancement of athletic performance. In: *Nutrition and exercise*, M. Winick (ed.), Wiley, New York, 67–97.

World Health Organization (1993) Drug use and sport. Current issues and implications for public health. WHO/PSA/93.3, 1–50.

Chapter 2

Drug use and abuse in sport

Michele Verroken

2.1 Historical perspective

The extensive use of medicinal products for the alleviation of the symptoms of disease can be traced back to the Greek physician, Galen, in the third century BC. Interestingly, it was Galen who reported that ancient Greek athletes used stimulants to enhance their physical performance. At the Ancient Olympic Games, athletes had special diets and were reported to have taken various substances to improve their physical capabilities. The winner of the 200 m sprint at the Olympic Games of 668 BC was said to have used a special diet of dried figs! (Finlay and Plecket, 1976). The Ancient Egyptians used a drink made from the hooves of asses, which had been ground and boiled in oil, then flavoured with rose petals and rose hips, to improve their performance. In Roman times, gladiators used stimulants to maintain energy levels after injury. Similar behaviour by medieval knights has also been noted (Donohoe and Johnson, 1986). In fact throughout history, there are examples that athletes have sought a magic potion to give them that extra edge, to help them take a short cut to achieving a good performance or to enable them to compete under circumstances when otherwise it might not have been possible, such as injury or illness. Today's athletes may simply be following previous traditions.

The use of drugs is not restricted to humans, horses were also found to have been doped. The intention was not always to improve performance, it may have been to 'nobble' the opposition. Doping of horses was prohibited in 1903, however it was not until saliva testing was used effectively in 1910 that horse doping could be proven. Subsequent improvements in technology to identify the vast range of substances prohibited in equestrian sports has led to blood and urine testing being carried out regularly at race meetings and more recently at no notice at stables.

In the nineteenth century, swimmers in the Amsterdam canal races were thought to have used some form of stimulant, as were cyclists in the endurance events. Caffeine, cocaine, strychnine, ether, alcohol and oxygen were reported to have been used alone and in combination (Goldman, 1992).

Probably the first reported drug-related death in sport was the cyclist Arthur Linton in 1896, who was reportedly administered strychnine by his coach. Although later reports suggest that Linton died of typhoid fever, his coach had been banned from the sport, presumably for his part in doping. Another British athlete, Thomas Hicks came close to death after winning the 1904 Olympic Marathon in St Louis USA, following the use of strychnine and brandy. His life was probably saved by the actions of doctors at the finish.

Up to the middle of the nineteenth century, there was little documentary evidence available to substantiate the hypothesis that drugs had been used in sport. Whilst there were no control mechanisms in place in sport, the Dangerous Drugs Act was introduced in 1920 to restrict the availability of cocaine and opium by prescription only. Perhaps the dearth of evidence for the abuse of drugs in sport up to the Second World War is reflective of the paucity of substances available, coupled with their low potency, when compared with the powerful chemicals of today. Around the time of the Second World War, the development of amphetamine-like substances reached a peak. These drugs were administered to combat troops in order to enhance their mental awareness and to delay the onset of fatigue. Not surprisingly, in the 1940s and 1950s, amphetamines became the drugs of choice for athletes, particularly in sports such as cycling, where the stimulant effects were perceived to be beneficial to enhancing sporting performance in sprint and stamina events.

Deaths of sportsmen from amphetamine abuse in the 1960s demonstrated how widespread drug abuse had become. At the 1960 Rome Olympics, the cyclist Knud Jensen died on the opening day of the Games as he competed in the 100 km team time trial. Two team mates were also taken to hospital. The post-mortem revealed traces of amphetamine and nicotinyl nitrate in Jensen's blood. In 1967, the death of the British cyclist Tommy Simpson during the Tour de France was televised across the world. Weeks later, it was revealed that traces of amphetamine, methylamphetamine and cognac were found in Simpson's body. Amphetamine was also found in the pocket of his jersey and his luggage. Two other deaths in cycling and football were recorded in the next year. Further evidence of the increase in amphetamine abuse came from the admission by the British athlete Alan Simpson that he has used them during the 1966 Commonwealth Games.

The phenomenon of drug use in sport must be seen in parallel with two other factors. First, the sixties heralded a more liberal approach to experimentation in drug taking, particularly among the followers of pop music. Second and of far greater significance, a 'pharmacological revolution' began in the 1960s. The search by pharmaceutical companies for more potent, more selective and less toxic drugs resulted in a vast array of powerful agents capable of altering many biochemical, physiological and psychological functions in the body. Not surprisingly some athletes saw, in these chemical agents, a means of enhancing performance beyond anything that they could achieve by hard work and rigorous training. Moreover, it offered a greater menu of choice for athletes to use. Athletes could simply select the most specific drugs to meet their particular needs for improving performance.

Originally athletes used amphetamines and other stimulants, mainly on the day of, or during, performance. There was growing evidence that these drugs might be linked with sudden collapse or death, usually from cardiac or respiratory arrest, particularly during competition, yet the long term side-effects on the body were regarded as minor. By comparison the drugs which emerged in the 1950s among body builders in America and later among athletes and weightlifters, the anabolic steroids, were a different story. These drugs, whilst increasing size and strength in some athletes, also cause significant side-effects. The advantage these drugs offered was their usefulness to an athlete in training, in preparation for a competition. This was especially important in the early days of testing programmes to control the use of drugs. The desire to enhance performance for national prestige and ideological supremacy dominated the sporting world in the 1970s and 1980s. The Stasi files documented the governmentally organized steroid doping of the German Democratic Republic (Franke and Berendonk, 1997); it is possible that other programmes may not have been as well documented or evident.

Drug misuse today has increased in sophistication, athletes are seeking out ways to improve performance using the most advanced technology. The former coach to Ben Johnson, Charlie Francis wrote 'There are thousands of possible synthetic permutations of the testosterone molecule. The great majority of these steroids remain an unexplored frontier . . . private laboratories stand ready to synthesise any number of these steroids – and keep the athletes ahead of the game' (Francis, 1990).

Unfortunately, evidence for the performance-enhancing properties of drugs is sparse. It has not been possible to undertake controlled trials, where drugs could be evaluated on large groups of individuals and compared with a placebo, preferably on a double-blind basis where neither the tester nor the individuals being tested are aware of whether they are taking the drug or the placebo. This approach would have been similar to that adopted by drug companies in order to establish whether new drugs are effective therapeutic agents. Clearly there are logistical and ethical reasons why such trials could not take place. Consequently, much of the rationale behind drug taking in sport is based on hypothetical performance-enhancing properties, speculation, misinformation from 'underground' booklets and sheer ignorance. In addition, little cognizance is taken of the side-effects associated with drugs and the potential adverse effect these may have on performance.

Statistics published by the IOC/WADA accredited laboratories since 1993 (Table 2.1) indicate anabolic steroids are the most frequently detected substance, consistently representing a significant percentage of the total findings.

Percentages of the detection levels of stimulants and anabolic steroids from \DA accredited laboratories 1993–2003

	1993	1994	1995	1996	1997	1998	1999	2000	2001	2002	2003
Stimulants	22.8	24.0	18.9	16.8	17.2	18.9	20.3	18.3	15.4	14.9	19.0
Anabolic steroids	59.9	50.5	47.8	49.6	46.8	39.3	37.1	38.1	40.1	36.8	32.1

Source: IOC/WADA Laboratory Statistics.

2.2 Definition of doping

The origin of the word doping is interesting, *dop* referred to a stimulant drink used in tribal ceremonies in South Africa around the eighteenth century. *Dop* first appeared in an English dictionary in 1889, it was described as a narcotic potion for racehorses to reduce their performance. Contemporary use has extended the definition to include the improvement of performance. As practice has developed, the definition also refers to maintenance of performance and manipulation of the testing procedures by the use of doping classes or methods.

So the word 'doping' is now used to describe not only the misuse of drugs by sportsmen and women, but also the use of other methods of improving performance or of attempting to manipulate the test. This definition is not without controversy. There are many different ways athletes attempt to improve their performance, for example, altitude training, diet, biomechanical analysis and psychological preparation. However, these techniques are generally accepted as a part of an athlete's training and preparation regime.

The doping definition of the IOC is based on the banning of pharmacological classes. Rule 29A of the Olympic Charter states: 'Doping is forbidden. The IOC Medical Commission shall prepare a list of prohibited classes of drugs and of banned procedures.' Further explanation of this approach is given in the introductory paragraph to the published list. 'The definition has the advantage that also new drugs, some of which may be especially designed for doping purposes, are banned'.

This definition demonstrates the concern for the increasing sophistication in chemical technology, as athletes and their scientists seek chemical agents to improve performance but which may not yet be covered by current regulations, a veritable competition between the testing regime and some athletes.

A comparison of initial attempts to define doping illustrates the difficulties of reflecting practice in words. An early definition from the International Amateur Athletic Federation (IAAF) referred to:

The administration of, or use by a competing athlete of any substance foreign to the body or any physiological substance taken in abnormal quantity or taken by an abnormal route of entry into the body with the sole intention of increasing in an artificial and unfair manner his/her performance in competition. When necessity demands medical treatment with any substance which, because of its nature, dosage, or application is able to boost the athlete's performance in competition in an artificial and unfair manner, this too is regarded as doping.

(*IAAF 1982, Rule 144*)

This definition could be challenged on many points; not all substances are foreign to the body, the issue of intention and the link with performance improvement.

Legal challenges have encouraged the progress of a definition of doping and most sports federations have adopted an absolute offence approach. The more recent definition of the IAAF states:

Doping is strictly forbidden and is an offence under IAAF rules. An offence of doping takes place when either

1. a prohibited substance is found to be present within an athlete's body tissue or fluids; or
2. an athlete takes advantage of a prohibited technique; or
3. an athlete admits having used or taken advantage of a prohibited substance or prohibited technique.

(*IAAF Handbook 1992–1993, Rule 55*)

Further explanations refer to metabolites of a prohibited substance and to a more detailed definition of prohibited techniques, including blood doping and use of substances to alter the integrity and validity of urine samples used in doping control. Ancillary offences such as failure or refusal to submit to doping control are indicated, as are assisting or inciting others to use a prohibited substance or technique.

Already the definition has been extended, not only to take account of a move from the analysis of urine to blood or other body tissues, but also to supporting evidence of doping, admission, supply and not submitting to a test. The British Athletic Federation originally tackled the issue of availability for testing by including a regulation about notification of address, if an athlete is absent from the home address for a period of 5 days or longer. This in itself may be regarded as a doping offence, and whilst it seems far removed from the misuse of drugs, it is further evidence of the need to reflect practice in the rules and procedures that control doping in sport. More recently the International Amateur Athletic Federation (now renamed the International Association of Athletic Federations) has reduced the period of absence requiring notification to 3 days.

One of the problems with a definition based upon a list of substances is that not all sports may adopt the same classification. The offence of doping may vary between sports. This situation occurred during the 1988 Tour de France, when the Spanish cyclist Pedro Delgardo tested positive for a substance banned by the IOC. However, because this substance was not banned by the International Cycling Union, no penalty could be imposed. A similar situation arose at the 1998 Nagano Winter Olympics when the Canadian snow boarder Ross Rebagliati tested positive for marijuana. The true construction of the IOC Rules regarded marijuana as a doping offence, however the absence of an agreement between the IOC and the relevant international sports federation about the status of this substance led the Court of Arbitration for Sport to rule that no specific prohibition had been made. (NAG OG/98/002 in Reeb, 1998). The majority of sports have adopted the list of prohibited classes published by the IOC and more recently taken over by the World Anti-Doping Agency (WADA). Differences still exist between the WADA list and the prohibited substances list of some international federations. Whilst the opportunity to create a more sports-specific list would make the testing more relevant, it might also presuppose a link between performance enhancement and the prohibited substances.

The most recent definition comes from the Olympic Movement Anti-Doping Code of 1999, which defines doping as

1. the use of an expedient (substance or method) which is potentially harmful to athletes' health and/or capable of enhancing their performance; or
2. the presence in the athlete's body of a prohibited substance or evidence of the use thereof or evidence of the use of a prohibited method.

This definition sets out clearly the basis for defining doping as a strict liability offence; it is the very presence of a prohibited substance that triggers the disciplinary process. Despite this, there have still been a number of challenges about the performance-enhancing effects of substances detected or the absence of any health consequences for the detection of a substance.

Defining doping as the use of prohibited substances places great emphasis on the role of a drug testing programme to detect banned substances. However, as discussed in the next section, not all banned substances are detectable. Legal challenges have led to more specific explanations within the regulations, including the presence of metabolites, the use of substances to alter the validity or integrity of the urine sample, refusal or failure to submit to doping control, and assisting or inciting others to use a prohibited substance or technique. This extension of the definition of doping to beyond the scientific evidence of substance misuse creates an even greater challenge of bringing sufficient proof.

2.3   A review of the WADA list of doping classes and methods

Doping classes

Since the IOC list of doping classes was first published in 1967, it has evolved gradually to its present form (Table 2.2) which is administered by WADA.

Table 2.2 WADA prohibited substances and prohibited methods – January 2005

I	Substances and methods prohibited at all times (in- and out-of-competition)		
	S1	Anabolic agents	
		1. Anabolic androgenic steroids (AAS)	
		2. Other anabolic agents	
	S2	Hormones and related substances	
		1. Erythropoietin (EPO)	
		2. Growth Hormone (hGH), Insulin-like Growth Factor (IGF-1), Mechano Growth Factors (MGFs)	
		3. Gonadotrophins (LH, hCG)	
		4. Insulin	
		5. Corticotrophins	
	S3	β_2-agonists	
	S4	Agents with anti-estrogenic activity	
	S5	Diuretics and other Masking Agents	
	M1	Enhancement of oxygen transfer	
	M2	Chemical and physical manipulation	
	M3	Gene doping	
II	Substances and methods prohibited in-competition		
	S6	Stimulants	
	S7	Narcotics	
	S8	Cannabinoids	
	S9	Glucocorticosteroids	
III	Substances prohibited in particular sports		
	P1	Alcohol	
	P2	Beta Blockers	
IV	Specified substances		

Source: www.wada-ama.org (January 2005).

The first IOC list included stimulants and narcotic analgesics. Anabolic steroids were first banned in 1974 by the IOC Medical Commission when the technology to detect these substances became available and in response to the concern about potential abuse during training. Although the addition of anabolic steroids to the list recognized their potential for abuse by athletes, testing was based at competitions, so the regime of drug use was not effectively addressed. The introduction of out of competition testing acknowledged the need to control substances both in and out of competition.

A detection method for testosterone was introduced at the 1982 Commonwealth Games in Brisbane. The inclusion of this substance in the IOC list in 1983 was significant as it was the first endogenous or naturally produced steroid to be banned. Up to that time banned substances were foreign to the body. Scientists were faced with the problem of determining limits for the concentration of a natural substance in the body, beyond which it could be determined doping had taken place. Detection of testosterone (T) was based upon a comparison of hormones in the body, luteinizing hormone (LH) secreted by the pituitary gland and epitestosterone (E) secreted by the testes. Originally the ratio for testosterone to epitestosterone (T/E) determination was set at 6:1, however in 1992 the IOC introduced evaluation criteria for T/E ratios above 6 and below 10. If the ratio exceeded 6 to 1, further investigations were recommended, including a review of previous tests, endocrinological investigations and longitudinal testing over several months. A doping offence would be reported, unless it could be determined that the ratio was due to a physiological or pathological condition. A ratio that exceeded 10 would be regarded as a doping offence. Challenges to the acceptability of the IOC specified level have criticized the arbitrary nature of the reporting level set by the IOC, especially as it is an endogenous substance. Confusion about responsibility and precise requirements for an independent medical examination to determine whether a medical condition is responsible for the unusual ratio have caused difficulty in cases where the governing body has been primarily for determining whether a doping offence has occurred.

A quantitative test for the stimulant, caffeine was introduced at the Olympic Games in Sarajevo and Los Angeles in 1984. The concentration level was originally set at 15 micrograms per millilitre (μg/ml). This was reduced to 12 μg/ml in 1988.

In 1985, the IOC added the classes of beta blockers and diuretics to the list. For the first time, the IOC acknowledged the need for greater sports specificity in the application of the doping classes. Supporting information for the class of beta blockers referred to the 'misuse of beta blockers in some sports where physical activity is of no or little importance'. This was unlikely to include endurance events. Some International Federations have adopted the IOC's list but have also taken an opportunity to apply the doping classes more specifically to their sport and set aside the inclusion of all the doping classes. Thus not all sports have included beta blockers and/or diuretics in their regulations. In 1993, the IOC moved beta blockers from the main section of doping classes to the 'Classes of drugs subject to certain restrictions', indicating that they should be tested for only in those sports where they are likely to enhance performance.

Probenecid and other masking agents were added in 1987, together with human chorionic gonadotrophin (hCG). Growth hormone (GH) and other peptide hormones were included in the 1989 list under the new class of peptide hormones. This class also includes corticotrophin (ACTH) and erythropoietin (EPO). The development of recombinant technology has increased the availability of GH in synthetic form. The evolution of the list is clearly indicative of the increasing sophistication of techniques to improve performance and a growing concern to regulate in the absence of unequivocal detection methods. The classifications have also been broadened by the term 'and related compounds' to the list of examples of each class.

Through this route the precursors of nandrolone were captured through tests as a metabolite of the anabolic steroid nandrolone.

Doping methods

Blood doping was banned in 1985 although no detection method existed at that time. Its inclusion came about as a result of admissions of blood doping from long distance runners and latterly from members of the US cycling team. Evidence emerged that US cyclists had received blood transfusions two days prior to the start of the Los Angeles Olympics. A detection method was not available, so early offences of blood doping rested on admissions from athletes. Only recently has the testing procedure in some sports been extended to allow for the collection of blood samples. Urine samples are also collected from athletes. The first blood testing was carried out at the 1988 World Ski Championship and continued in a limited way in skiing and track and field athletics. Blood testing at the Olympic Games was first carried out during the Winter Olympic Games in Lillehammer in 1994. The samples are investigated for evidence of homologous blood cells, i.e. blood other than the athlete's own. Current scientific knowledge is insufficient to confirm the use of autologous (same) blood, although scientists have made advances in detecting refrigerator-stored blood (Birkeland, 1994). Most recent advances in blood testing techniques have focused upon erythropoeitin and other plasma expanders. This has involved the testing of blood parameters, haemoglobin, haematocrit and reticulocytes. Athletes failing to achieve the required parameters from the blood sample provide a urine sample for more detailed analysis for the presence of blood doping.

Pharmacological, chemical and physical manipulation was also added to the list in 1985 in an attempt to control the growing trend of deception that had entered into the procedure. Anecdotal evidence of urine substitution, catheterization and in some cases actually having the sample provided by impostors threatened the effectiveness of the testing system. Athletes also tried to use substances to inhibit renal excretion, such as probenecid and to titrate testosterone/epitestosterone levels in the body. Where evidence of these manipulation techniques emerged the classification of doping methods enabled the sports authorities to act. Significantly, very few cases of manipulation are ever confirmed as doping offences, indicating perhaps the difficulty of presenting evidence. The most well-known case to have been heard was that involving Katrin Krabbe, Silke Muller and Grit Breuer, whose urine samples provided during a training session in South Africa bore such a similarity it led to the allegation that they had been provided by the same person. Evidence brought forward at the disciplinary hearing in London in June 1992 concluded that the same individual probably had provided the samples and that an opportunity had existed for the athletes to catheterize urine from another person prior to the sample collection. The offences could not be pursued as the doping regulations of the German Athletic Federation (DLV) did not provide the authority to collect samples out of competition abroad (IAAF Arbitration Panel Statement, June 1992).

Gene doping was added to the list of prohibited methods in January 2004. It includes the non-therapeutic use of cells, genes, genetic elements or the modulation of gene expression.

Substances prohibited in certain sports

In addition to the doping classes and methods noted above, there are restrictions on specific pharmacological classes in certain sports. The responsibility is with the international federation to determine whether controls on these substances are necessary. Within this group, alcohol and beta blockers are prohibited. Alcohol may be tested for by breath or blood testing; actual levels may vary between sports that restrict the use of alcohol. Control of the abuse of alcohol has taken on a different dimension with the timing of breath testing prior to a competition in order that offenders may be withdrawn.

Specified substances

In January 2005, WADA introduced a section of the prohibited list headed 'Specified Substances'. This section includes drugs from various sections of the prohibited list, such as over-the-counter stimulants (e.g. ephedrine), cannabinoids, inhaled β_2-agonists, glucocorticosteroids, beta blockers and alcohol. WADA (2005) states that:

> these drugs are particularly susceptible to unintentional anti-doping rule violations because of their general availability in medicinal products or which are less likely to be successfully abused as doping agents. A doping violation involving such substances may result in a reduced sanction provided that the athlete can establish that the use of such a specified substance was not intended to enhance sport performance.

Therapeutic Use Exemption (TUE)

Athletes and their physicians can apply for permission to use certain prohibited substances for therapeutic purposes. Examples of such drugs included β_2-agonists and glucocorticosteroids. Criteria for granting a TUE include:

- there is no reasonable therapeutic alternative;
- the athlete would experience a significant impairment in health if the prohibited substance or method were to be withheld;

- the substance or method would produce no additional enhancement of performance other than a return to a state of health.

Monitoring programme

WADA established the monitoring programme in 2004, in relation to a number of drugs that they had withdrawn from the prohibited list in that year. The list includes a number of stimulants such as caffeine and drugs that are commonly found in cough and cold medicines that can be purchased over-the-counter. These include phenylephrine, phenylpropanolamine, pseudoephedrine and synephrine. The programme is intended to continue to monitor these drugs in order to detect patterns of misuse in sport.

Summary

Sport has now inherited a substantial list of prohibited substances that reflects, in part, the practices of athletes, but also the concerns of pharmacologists that loopholes might exist in the regulations that would allow athletes to design their own doping substances. Whilst the IOC was the originator of a general list for sports (that has been welcomed with different degrees of acceptance by some sports), WADA has taken on the task of developing a list that can be generally applied and yet has sport's specificity. The first WADA list was published in January 2004. There is considerable debate among the medical profession and sporting fraternity as to whether some of the drugs should remain on the list. Much will depend upon the agreed definition of doping. However, the justification for inclusion of substances is not simply based on their potential for performance enhancement. Unfortunately, the list of doping classes has also become a reference point for those considering using drugs to improve performance, without any real understanding of why they are prohibited or what their effects are.

The mere presence of one of the banned drugs, or their metabolites, in a urine sample collected as part of an authorized testing programme may constitute an offence. In the case of testosterone, a quantitative analysis of the urine is required. This will determine whether the drug is present in the urine in quantities significantly greater than those 'normally' found in urine.

Initially, the IOC list only included drugs for which a specific, conclusive testing procedure was available. However, in recent years blood doping and peptide hormones have been included, for which confirmatory tests were unavailable. Research into definitive detection methods is on-going and likely to catch athletes unaware. The use of blood rather than urine sampling would significantly assist testing of these substances; however, there are ethical, legal, procedural and medical issues to be resolved before this form of testing becomes more widely accepted and useful. Donike et al. (1994) have suggested that 'blood sampling is less meaningful when performed after a competition; blood sampling should be performed before competition and in the training periods'. This hypothesis continues to have a major impact upon the perceived effectiveness of blood testing.

Changing trends in the misuse of drugs in sport have been reflected in the periodic revision of the list of doping classes and methods. Unfortunately the absence of a strict timetable for this revision has led to confusion in the past. This caused some delay in the implementation of revised regulations or the rapid introduction of regulations without warning. WADA has clarified the timetable for revising and publicizing the list. It now operates an annual revision and specified introduction date.

For each of the classes of drugs, the prohibited substances classes are supported by lists of examples of the drugs that fall within that group. The lists are not comprehensive and any drugs that are related to that class by their pharmacological actions and/or chemical structure are also banned. This explanation was added to the 1993 IOC list. The principal reason for giving such a broad definition is to ensure that any new drug which is introduced on to the market and which belongs to a prohibited class is automatically included in the list. This avoids the need for a continual up-date of the lists and prevents an athlete from claiming the substance they have taken is not covered by the regulations. The drugs are listed under their generic name, which identifies the particular chemical substance(s) the drug contains. However, the same drug may be manufactured and sold by several different drug companies throughout the world and each company will use their own commercial name to describe that drug; for example, the analgesic paracetamol (generic name) can be bought under the commercial names Panadol, Disprol, Paldesic and Calpol. Paracetamol is permitted under current doping regulations.

2.4   The rationale for drug misuse in sport

As the motivation for drug misuse cannot be determined from the analysis of the urine sample, it requires further investigation with the athlete and of their environment. The opportunity to do this is not provided for within the rules of many sports federations. Investigations into the environment in which doping has taken place have primarily been led by governments or the judiciary, rarely has sport been able to undertake the thorough investigations required. The introduction of an independent observer system under WADA and certified quality systems helps to normalize external monitoring, investigation and reporting.

> Have we . . . lost track of what athletic competition is about? Is there to much emphasis by the public and by the media on the winning of a gold medal in Olympic competition as the only achievement worthy of recognition?
>
> (*Dubin, 1990*)

The substances that have been prohibited or restricted for sportsmen and women are only a minority of the number of drugs and medications available. The reasons why they may be misused by athletes are many and various, however the justification for controlling the use of drugs is simply explained: 'the use of doping agents in sport is both unhealthy and contrary to the ethics of sport' (IOC, 1990).

There may be many reasons why an athlete uses drugs in sport. If the motivation is performance enhancement, the type of drug used will depend on its pharmacological action and the sporting activity the athlete is involved in. To understand why athletes may use prohibited or restricted substances, the effects and perceived benefits to athletes of doping substances are explained in the following section. However, there are athletes who combine substances in an attempt to increase their effects or to counter side-effects.

Stimulants

By comparison with other classes of drugs, stimulants have probably been misused in sport over the longest period of time. Their main purpose has been to improve performance by the general action of stimulation of the central nervous system. Athletes may use stimulants to reduce tiredness, or to increase alertness, competitiveness and aggression. They are considered to have a performance-enhancing effect on endurance events as well as on explosive power activities because of an increased capacity to exercise strenuously and a reduction in sensitivity to pain. Probably one of the earliest reasons for the use of stimulants was to help athletes through 'the pain barrier'. Stimulants are more likely to be used on the day of a competition; however, it seems likely that athletes now consider the use of stimulants in training to allow the intensity of the training session to be increased. There is, however, little scientific evidence available to suggest that stimulants do improve performance. As stimulants could increase an athlete's aggression towards other competitors or officials, there are potential dangers involved in their misuse in contact sports.

The stimulant class includes psychomotor stimulants, sympathomimetics and miscellaneous CNS stimulants. Examples of this class include the amphetamines, ephedrine and cocaine.

Caffeine used to be banned, was removed by WADA in 2004, but its use in sport continues to be monitored by WADA. Caffeine is the pharmacologically active substance which occurs in social drinks such as tea, coffee and cola. The amount which normally occurs varies according to the type of drink and the way it has been prepared. Relatively high doses are needed to reduce fatigue and the side-effects of tremor may be detrimental. According to one study, doses of about 1000 mg would be needed to produce caffeine levels exceeding 12 µg/ml in the urine, the quantitative level set previously by the IOC (van der Merwe *et al.*, 1988). Concentrations found in tea and coffee are, on average, 50–80 mg and 80–150 mg, respectively. In addition, caffeine is a constituent of some medications such as cold preparations and migraine treatment, usually in quantities of less than 100 mg per dose. Caffeine produces a mild central stimulation, similar to amphetamine, reducing fatigue, increasing concentration and arousal. Physiological effects include increased heart rate and output, increased metabolic rate and urine production. High doses can cause anxiety, insomnia and nervousness.

Amphetamines are a controlled drug under the UK Misuse of Drugs Act 1971. Although they have been prescribed as appetite suppressants and for the treatment of narcolepsy, amphetamines are known to produce dependence, often in increasing doses. Athletes have probably used amphetamines to sharpen reflexes, reduce tiredness and increase euphoria. However, competitors have also died as a result of amphetamine misuse, as they raise blood pressure which, with increased physical activity and peripheral vasoconstriction, makes it difficult for the body to cool down. If the body overheats and is unable to cool down, it dehydrates and blood circulation decreases. The heart and other organs are unable to work normally.

The sympathomimetic drug, ephedrine, has been used in cold treatments and originally in bronchodilation for asthmatics. However, it is now regarded as less suitable for use as a bronchodilator having been linked with cardiac arrhythmias. Ephedrine is likely to be misused for its euphoric effect, but could also be used inadvertently as an over-the-counter medication to treat cold or influenza symptoms. Because of the possibility that inadvertent use could be argued, it is likely that athletes would try to misuse ephedrine to obtain an amphetamine-like euphoria.

Cocaine has been used in a variety of treatments for many years; it even appeared as an original ingredient in Coca-Cola until it was removed in 1903. Its therapeutic indication is as a local anaesthetic, though it is likely to be misused for its euphoric effects and feeling of decreased fatigue. Moreover it has the potential for use as a recreational drug arising from the lifestyle some athletes engage in. Cocaine has been directly linked to the deaths of US basketball player Len Bias and American footballer Don Rogers. In sprint-trained athletes, cocaine is likely to increase heat and lactic acid formation, which coupled with the vasoconstriction effect contributes to fatal cardiac damage.

β_2-agonists

One of the more controversial groups of stimulants are the β_2-agonists, which are frequently used in medicine as an anti-asthmatic treatment. Up to 1993, the IOC permitted the following β_2-agonists by inhalation only: bitolterol, orciprenaline, rimiterol, salbutamol, terbutaline. In 1993, this group was reduced to salbutamol and terbutaline. Currently, salbutamol, terbutaline, formoterol and salmeterol are permitted for use by inhalation provided the athlete obtains an Abbreviated TUE. Concerns about the potential mild anabolic effects of β_2-agonists have led to a special section for this particular group of drugs under the class of anabolic agents (see below).

Sports are also beginning to regulate potential misuse of asthma inhalers in a different and more applicable way. Rumours circulated that use of asthma inhalers just prior to competing would improve performance. This appeared to have gained credence among competitive swimmers who believed that use of an inhaler would enable them to take in more air before diving into the water, to stay underwater for longer and therefore to experience less resistance. Reduction of resistance might provide the split second advantage needed to win. To counter this, the governing body has ruled that an athlete must move away from the pool-side to receive treatment and to allow time for recovery.

Narcotic analgesics

Pain relief was one of the earliest medical uses of drugs. Narcotic analgesics act on the brain to reduce the amount of pain felt from injury or illness. In sports, the use of powerful pain-killing drugs might enable an athlete to exert themselves beyond their normal pain threshold. There are considerable dangers in this to the health of the individual athlete, who may try to compete or train despite an existing serious injury which could lead to further injury, permanent damage or to physical dependence on the drugs themselves.

Narcotic analgesics have strong addictive properties and, as such, are tightly controlled by legislation in most countries. The WADA regulations apply specifically to the opiate analgesics including derivatives such as morphine, heroin, pethidine and dextropropoxyphene. Particular mention is made in the WADA regulations of those substances which are permitted, dextromethorphan, pholcodeine and diphenoxylate. One of the milder forms, codeine, was previously prohibited for use. Codeine is widely available in a variety of medicines, analgesics, diarrhoea suppressants, cough mixtures and cold remedies, over-the-counter. The level of codeine present in these medicines is too low to induce the serious adverse effects associated with narcotic analgesics but its availability may have caused difficulties in self-medication without contravening doping regulations. In 1993, the IOC removed codeine from the list of examples of prohibited substances and initially indicated that it was now permitted for therapeutic use. (A revised version of the IOC list which appeared later in the year did not contain this advice.) Whilst this move is likely to be welcomed by athletes, it does, however, cause difficulties for testing, since codeine is metabolized to morphine, among other substances, in the body. Not all sports federations had agreed with the IOC's previous ruling prohibiting codeine; track and field athletics, for example, had permitted the therapeutic use of codeine. In terms of treatments for pain, non-steroidal anti-inflammatory drugs, such as aspirin, remain permitted.

Anabolic agents

In March 1993, the IOC changed its classification of anabolic steroids to anabolic agents and created two subgroups: androgenic anabolic steroids and other anabolic agents and β_2-agonists (e.g. clenbuterol). This realignment of anabolic agents within a broader group was a further clarification of the IOC's position in respect of clenbuterol. Apparent confusion about its status may have led to use by athletes and body builders for performance enhancement reasons. In particular, a rather acrimonious and lengthy debate followed reports of clenbuterol use by athletes prior to the 1992 Barcelona Olympics and the classification of clenbuterol as an anabolic agent as well as a stimulant. The reports, having arisen from out-of-competition testing which concentrates primarily upon anabolic agents, masking agents and peptide hormones, have been challenged by the athletes concerned and the matter remains unresolved. Clenbuterol has been shown in animal studies to increase skeletal muscle mass and reduce body fat (Matlin *et al.*, 1987). It was described in the *Underground Steroid Handbook* (Duchaine, 1992) as 'the hottest drug on the steroid black market . . . It has changed body building forever' and has been reported to have been found in athletes' urine despite not being licensed for therapeutic use in the country of the athletes concerned.

The trend away from the relatively short term use of stimulants towards longer term administration of androgenic anabolic steroids (AAS) aimed at increasing performance by modifying muscle size or nature marks a serious departure into planned and organized drug misuse. The steroid drugs currently in use are largely chemically derived alternatives to naturally occurring testosterone. Contrary to popular belief, oral administration of androgenic anabolic steroids is more dangerous than injection of these drugs. Oral forms have to be broken down in the liver first, creating risks of liver disease; injectable forms are oil based and fat soluble making their release into the body system slower, as fat stores are broken down. Orally active AAS are water soluble and are likely to have a shorter clearance time in the body, making their use more popular among athletes subject to drug testing. However, clearance times are also likely to be dose related and are difficult to calculate with any certainty. The use of androgenic anabolic steroids by athletes from certain sports has become widespread in particular in strength, power, body-building and stamina activities. Whilst the pretext for using AAS is to increase muscle development, there is no strong evidence to show that AAS exert a direct growth-promoting effect on muscles. The exception here would be in female athletes and pre-pubescent males.

Attempts to interfere with the ageing process have been made since the first use of 'monkey glands' 100 years ago. Emphasis has mainly been on the male sex hormones, such as testosterone, and their ability to improve the quality of life. The protein-building properties of anabolic steroids had led to the hope that they might be more widely useful in medicine, but this has not been realized due to the adverse side-effects reported. The side-effects associated with androgenic anabolic steroids are extremely serious, particularly the consequences of long-term or high dosage. Regrettably these side-effects do not seem to have deterred athletes, in particular body builders, from misusing steroids (and other drugs to counter some of the side-effects). Anabolic steroids are discussed in greater detail in a subsequent chapter, the following summarizes some of the main reasons why athletes would use androgenic anabolic steroids and why there are concerns about their use.

The side-effects associated with these drugs are extremely serious, particularly the consequences of their long-term use. Dr Robert Voy (1991) warned 'there is absolutely no anabolic-androgenic steroid that affects an athlete anabolically without also affecting him or her androgenically . . . There isn't an anabolic-androgenic steroid an athlete can take to increase muscle mass, endurance, or speed without risking dangerous hormonal side-effects.'

To overcome the difficulties of administering testosterone orally, the chemically derived versions attempted to separate the androgenic properties (masculinization in females, acne, suppression of testicular function) from the anabolic effects of increased muscle mass and body weight, positive nitrogen balance and the general feeling of well being. This separation has not proved possible, so athletes who wish to use these drugs have to accept the androgenic and anabolic effects. Use of steroid drugs alone will not improve performance. An athlete would require a high protein intake and intensive training if gains in performance are to be achieved. Research suggests that physical performance is enhanced in a limited way, for example as increased strength but not endurance (Haupt and Rovere, 1984). However, another effect of androgens in the body is to stimulate the production of endogenous erythropoietin, which would lead to an increase in the number and stability of red blood cells (Royal Society of New Zealand, 1990).

It is in the two groups of individuals who are most likely to derive benefit from muscular development that the greatest risk of toxic side-effects occurs. Females will undergo masculinization resulting in hair growth on the face and body, irreversible voice changes and serious disturbances to the menstrual cycle. Adolescent males may experience stunting of growth. All users are likely to experience severe acne on the face and body. In males, depending on the types and doses, the side-effects may include gynaecomastia, heart disease, hypertension, liver toxicity and premature baldness.

Users seem likely to ignore these side-effects, particularly as they may not be obviously apparent. The side-effects which are more serious and potentially fatal are side-effects such as atherosclerosis and fluid retention, both of which may lead to cardiovascular problems, and the increased risk of developing cancer of the liver and kidneys. Another important point to remember is that some reported adverse side-effects may coincide with other factors. Body builders, for example, use a wide variety of other drugs to achieve their body image, such as diuretics, insulin, thyroid hormone and growth hormone in addition to steroids. They also ingest many nutritional supplements and sports supplements which are unregulated and may contain contraindicated substances. Yesalis (1993) suggests that some of the effects (e.g. thrombotic stroke) may be uniquely related to the extraordinary doses used by athletes. In fact, he indicates that for some the only limit seems to be cost and availability of the drugs.

Unfortunately the reputation of anabolic steroids as performance-enhancing drugs has achieved a considerable level of notoriety among athletes, whilst the adverse effects, being more long term, have been ignored. It is debatable whether an extensive programme of education and information to warn athletes of the consequences of androgenic anabolic steroid use in a non-therapeutic manner would bring about a change in behaviour and attitude. Angela Issajenko, Olympic silver medallist, confessed to taking anabolic steroids, hCG and testosterone (BBC, 1989).

> I came to the conclusion that people I'd compete with in Moscow were also on anabolics so I decided that was the way to go. People are not concerned with the side-effects, or so called side-effects, with anabolic use. They don't believe it. First and foremost what comes to mind is this is going to help me be the best in the world. Whatever comes later, comes later.

Charlie Francis, Ben Johnson's former coach, speaking at the Dubin Inquiry (Dubin, 1990) stated 'It's pretty clear that steroids are worth the price of a metre at the highest levels of sport' (BBC, 1989).

The introduction of an out-of-competition testing programme has added a potential deterrent to steroid use for those subject to a testing programme; however, the programme is not implemented on any large scale world-wide and certainly lacks the necessary co-ordination.

Diuretics and other masking agents

Diuretics have the pharmacological effect of elimination of fluid from the body. As such they have a medical use in removing excess fluid due to heart failure, and in lower doses to reduce blood pressure. These drugs may, however, be misused by sportsmen and women for three main reasons. First, they may be taken to effect acute reduction of weight to meet weight-class limits. In this respect they may offer a potential advantage in sports such as boxing, judo or weightlifting where competition is in weight categories. Second, diuretics may be used to overcome fluid retention induced by androgenic anabolic steroids. This could be useful to body builders trying to obtain a 'cut' look. Third, athletes may use diuretics to modify the excretion rate of urine and to alter urinary concentrations of prohibited drugs. An athlete likely to be selected for drug testing might attempt to increase the volume of urine and to dilute the doping agent, or its metabolites in the urine. The sophistication of detection techniques means that this form of manipulation is unlikely to be effective (Delbeke and Debackere, 1986).

Diuretics are controlled in competition because of their weight reduction potential. Out of competition there is careful monitoring of their use as a manipulation technique. Before, during and after exercise, athletes should take in considerable amounts of fluid. Competitors who misuse diuretics could suffer from dehydration; insufficient fluid in the body may cause faintness, muscle cramps, headaches and nausea. Losing too much water could also cause the kidneys and heart to stop working.

There may also be some additional benefits to the use of some diuretics which might support a claim of therapeutic use. The systemic diuretic acetazolamide appears to reduce mountain sickness and improve exercise performance at high altitude (Bradwell et al., 1986). Research suggests it can also produce an alkaline urine and so decrease the urinary output of some drugs for short periods of time; however, drugs remained in the urine for longer.

Probenecid has also been used by athletes in an attempt to mask the presence of drugs or their metabolites because of its ability to inhibit movement of molecules across kidney tissue. Use of probenecid first came to light in the Delgado affair, suspicions were alerted when a treatment for gout appeared in the urine of a seemingly healthy, active cyclist in competition. The combination of gas chromatography and mass spectrometry in the analytical procedure ensures that probenecid use no longer prevents detection (Royal Society of New Zealand, 1990).

Hormones and related substances

The increasing availability of hormone substances has led to greater use by athletes. Moreover the difficulties in detecting levels of abuse make them an attractive drug for athletes subject to testing. Corticotrophin (ACTH) increases adrenal corticosteroid levels in the body. The powerful anti-inflammatory action of corticosteroids may be a useful aid to recovery from injury. Athletes might also seek the testicular stimulatory function of the gonadotrophins as a way to counter androgenic anabolic steroid effects.

Growth hormone would be used, presumably, for its anabolic properties to increase size, strength or ultimate height, depending on the age of the user. As an injectable drug, there are risks associated with shared needles and syringes. Prior to the availability of synthetic growth hormone, use of cadaver pituitary gland infected with the Creutzfeldt–Jakob virus led to the development of Creutzfeldt–Jakob disease. Athletes are also using amino acid supplements in an attempt to stimulate their own growth hormone production, this is not currently prohibited.

Erythropoietin (EPO) is a peptide hormone which is used by athletes. Usually released from the kidneys, EPO has more recently become more readily available due to recombinant DNA technology. EPO is the major hormone regulator of red blood cell production, used in medicine in cases of kidney failure. The long-term effects of use in medicine or misuse in sport are unknown, however overload of the cardiovascular system is likely where there is no medical need.

Enhancement of oxygen transfer

Enhancement of oxygen transfer includes blood doping, a unique form of performance enhancement, as it does not involve the administration of drugs. Red blood cells or blood products containing red blood cells are administered intravenously in an attempt to gain unfair advantage in competition. The intravenous administration of red blood cells (either from the same individual or from a different but blood-type matched person) would increase the oxygen-carrying capacity of the blood. Competitors in endurance activities such as marathon and long-distance running, cycling and skiing might use blood doping to increase the oxygen-carrying capacity of the blood. Similar effects are reported from training at altitude.

Blood doping carries considerable risk to the athlete. Injection of an additional volume of blood can overload the cardiovascular system and induce metabolic shock. The use of an athlete's own blood can be safer in terms of cross-infection; however, adverse effects can be compounded if blood from a second individual is used. There may be a potentially fatal haemolytic reaction with kidney failure resulting from mismatched blood or allergic reaction. There is also an increased risk of contracting infectious diseases such as AIDS or viral hepatitis.

An alternative prohibited method of increasing blood haemoglobin and/or haematocrit is the use of erythropoietin (EPO) (see above). Oxygen transfer may also be enhanced by the use of modified haemoglobin products and perfluorochemicals, all of which are prohibited.

Beta blockers and other drugs with sedative action

Among the range of drugs which may be misused are those whose actions are the opposite to the stimulant drugs. Certain sports require a steady action and an ability to control movements, such as archery and shooting.

If an athlete was seeking a drug which might help to improve performance, where a steady action was required, beta blockers have the potential to enhance this type of performance. By moderating the cardiac output and muscle blood flow caused by the nervous system's response to stress and arousal, beta blockers would generally reduce ability to perform strenuous physical sports. However, one of the side-effects noted in the treatment of cardiac arrhythmias was an ability to reduce muscle tremor. This would be of benefit in accuracy events and those where extraneous movement had to be kept under control.

The inclusion of beta blockers in the list of doping classes has not been without controversy. Their primary therapeutic use is in diseases of the cardiovascular system, due to their actions in reducing heart rate and cardiac output. This cardiodepressant effect can be useful. However, other side-effects such as cold hands and sleep disturbances may militate against their use in sport.

It is significant that early attempts to monitor their use were made by requiring a declaration of the medications and a doctor's certificate stating the reasons why they were required. At the 1984 Los Angeles Olympics, team doctors came forward with certificates to cover the whole team. The inclusion of beta blockers on the list of doping classes in 1985 was only one method to control their misuse. Officials in the sport of modern pentathlon tried to amend the competition timetable to hold the shooting event on the same day as the cross-country event. It was hoped that although beta blockers might be an advantage for the shooting event, they would be a positive disadvantage for running. In response, athletes simply moved to beta blockers with a shorter life which were metabolized before the running event began.

Fears that beta blockers may be misused in professional snooker have led to their inclusion on the list, but under pressure to address cases of medical need, the World Professional Billiards and Snooker Association have taken the unusual step of permitting, under certain circumstances and with prior permission, the use of cardioselective beta blockers for a heart condition. Applications for consent may require an independent medical examination and presentation of the full medical history. The introduction of this procedure reflects a growing trend towards acceptance of therapeutic drugs but a need to maintain control over potential misuse.

Beta blockers were moved to the 'Classes of drugs subject to certain restrictions' section of the IOC list in 1993, to indicate their specific application to certain sports. WADA now lists the particular sports in which beta blockers are prohibited. These include, amongst others, archery, automobile, motocycling, bobsleigh, ski jumping, modern pentathlon and gymnastics.

Obviously there are difficulties in trying to separate therapeutic use from misuse. With the increasing emphasis on scientific support for athletes, it is now possible to control anxiety without the use of drugs, calling on mental rehearsal and relaxation techniques.

Local anaesthetics

Local anaesthetics, apart from cocaine, are permitted. Local anaesthetics may be used to treat local injury but their use to block pain to enable an athlete to continue participating beyond the normal pain barrier is to be deprecated. There is a high risk of greater injury if the body's normal pain threshold is masked.

Glucocorticosteroids (corticosteroids)

Corticosteroids are potent anti-inflammatory substances. In their naturally occurring form they are released by the adrenal gland during stress activity. The synthetically produced versions are used in medicine as analgesics and anti-inflammatories. In addition, corticosteroids are used in the treatment of asthma, a disease characterized by inflammation of the respiratory tract. Athletes seeking to open up the airways or, in larger doses, to mask injury or to increase training ability might misuse corticosteroids. They should not be confused with anabolic steroids. Serious toxic effects can occur if corticosteroid use is prolonged or under inadequate medical control. Topical administration of corticosteroids is used in medicine wherever possible in preference to systemic treatment as adverse side-effects are less likely. Originally the IOC attempted to restrict their use in competition by requiring a declaration from doctors. However, because it became known that corticosteroids were being used non-therapeutically by the oral, rectal, intramuscular and even the intravenous route in some sports, stronger measures were introduced. The use of corticosteroids is now prohibited except for dermatological use. All other routes of administration, such as inhalation therapy (asthma, allergic rhinitis) and local or intra-articular injections require a TUE.

Alcohol

For most sports the use of alcohol would be detrimental to performance, so it is logical that alcohol falls into the category of 'substances prohibited in particular sports'. In low doses, alcohol (or ethanol) has some sedative effects. Higher doses can cause poor co-ordination, increased reaction time and mental confusion. As a potential doping substance to reduce anxiety, the dose would have to be carefully controlled. In sports such as archery or shooting, the use of alcohol may stabilize tremor but could adversely affect reaction time and increase the unsteadiness of the arm when aiming. Because of the degree of euphoria alcohol can produce, it might also be used to overcome nervousness in other sports such as motor racing. Alcohol is also restricted for referees and umpires at international volleyball competitions.

Chemical and physical manipulation

As the testing programmes to control the use of doping substances have increased in sophistication, one response from athletes has been to try to manipulate the test in some way; the purpose being to invalidate the sample given or to secure the collection of a clean sample. Athletes have attempted to use other substances like vinegar to influence the quality of the urine. More often an athlete would try to provide a clean urine sample which had been obtained from another person during the procedure. The clean sample is then secreted around the body and voided in place of the athlete's own urine. Tightening of the collection procedures, particularly in relation to the time between notification and collection of the sample have helped to control this practice. The collection procedures have also been challenged by an individual masquerading as the athlete presenting themselves for testing. Checks on the identity and confirmation by official documentation are the only way to control this. Other forms of physical manipulation involve collusion between the athletes and the officials in the safe custody of the samples, the analysis of the samples at a laboratory which is not subject to independent monitoring or the manipulation of results. Rumours of these forms of manipulation were noted in several governmental or sports federation inquiries into drug abuse in sport (Moynihan and Coe, 1987; Amateur Athletic Association Coni Report, 1988; Senate Standing Committee (The Black Report), 1989 and 1990; Dubin, 1990; Voy, 1991). Evidence of state-controlled drug-taking programmes, with and without the knowledge of the participants has emerged from former Eastern European countries.

Summary

In summary, it is sometimes difficult to justify scientifically why a substance has been included in the list of doping classes, it is not always for performance enhancement reasons. Many of the drugs which appear could possibly be removed; however, one of the complexities is that in the minds of athletes the drugs do work. A further complication is the tendency for athletes to engage in polypharmacy and supplementation emphasizing the belief that there are drugs which will improve performance, and that more is better.

2.5   Attitudes towards drugs in sport

> The overwhelming majority of athletes I know would do anything, and take anything, short of killing themselves to improve athletic performance.
> (*Harold Connolly, 1956 Olympic hammer-throw champion, testifying to a United States Senate Committee in 1973*)

There are many reasons why an athlete may take a drug, other than for legitimate therapeutic purposes. Previous experiences, at school or college, may prompt further experimentation with drugs within a sporting context.

This approach may easily be fuelled by an athlete reading about drugs and their effects in popular magazines or even in serious scientific journals. Unfortunately, too many people involved in sport, at all levels, are prepared to speculate through television, newspapers or other media on the problem of drug abuse in sport. Too often these unsubstantiated reports lead to accusations and counter-accusations between those involved in the practice and administration of sport. Such activities do little to enhance the reputation of sport and inevitably lead to confusion in the minds of the majority of sportsmen and women who do not take 'performance-enhancing' drugs. This uncertainty presents the greatest danger to those younger athletes who either become disenchanted with their chosen sport or are misled into believing that drug taking has become a necessary part of the route to sporting success.

Other athletes may experience pressure from peer groups, particularly fellow athletes from their own or other sports. This pressure may result from a desire to conform with the 'in-crowd'. Alternatively, it may be a fear of competing, on unequal terms, with athletes who are suspected of taking drugs. Peer pressure may also be exerted through fellow athletes encouraging an individual to participate in drug taking. Certainly drugs have become readily available and black market prices ensure that drug peddlers can make a handsome profit at the expense of athletes.

A different type of psychological pressure may be involved in another group of athletes. For these athletes, drug taking may be the last resort for the improvement of performance, having reached their apparent limit of capability by conventional methods of training.

The motivating factors for drug misuse do not necessarily lie in the hands of the athlete. It is an unfortunate fact that certain athletes are coerced into taking drugs by someone in authority. This person may be their coach, trainer or team doctor. The directive may even have originated from a country's governing body. Such pressures are obviously extremely difficult to resist, particularly where team selection is at stake. Evidence of the direct involvement of the government in the German Democratic Republic demonstrated not only the complicity of those in positions of trust but also the way the athletes themselves, in particular females, unknowingly took substances and have suffered the consequences (Franke and Berendonk, 1997).

Many studies have been carried out using questionnaires to ascertain attitudes towards drugs in sport. From these studies, the majority of athletes, coaches, medical practitioners and others involved in sport do not favour the use of performance-enhancing drugs. However, these results may reflect the respondent's ethical and moral attitudes to the problem, but in practice the pressures of competition may compel them to take a more pragmatic approach to drug taking. This denial of drug taking is a common feature among alcohol and drug abusers and further hinders any attempt at tackling the problem. Potentially more damaging is the type of athlete who

openly admits to taking drugs and by so doing provides a model for the younger, more impressionable athletes to follow.

The blame for taking drugs does not, of course, always lie entirely with the athlete. There is often a body of so-called 'enablers' such as friends, family, and coaches who either actively encourage the athlete to participate in drug taking or vehemently shield the user from the need to deal with the problem. The reasons for this attitude are not always clear but in most cases involve self-interest. Conversely, those closely associated with the athlete may be unaware of their drug-abusing habits. This may, to a large extent, be due to a lack of knowledge and understanding of the drugs used and of their pharmacological effects.

It is clear that the majority of those involved in sport, both administrators and participants, are against the misuse of drugs in sport. It is equally clear that there is too little understanding of both the motivating factors that lead an athlete to take drugs and also the effects that those drugs can induce. It is vital that a wider knowledge of drugs and their adverse effects is achieved so that the current problem of drug abuse in sport can be contained and that future generations can be educated and persuaded against such misuse.

2.6   Ethical issues associated with drug use in sport

the use of doping agents in sport is both unhealthy and contrary to the ethics of sport, . . . it is necessary to protect the physical and spiritual health of athletes, the values of fair play and of competition, the integrity and unity of sport, and the rights of those who take part in it at whatever level.

(IOC, 1990)

Drug use in sport is contrary to the very principles upon which sport is based. Sport is considered as character building, teaching 'the virtues of dedication, perseverance, endurance and self-discipline' (Dubin, 1990). If, as Justice Dubin observes: 'sport helps us to learn from defeat as much as from victory, and team sports foster a spirit of co-operation and interdependence . . . import(ing) something of moral and social values and . . . integrating us as individuals, to bring about a healthy, integrated society' drug abuse would have no place in sport. Justice Dubin goes on to ask 'how has it come about, then, that many athletes have resorted to cheating. Why are the rules that govern sport often regarded as obstacles to be overcome or circumvented rather than as regulations designed to create equality of competitive opportunity and to define the parameters of the sport?'

Using drugs in sport for the purpose of gaining an unfair advantage presents an ethical dilemma for athletes, coaches, doctors and officials. It is clearly cheating, moreover it may put the health of the athlete at risk. Furthermore it may also be calculated cheating, when quantities and substances are carefully monitored in an attempt to cheat the rules on drug testing. It has been argued that the ethical dilemma has emerged for many reasons:

- media pressure to win;
- the prevalent attitude that doping is necessary to be successful;
- public expectations about national competitiveness;
- huge financial rewards of winning;
- the desire to be the best in the world;
- performance-linked payments to athletes from governments and sponsors;
- coaching which emphasizes winning as the only goal;
- unethical practices condoned by national and international sports federations;
- competitive character of the athlete;
- infallibility of the 'medical' profession to cure and improve performance;
- psychological belief in aids to performance – the magic pill;
- the development of spectator sport; and
- a crowded competition calendar.

The majority of these reasons were cited in the Dubin Inquiry itself, as explanations were sought for the context in which five Canadian athletes (four weightlifters and one track and field athlete) came to be disqualified for anabolic steroid use at the Seoul Olympics.

René Maheu (1978) has noted that development of spectator sport has turned attention away from the moral value of sport for the individual towards its entertainment potential. 'The success of spectator sport and the importance it has come to assume in everyday life are unfortunately too often exploited for purposes alien to or even opposed to sport – commercialism, chauvinism and politics – which corrupt and deform it.'

Dubin, however, whilst acknowledging the existence of all the influences and their undoubted effects which might lead to drug misuse in sport, argued first that there can be no justification for athletes to cheat in order to win, and second that the pressures and temptations are the same for all athletes yet most show greater character and do not succumb. He concluded the problem is not educational, economic or social but, essentially, a moral problem.

The sporting contest is seen to have been replaced by a competition between doctors and biochemists on the one side and the regulating authorities on the other. The athlete becomes the puppet of this technology, health risks are simply ignored and other competitors cannot participate in the competition unless they, too, are prepared to use substances to improve performance. In an era where genetic and chemical manipulation has become commonplace it is hardly surprising that some athletes no longer rely on their natural abilities and skills.

In 1892 at a conference at the Sorbonne, Baron de Coubertin, founder of the modern Olympics said: 'Before all things it is necessary that we should preserve in sport these characteristics of nobility and chivalry which have distinguished it in the past, so that it may continue to play the same part in the education of the peoples of today as it played so admirably in the days of ancient Greece.' This may have been so at the turn of the twentieth century and the emergence of the modern day Olympic Games, yet in present day sport, the pressures on all concerned are immense. An athlete is faced with the pressures of winning, of competing, of meeting the expectations of the coach, team-mates, family and friends. Coaches are under pressure to produce the winning combination, of coping with fitness levels and of making demands on individual competitors, which may give the wrong signals in respect of drug misuse. Doctors may be faced with the dilemma of prescribing drugs for athletes and monitoring their effects as a safe way of containing drug misuse rather than know an athlete will seek black market sources and advice. The doping regulations may also apply to others who assist or incite an athlete to commit a doping offence.

Occasionally, criticisms of the drug-testing procedure itself are made: in particular the suggestion of invasion of privacy and impropriety in observing a person urinating. Athletes are looking forward to the advent of blood testing as a sophisticated progression towards comprehensive doping control. However, it is likely to be some time before scientists are willing to move from urine analysis because of the range of substances which can be detected. Blood testing offers a limited opportunity for detection of prohibited substances at present.

There is also another perspective, that of 'what constitutes drug misuse?'. Some banned substances actually originate in the body and it is an excessive level which has been deemed to be a doping offence. Critics would argue this level has been arbitrarily set. Other substances, such as ephedrine, commonly occur in over-the-counter medications, herbal preparations and even in social drinks. Do they actually improve performance? There is no doubt that athletes are prepared to make use of these substances to assist their performance. In terms of drugs with a therapeutic purpose there is also considerable abuse of medications by athletes who have no therapeutic indication. Given this array of drug misuse by sportsmen and women, it is hardly surprising that anti-doping rules have been introduced.

The definition of doping has to begin somewhere. The time may have come for the critics and the sports regulators to work together to achieve a practical set of rules, a realistic competitive calendar, an efficient support system and greater controls on the commercialization of sport. Elite athletes have become the focus of a considerable amount of media attention, with stories about their injuries and illnesses filling column inches. Moreover, speculation and reporting about the lifestyle of professional athletes has given rise to an image totally out of step with the dedication, training and motivation required to survive the sporting calendar. In many sports, increasing commercialism has seen a price put on an athlete's head; some cope better with this than others.

2.7   An international policy perspective/government action and policy

Drug use and abuse by athletes has now become a frequent feature of sport. It is clear that if drug use and abuse in sport is to be treated seriously it will require consolidated action, a joint commitment by sport, governments and others. In the words of Justice Dubin 'The resolution of this problem cannot simply be left to those who govern sport nationally and internationally.'

Initially, sport attempted to put its own house in order, and it was the international sports federations and the IOC who were the first bodies to introduce testing. Concern that the commitment required to achieve effective controls was lacking led to the involvement of governments. Testing had been limited to major competitions such as the Olympic Games and world championships; the regulations of the international sports federations introduced testing in a limited way. The IOC created a reference list of prohibited substances and proceeded to amend it to reflect doping practices. Testing programmes rested on accurate analysis. The IAAF and the IOC undertook the accreditation of laboratories for the analysis of urine samples. In many ways the progress being made to control drug misuse was not sufficient to demonstrate a real commitment to resolving the problem. The limitations and potential conflicts of interest which developed in the way testing programmes were delivered did nothing to reassure governments that action taken was sufficient and others began to take a close interest in the control of drugs in sport.

Governments became the other key players in the fight against doping. Sport is played on a national level throughout the world and governments were concerned about the ineffectiveness of the inconsistent actions of sports bodies, some had regulations – some did not. In 1967, prior to the first testing at an Olympic Games, the Committee of Ministers of the Council of Europe adopted a resolution on doping in sport, the first international text of its kind. The resolution stressed the moral and ethical principles at stake for sport, and the health dangers for athletes. The resolution explicitly referred to doping as cheating and included a broad definition of doping, including doping methods as well as the misuse of drugs. Governments were recommended to persuade sports organizations to take the necessary steps to have proper and adequate regulations and to penalize offenders. Finally the resolution recommended governments to take action themselves if the sports organization did not act sufficiently within 3 years. Anti-doping legislation was introduced in several European countries in response to this resolution.

Having continued to monitor the situation for 11 years, sports ministers adopted a further resolution in 1978, which called for governments to provide a co-ordinated policy and an overall framework in which the doping controls of sports organizations could take place. A European Charter, a statement of principles, anti-doping strategies and policies was adopted in 1984. It is significant that the chairman of the drafting group was the Chairman of the IOC Medical Commission, Prince Alexandre de Merode and that the Charter received the support from international sports organizations. It was obvious that sport alone would be unable to contain the problem; the Charter provided the first opportunity for governments to drive the agenda with the sports bodies, many of whom appeared to be above the law in the way they dealt with doping matters. Although the Charter received support from international sports organizations it was not binding upon governments, but would have 'moral, political and practical impact' (Council of Europe, 1989).

Anxious to keep up the momentum, the Council of Europe Committee of Ministers pressed for testing out of competition without prior warning to the athlete. Ministers also sought to secure a commitment to international harmonization, not only among sports but also among countries. Ministers agreed to the drafting of an anti-doping convention in 1989 that would be binding on governments. The key significance of this document was the recognition of political will to address the problem of doping. The Convention also provides a number of common standards – legislative, financial, technical and education, for implementation by all the bodies concerned with the state, by governments themselves and by government in support of sports organizations. Governments have embraced the standards being agreed through the Convention, although not wholeheartedly supported by the international sports organizations. In some countries the Convention has been adopted as the national legislation.

Progress towards a uniform international anti-doping policy took a further step forward when the IOC, international sports organizations and national governments came together at the First Permanent World Conference on Anti-Doping in 1988. The conference was held in Canada (later that year to discover first hand the problem of drug misuse among its athletes at the Seoul Olympics). The outcome of this conference was the development of the International Olympic Charter against Doping in Sport. This important document identified the policies and practices required to counter doping and was relevant mainly to national policies and practice. Its adoption as an IOC Charter was crucial to its success and influence, although the full support of the sports movement was not evidenced in the anti-doping programmes of that time. A second world conference the following year in Moscow helped to take forward some practical issues such as the operating standards for out-of-competition testing. However, a third world conference in London in 1993 focusing on the planning of testing programmes, national organization of anti-doping programmes, ethics and education showed the broader agenda still in need of attention. After that conference the sport/government partnership appeared to falter.

Whilst recognition of the need for a symbiotic relationship between sports organizations and governments was noted in the IOC/IF Agreement against Doping in Sport in June 1993, the identification of roles may be illustrative of underlying tensions. In seeking ways to 'intensify the prevention of, education and fight against doping in sport', the IOC and International Sports Federations agreed to 'develop the co-operation between the IOC, The International Sports Federations, the National Olympic Committees, the National Federations and the governmental or other organizations concerned in order to combat the trafficking of doping substances'. Interestingly, International Sports Federations were invited 'to adopt each year as a basic minimum document, the list of banned classes and methods established by the IOC Medical Commission and to undertake the appropriate controls for each sport'. Sport was clearly indicating the role for governments in the regulation of supply and availability of drugs, whilst reserving the actual controls in sport for the sports movement.

In the 1990s actions to control drug misuse in sport were numerous. Initially the IOC took control of the doping in sport agenda. Harmonization was the theme of a conference called in Lausanne in 1994 for the IOC Associations of Summer and Winter Olympic Federations, National Olympic Committees and athlete representatives and led to the publication of more unified rules and procedures in the document *Preventing and fighting against doping in sport* (IOC, 1994). The very next year the IOC published the IOC Medical Code, bringing together the IOC anti-doping rules and regulations in one document for the first time in 1995. However, the sports federations were slow to adopt the IOC standards, and differences in the lists of prohibited substances, the sanctions to be applied, and waiver in respect of minor procedural irregularities were evident. The compilation of directories of international sports federations' anti-doping regulations by UK Sport (1991, 1993, 1995), demonstrated that essential differences between sports remained, notably in the definition of doping itself.

Governments have continued to be critical of the lack of action by sports organizations themselves to address the problem seriously from within. In 1987 the then UK Sports Minister Colin Moynihan and former Olympic athlete Sebastian Coe co-authored a report that noted 'Within the present arrangements there appear to be too many loopholes, and perhaps insufficient security for satisfactory levels of effectiveness and confidence to be achieved . . . there is too much potential for evasion, leading to public concern and also to frustration among administrators and sportsmen and women.'

Similarly the Commission of Inquiry into the Use of Drugs and Banned Practices intended to Increase Athletic Performance in Canada in 1990 pointed to the failure of leadership among sports organizations and to the involvement and compliance of officials in drug use. 'The evidence of those witnesses at this inquiry who admitted their use of banned substances was in large part instrumental in uncovering the scandalous and pervasive practice of doping in sport that until then has hidden from public view, although not from the view of national and international sports federations.'

The action taken by sport itself, whilst an important contribution, can only be strengthened by a concerted world-wide effort supported by governments. Regrettably there have also been incidents of testing programmes actually being used to cover-up drug misuse. Testing of athletes prior to a major event to determine whether they would pass the competition test has been admitted in several former Eastern bloc countries. Covering-up results from major competitions has also been revealed. Robert Voy, formerly Chief Medical Officer to the United States Olympic Committee explained how problematic this is: 'Allowing National Governing Bodies (NGBs), International Federations (IFs) and National Olympic Committees (NOCs) such as the United States Olympic Committee to govern the testing process to ensure fair play in sport is terribly ineffective. In a sense it is like having the fox guard the hen house' (Voy, 1991). Independence of the testing programmes and an openness of information would seem to be the only way forward, if public confidence and in particular the confidence of athletes is to be restored.

It is significant that the IOC's own role at that time indirectly extended outside the Olympic Games through the accreditation of laboratories, the establishment of the list of doping classes, a financial assistance programme for IFs who need help to intensify their anti-doping controls and encouragement to Olympic sports to comply with the principles of the agreement. Yet their role was dogged with suggestions and innuendos about conflicts of interest, even direct actions to cover-up doping issues within the Olympic family.

Co-operation between international and national sports federations and the newly created national anti-doping organizations has the potential to provide one of the strongest practical deterrents to drug misuse. However, the authority of international sports federations and of national policies and legislation can sometimes lie uneasily together. Some sports have interpreted the intervention of governments in anti-doping matters as threatening their independence and challenging their abilities to undertake urine sampling. As the majority of testing and especially laboratory expertise is government funded, a mutually supportive relationship between sports organizations and governments is crucial to the ongoing success of anti-doping activities.

The response of governments and international organizations to the whole issue of doping in sport has been significant and interesting. Government-initiated enquiries in Australia, Canada, New Zealand and the UK have acted as a catalyst for progress in anti-doping activities, creating the International Anti-Doping Arrangement (IADA), in 1990, an intergovernmental agreement on consolidated actions in the fight against drug misuse. Originally founded by the countries of Australia, Canada and the UK, this alliance was soon joined by the countries of Norway, New Zealand, Sweden, Netherlands, Denmark and Finland. At about the same time the Nordic Convention between the Scandinavian countries opened up the borders to reciprocal testing and mutual recognition of results, working directly with their sports federations, sometimes adopting a stronger position than the international federation. The strong alliance of the IADA countries has led to the achievement of the most significant development in standardization of anti-doping procedures, the International Standard for Doping Control, a quality assured standard for the planning, implementation and monitoring of results of testing. Several international forums have now endorsed this standard as the accepted standard for anti-doping programmes and the International Standards Organization are presently considering its transfer to an ISO certified standard.

In an article published in 1992, the Chairman of the IOC Medical Commission acknowledged the strategy of a common policy to be the most effective, he stated: 'A commonly accepted international policy is necessary for the elimination of doping in sport. Such a policy would lead to an improved and more consistent approach and would contribute to equality and equity in the international sporting community. Both public authorities and the independent sports organizations have separate but complementary responsibilities and should work together for this purpose at all levels.'

Legislation has become a major problem for sport as athletes turned to the law to address perceived inconsistencies in the rules of sport, Katrin Krabbe, Harry (Butch) Reynolds and Diane Modahl were only some of the high profile cases that challenged the reliability of testing procedures and resulted in significant financial pressure upon the national federations. Governments also added to the pressures by making funding of sport conditional upon minimum anti-doping programmes, as required by the 1989 Anti-Doping Convention, which was gathering speed as more countries adopted its articles into their national policies and laws. In some countries the requirements for an effective anti-doping response were enforced through legislation. The direct action taken by the French Government to intervene during the 1998 Tour de France and reveal evidence of blood doping and drug misuse shocked the sporting world but won the admiration of athletes. The International Cycling Federation, previously considered one of the more responsible federations in anti-doping procedures, was exposed as failing to address the extensive drug misuse in this premier event. These events were undoubtedly the catalyst for the IOC response in February the following year. The ongoing tensions surrounding the allegations of cover-ups in the testing at the 1996 Atlanta Games, the scandals of corruption and bribery over Olympic bidding and increasing interest of the European Union to intervene more directly culminated in the most significant opportunity for drug-free sport finally to become a possibility.

In 1999 the IOC called a World Conference on Anti-Doping in Sport in Lausanne. This conference attended by sports federations and the IOC also attracted a number of government ministers. In particular the Director of the United States Office on National Drug Control Policy Barry McCaffrey and UK Sports Minister Tony Banks were vociferous in their criticism of the IOC. Support for a new independent world agency spread and was evident among many of the athletes and sports federations present. The debate demonstrated the strength of feeling among the governments to require the sports movement to clean up their sports or face government intervention. Initial suggestions to form an international anti-doping agency, 'headquartered in Lausanne, governed by a council presided over by the IOC President' were rejected. The conference culminated in an agreement to form the World Anti-Doping Agency, 'to be fully operational in time for the XXVII Olympiad in Sydney in 2000' as an equal partnership between sport and governments. In the years following there has been an uneasy struggle to find a basis for the formal establishment and operation of the World Anti-Doping Agency (WADA) in a way that would ensure mutual ownership but not surrender control to either sport or government. The IOC originally offered funding with an expectation that governments would pay their share and the bidding process for a permanent home began in earnest. The government side has developed regional co-ordination across the world under the umbrella of the 'International Intergovernmental Consultative Group on Anti-Doping'. Meetings have been held in Montreal, Oslo, Cape Town and Kuala Lumpur involving an increasing number of governments in the fight against doping.

WADA has sought greater legitimacy in promoting drug-free sport. Among its responsibilities are 'expanding out of competition testing, co-ordinating research, promoting preventive and educational actions and harmonizing scientific and technical standards and procedures for analyses and equipment' (WADA, 1999). A WADA programme of testing out of competition has been initiated through a contracted arrangement with a consortium of government-sponsored national anti-doping agencies. Debate about the additional testing in countries where there are strong independent national programmes has led to some criticism of WADA's ability to meet its principal objectives. Duplication of testing by international federations and national agencies as well as the Australian government prior to the Sydney Olympics demonstrated the need for greater co-ordination, although the question of who would give up the authority to test remains a vexed question. The Sydney Olympics marked a turning point in the accountability for testing under the control of the IOC, when the WADA observer programme was introduced.

Unexpectedly, the voting of the Foundation Board led to the WADA headquarters being located in Montreal. The offices opened in April 2002. WADA's World Anti-Doping Code was accepted at the Copenhagen Declaration in 2003. The majority of stakeholders, including athletes, sport federations and governments, have subsequently signed up to the code. The prohibited list has been under the control of WADA since January 2004.

2.8 References

Amateur Athletic Association (1988) *The Coni Report*, September, London, England.

Birkeland, K. (1994) Towards blood sampling in doping control – the road ahead. In: *Blood samples in doping control* (eds P. Hemmersbach and K. Birkeland), On Demand Publishing, Oslo.

Bradwell, A.R., Dykes, P.W., Coote, J.H., *et al.* (1986) Effect of acetazolamide on exercise performance and muscle mass at high altitude. *Lancet*, **1** part 2, 1001–1005.

British Broadcasting Corporation (1989) *On the Line*, BBC2 production.

Delbeke, F.T. and Debackere, M. (1986) The influence of diuretics on the excretion and metabolism of doping agents. *Drug Res.*, **36**, 134–137, and 1413–1416.

Donike, M., Geyer, H., Gotzmann, A., *et al.* (1994) Blood analysis in doping control – advantages and disadvantages. In: *Blood samples in doping control* (eds P. Hemmersbach and K. Birkeland), On Demand Publishing, Oslo.

Donohoe, T. and Johnson, N. (1986) *Foul Play: drug abuse in sport*. Blackwell, Oxford.

Dubin, C.L. (1990) *Commission of Inquiry into the Use of Drugs and Banned Practices Intended to Increase Athletic Performance*. Canadian Government Publishing Center, Ottawa.

Duchaine, D. (1992) *Underground Steroid Handbook*. Power Distributors, Venice, California, USA.

Finlay, M. and Plecket, H. (1976) *The Olympic Games: the first hundred years*. Chatto and Windus, London.

Francis, C. (1990) *Speed Trap*, Lesters, Orpen, Dennys, Toronto, Canada.

Franke, W.W. and Berendonk, B. (1997) Hormonal doping and androgenization of athletes: a secret program of the German Democratic Republic government. *Clin. Chem.*, **43**, 1262–1279.

Goldman B. (1992) *Death in the Locker Room/drugs and sports*. Elite Sports Medicine Publications, Illinois, USA.

Haupt, H.A. and Rovere, G.D. (1984) Anabolic Steroids: a review of the literature. *Am. J. Sports Med.*, **12**, 469–484.

IAAF (1982) *IAAF Doping Control Regulations and Guidelines for Procedures*, London.

IOC (1990) International Olympic Charter against Doping in Sport, Medical Commission, IOC. www.olympic.org

IOC (1993) IOC/IF Agreement against Doping in Sport, June 1993. Medical Commission, IOC. www.olympic.org

IOC (1999) Lausanne Delaration on Doping in Sport, Lausanne, www.olympic.org

Maheu, R. (1978) L'Education et le sport. In: *Sport, A Prison of Measured Time* (ed. J.M. Brohm), Inklinks, London.

Matlin, C., Delday, M., Hay, S., Smith, F., Lobley, G. and Reeds, P. (1987) The effect of the anabolic agent, clenbuterol, on the overloaded rat skeletal muscle. *Biosci. reports*, **7**, 143–148.

Moynihan, C. and Coe, S. (1987) *The misuse of drugs in sport*. Department of the Environment, London.

Olympic Movement Anti-Doping Code (1999), www.olympic.org

Reeb, M. (ed.) (1998) *Digest of CAS Awards 1986–1998*. Berne, Switzerland.

Royal Society of New Zealand (1990) *Drugs and Medicines in Sport*. Thomas Publications, Wellington.

Senate Standing Committee on Environment, Recreation and the Arts, Australia (1989) *Drugs in Sport*, Interim Report (The Black Report), Australian Government Publishing Service, Canberra.

Senate Standing Committee on Environment, Recreation and the Arts, Australia (1990) *Drugs in Sport*, Second Report (The Black Report), Australian Government Publishing Service, Canberra.

van der Merwe, P.J., Muller, F.R. and Muller, F.O. (1988) Caffeine in sport: urinary excretion of caffeine in healthy volunteers after intake of common caffeine containing beverages. *S. Afr. Med. J.*, **74**, 163–164.

Voy, R. (1991) *Drugs, sport, and politics*. Human Kinetics Publishers, Illinois, USA.

World Anti-Doping Agency (WADA) Constitutive Instrument of Foundation, Lausanne 1999, www.wada-ama.org

World Anti-Doping Agency Independent Observers Report, Olympic Games 2000 – Sydney, Australia (2000) WADA, Switzerland.

WADA (2005) The World Anti-Doping Code 2005 Prohibited List. Available at http://www.wade-ama.org/ (accessed 02/02/05).

Yesalis, C.E. (1993) *Anabolic Steroids in Sport and Exercise*. Human Kinetics Publishers, Illinois, USA.

Chapter 3

Central nervous system stimulants

Alan J. George

3.1 Introduction

Various drugs which stimulate the central nervous system (CNS) have been known for over 2000 years. A simple classification of these substances is complicated by their combination of central and systemic effects. Thus, though the compounds mainly stimulate CNS activity, many central stimulants have, in addition, direct effects on cardiovascular functions and on the sympathetic nervous system.

CNS neurophysiology

To understand the various mechanisms by which CNS stimulants produce their effects, it is necessary to understand the basic functioning of neurones in the CNS (Figure 3.1). The stimulant drug must pass from the circulation, across the blood–brain barrier and into the brain tissue spaces. Once in the brain it may: (a) increase neurotransmitter release on to receptors (e.g. amphetamine and ephedrine); (b) directly stimulate the post-synaptic receptors (e.g. ephedrine and caffeine); or (c) inhibit neurotransmitter re-uptake (e.g. cocaine and amphetamine).

CNS stimulants are thought to act mainly on the dopamine (DA), noradrenaline (NA) and 5-hydroxytryptamine (5HT) (serotonin) neurotransmitter systems. Caffeine is thought to affect adenosine neurotransmission.

3.2 Amphetamines

Several structurally related drugs are known as 'amphetamines' and include dextroamphetamine, methamphetamine, phenmetrazine and methylphenidate. In this chapter the word amphetamine will refer to dextroamphetamine, the structure of which is shown in Figure 3.2.

Amphetamine is a phenyl isopropylamine (Figure 3.2) and was first synthesized in 1920. It was originally prescribed for the treatment of nasal congestion – inhalation of an amphetamine spray through the nose induced

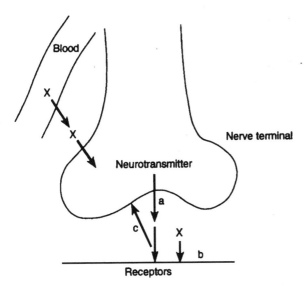

Figure 3.1 Sites of action of CNS stimulants (a) amphetamines; (b) caffeine; (c) amphetamine and cocaine.

nasal vasoconstriction which resulted in decongestion. In 1935, amphetamine was first used to treat the neurological condition narcolepsy, and its use in the treatment of depression, anxiety and hyperactivity in children followed from this. Amphetamine was used widely during the Second World War to reduce fatigue and increase alertness, particularly amongst naval and airforce crew on patrol duties. Reference to this was made in 1974 in Ludovic Kennedy's account of the pursuit and sinking of the German battleship *Bismarck*. The rapid development of tolerance to amphetamine and the insidious occurrence of dependence have led to the drug being withdrawn from clinical use, except in certain controlled circumstances, in both Britain and the USA.

The effect of amphetamines on human mood and performance

The desire to enhance mood or performance or both is usually the main reason for taking amphetamines. In their comprehensive review of amphetamines Weiss and Laties (1962) agreed that amphetamine does produce an enhanced performance in many tasks and does not simply normalize fatigue responses. They examined various tasks such as (a) work output by subjects on a bicycle ergometer, (b) performance on arduous military exercises, and (c) performance during flying or driving missions. Apparent improvements in athletic performance in events as diverse as shot put, swimming and

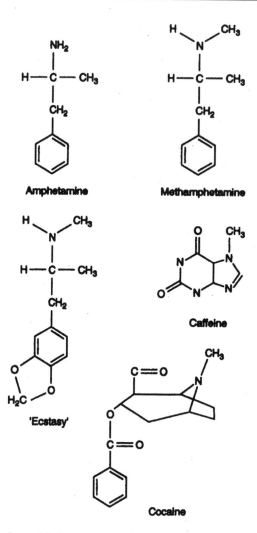

Figure 3.2 Some central stimulants.

running are produced by amphetamines as well as a reduction in reaction time and increased co-ordination and steadiness. These aspects will be discussed in detail later. Intellectual performance does not seem to be improved by amphetamines, unless the performance has been degraded by boredom and fatigue (Brookes, 1985). In the short term, amphetamine increases the speed of learning of new tasks. The effects of amphetamine on judgement are uncertain and several conflicting studies have been published (Brookes, 1985). There is general agreement that amphetamines cause a mild distortion of time perception which may lead to misjudgement in planning manoeuvres or in manipulations such as driving a car. Active avoidance learning is facilitated by amphetamine. Although there is considerable inter-individual variation in the effects of amphetamine on mood, the general effects are of positive mood enhancement. These positive effects include an increase in physical energy, mental aptitude, talkativeness, restlessness, vigour, excitement and good humour. Subjects taking amphetamine also report that they feel confident, efficient, ambitious and that their food intake is reduced. Many athletes report that they feel most aggressive when taking amphetamines and are unlikely to report or complain of injuries (Laties and Weiss, 1981).

Some 'negative' effects of amphetamine include anxiety, indifference, slowness in reasoning, irresponsible behaviour, irritability and restlessness, dry mouth, tremors, insomnia and following withdrawal, depression. These effects of amphetamine on mood are dose-dependent and are thought to be produced by the stimulation of dopamine and adrenergic receptors.

Tolerance and dependence

Tolerance develops rapidly to many of the effects of the amphetamines. Tolerance is said to be present when, over a period of time, increasing doses of a drug are required to maintain the same response. Brookes (1985) has reported several cases of subjects requiring as much as 1 g of amphetamine per day to produce the same effect on mood as a new taker of amphetamines who may require only 10–30 mg. There is much evidence to show that amphetamines induce drug dependence and the amphetamine-dependent person may become psychotic (see Toxicity, below), aggressive and anti-social. Withdrawal of amphetamines is associated with mental and physical depression. Recent evidence by Comer's group in New York suggests that tolerance to the positive effects of methamphetamine does occur over time at least in new abusers while the severity of the negative effects increases over time (Comer et al., 2001). Another study by the same group showed that methamphetamine is a powerful, positive reinforcing agent in humans as well as animals (Hart et al., 2001).

Therapeutic use

The many varied uses of amphetamine following its original introduction are now largely discredited. It is interesting to compare the initial enthusiasm for amphetamine as the 'cure-all' for numerous mental problems with that for the use of cocaine some 50 years previously.

Until quite recently amphetamine was used to treat narcolepsy, but its use is now limited to the treatment of hyperactivity in children. A rare use of amphetamines is as a diagnostic aid in determining which patients are unsuitable for a particular anti-manic or anti-schizophrenic treatment.

Toxicity

The major side-effects of amphetamine administration (excluding those following withdrawal of the drug) include (a) many of the negative effects described previously; (b) confusion, delirium, sweating, palpitations, dilation of the pupil and rapid breathing; and (c) hypertension, tachycardia, tremors, muscle and joint pain. Though amphetamines may initially stimulate libido, chronic amphetamine use often leads to a reduction in sex drive. Chronic amphetamine administration is also associated with myocardial pathology and with growth retardation in adolescents. Usually the personality changes induced by chronic low doses of amphetamine are gradually reversed after the drug is stopped. However, high chronic doses may lead to a variety of persistent personality changes. Possibly the most serious of the severe psychiatric disorders induced by amphetamine is the so-called amphetamine psychosis described by Connell in 1958. The frightening array of psychiatric symptoms he described in patients presenting with amphetamine psychosis include many commonly found in paranoid-type schizophrenics. An important distinction between amphetamine psychosis and schizophrenia is that amphetamine induces a preponderance of symptoms of paranoid and of tactile hallucinations.

The mode of action of amphetamine

There are four mechanisms by which amphetamine may produce its effects. These are (1) release of neurotransmitter – dopamine (DA), noradrenaline or 5HT – from their respective nerve terminals; (2) inhibition of monoamine oxidase activity; (3) inhibition of neurotransmitter re-uptake; and (4) direct action on neurotransmitter receptors. Of these four possibilities, neurotransmitter release appears to be the most important (Brookes, 1985).

Amphetamine stimulates DA release by reversing the neuronal membrane uptake transporter (Seiden et al., 1993). It also inhibits the activity of the enzyme monoamine oxidase (Seiden et al., 1993). It seems that several major behavioural changes induced by amphetamine are most closely mimicked by stimulation of central noradrenaline-releasing neurones. Thus, the amphetamine-induced locomotor activity and self-stimulation seen in animals and the increased alertness and elevation of mood produced in humans are closely related to increases in noradrenergic activity. Amphetamine is a potent anorectic and elevates plasma free fatty acid levels. Body temperature is also elevated. The cardiovascular, gastrointestinal and respiratory effects of amphetamine are sympathomimetic in nature. However, both animal and clinical experiments suggest that the effects of amphetamine are mediated by the release of at least two neurotransmitters, NA and DA, and that in the rat the development of tolerance to amphetamine involves the release of 5HT. However, the stereotyped behaviour induced in the rat by amphetamine administration appears to depend on DA release. The euphoriant action of amphetamine can be abolished by the DA receptor antagonists such as haloperidol and pimozide. There is some evidence to suggest that the positive behavioural effects of amphetamine may be mediated by DA while the effect of amphetamine on food intake may be mediated by NA. However, Silverstone and Goodall (1985) produced conflicting evidence of this.

Pharmacokinetics

Amphetamines are readily absorbed, mainly from the small intestine and the peak plasma concentration occurs in 1–2 hours following administration. Absorption is usually complete in 2.5–4 hours and is accelerated by food intake.

The metabolism of amphetamines has been difficult to investigate because of the wide variation between species in the metabolic effects of amphetamines. The principal amphetamine metabolites are p-hydroxyephedrine and p-hydroxyamphetamine. Both these metabolites have similar pharmacological effects to the parent amphetamine. Amphetamine is lost from the blood by renal filtration. An acid urine and treatments which increase the acidity of urine enhance amphetamine loss – a reaction which is useful in the treatment of amphetamine overdose.

The effects of amphetamines in sport

In the USA, the increasing use of amphetamines in all sports led the American Medical Association to initiate research projects to test the effects of amphetamine on sports performance and the incidence of side-effects associated with the drug. One of these studies (Smith and Beecher, 1959) reported that 14–21 mg of amphetamine sulphate per kg body weight when administered 2–3 hours prior to running, swimming or weight throwing, improved performance in 75 per cent of the cases investigated. This was a double-blind study in which 14 out of 15 swimmers and 19 out of 26 runners showed a statistically significant improvement in performance after amphetamine administration. However, the improvements demonstrated were quite small (usually 1 per cent). This study also demonstrated that the performance of athletes in throwing events was improved by an average of 4 per cent following amphetamine administration. Criticism of the study soon followed because the athletes were sometimes allowed to time themselves, there was little control for weather conditions, a wide range of distances (600 yards to 12 miles) was used to test the athletes and a minor dosage of amphetamine was administered. Chandler and Blair (1980) reported that amphetamine improved athletic performance in terms of acceleration, knee extension strength and time to exhaustion but that it had no effect on sprinting speed. Haldi and Wynn (1959) reported that 5 mg of amphetamine 90 minutes before a 100-yard swim had no effect on the time of the swim. A more sophisticated double-blind investigation of amphetamine was carried out by Golding and Barnard (1963) using a treadmill. They studied the effect of amphetamine on treadmill running in trained and untrained subjects. Each subject undertook an initial run followed 12 minutes later by a second 'fatigued' run. Thus, the effects of amphetamine on initial performance and fatigue could be examined in the same subject. Their subjects showed that amphetamine had no effect on performance during the initial and fatigued runs in either the trained or the untrained athletes. During the fatigued runs, amphetamine retarded the recovery rates for heart rate and blood pressure. Only one of the subjects was able to tell that he was receiving amphetamine. Many of the studies on the effects of amphetamine on athletic performance have been carried out on cyclists. One reason for this is that there are numerous examples of fatalities arising from the use of amphetamines by cyclists, notably the incidence of death from heat-stroke. Wyndham et al. (1971) carried out a wide-ranging placebo-controlled biochemical and physiological investigation on two champion cyclists exercising on a bicycle ergometer. Whilst working at rates between 12 000 and 16 000 ft/lb.min there was no difference between amphetamine and placebo in terms of submaximal or maximal oxygen uptake, heart rate or minute ventilation; however, there were significant increases in blood lactate levels. The authors concluded that amphetamines have no effect on the ability to do aerobic work but they insignificantly increased the cyclists' ability to tolerate higher levels of anaerobic metabolism. The dangers inherent in these results are that an athlete taking amphetamine might be better able to ignore the usual internal signals of over-exertion and heat stress, which may therefore explain the incidence of heat-stroke and cardiac problems in cyclists who take amphetamines during long-distance cycling events.

Since amphetamine was reviewed in this book in 1996 (George, 1996) there have been no significant new findings relating to the ergogenic effects of amphetamine. This has been attributed to a decline (in the USA) in the abuse of amphetamine by athletes and by the general public, following increased controls on its prescription and availability (Wadler and Hainline, 1989). Several reviewers, including Conlee (1991) have remarked on the considerable inconsistency of amphetamine effects in humans, particularly with regard to ergogenicity. A poorly explored feature of amphetamine action is its effect on fatigue. Most studies have concentrated on the central aspects of fatigue while neglecting peripheral contributions. However, the few studies of amphetamine effects on muscle glycogen stores before and during exercise have been contradictory (Conlee, 1991).

Since no significant improvement in performance is associated with amphetamine use, why does it continue to be taken? The answer could be an effect on mental attitude in terms of improved mood, greater confidence and optimism and increased alertness. It should also be remembered that, like anabolic steroids (Chapter 5), amphetamine could be abused for different reasons by different athletes. Thus, baseball and football players may use them to increase alertness and concentration, runners or swimmers to increase energy and endurance (Smith and Perry, 1992).

An interesting insight into the differential abuse of amphetamine in an American football team has been provided by Mandell *et al.* (1981). They reported that amphetamine dosage would be adjusted according to the players' position in the team. The lowest doses of 5–15 mg per man per game were given to those players, such as wide receivers, whose concentration needed to be heightened while maintaining near normal perception. The high doses of 10–60 mg per man per game (line-backers) and 30–150 mg per man per game (defensive linemen) went to those players in whom aggression was paramount.

It is also possible that amphetamine might increase preparedness and make the athlete more keyed up for his event. To examine this possibility the effects of amphetamine sulphate were compared with the tranquillizer meprobamate and with placebo control in 126 male medical students. The results showed that none of the students was able to tell which drug he was taking and also there was no correlation between either subjective feelings of increased alertness in those taking amphetamine or lethargy in subjects on meprobamate, with any change in reaction time or manipulative skills (Golding, 1981).

Several studies thus indicate that the effect of amphetamine on the psychological state of athletes might be self-induced and occurs as a result of the athlete expecting to perform better and be more alert. These and other aspects plus confounding influences in psychostimulant results have been reviewed by Clarkson and Thompson (1997). They quoted two studies carried out in the 1940s in which all the subjects on active drug (amphetamine) perceived that they had done more work on a cycle ergometer than was actually measured. In their review they also question the validity of some of the earlier experiments in terms of clinical methodological vigour (blindness), statistical inference and control. Several studies quoted have low numbers of participants and the detection of active drug by the subject was not controlled.

Another feature of most studies is the failure to control for trained or untrained subjects, a confounding feature of many anabolic steroid studies (see Chapter 5). This is very important if we are considering that amphetamine may have an effect on motivation, as trained athletes often exhibit higher motivational levels than the untrained and the untrained therefore may not exercise fully to exhaustion (Clarkson and Thompson, 1997).

Side-effects of amphetamine in relation to sport

Some side-effects of amphetamine are particularly important in athletes and have often only been revealed in individuals undertaking extremely arduous training or sporting schedules.

One of the most widely publicised side-effects of amphetamine from which a number of fatalities have occurred is heat-stroke. This has been most prominent in cyclists owing to the intensity of their exercise, the endurance required and the high ambient temperatures at which the exercise often occurs. Amphetamine causes a redistribution of blood flow away from the skin, thus limiting the cooling of the blood. As a result of this, two cyclists (Jensen and Simpson) who had both been taking amphetamine died of heat-stroke and cardiac arrest, respectively, during gruelling road races. The former occurred in the intense summer heat of Rome, the latter whilst climbing the infamous Mont Ventoux during the 1967 Tour de France.

The ability of amphetamines to obscure painful injuries has enabled many American footballers to play on and exacerbate injuries which would normally have resulted in their withdrawal from play, and soldiers to continue marching while they have foot blisters (Clarkson and Thompson, 1997).

The side-effects of amphetamine on behaviour are also important in sport. Mandell (1979) has investigated amphetamine abuse amongst American footballers and found extensive abuse amounting to 60–70 mg average dose per man per game. In this sport, amphetamine was administered apparently to promote aggression and weaken fatigue in the footballers. However, there are several accounts quoted by Golding (1981) in which the euphoriant effects of such doses have rendered the takers unaware of the errors and misjudgements they were making on the pitch.

Why take amphetamines?

Why take amphetamines when the chance of increased injury, dependence, heat-stroke and cardiac arrest is enhanced by these drugs and the actual improvement on performance, if it does occur, is so small – in the order of 1 or 2 per cent? The simple answer to this was proposed by Laties and Weiss (1981) who examined the improvements in world records in athletic events over the past 100 years. As an example, the 1500 m world record has improved by only 15 per cent since 1880 and on average in the past 50 years it has improved by only 1 per cent in every 7 years. Thus, they concluded that a top athlete who could consistently maintain a 1 per cent improvement in performance would be at an advantage over competitors. This advantage they termed 'the amphetamine margin'.

Conclusion

The prescription and administration of amphetamines are strictly controlled by law in most developed countries. They produce powerful stimulating effects on the CNS, which include euphoria, excitation and increased aggression and alertness. These effects are achieved at the expense of judgement and self-criticism. Amphetamine administration may be followed by severe bouts of depression and dependence. Increases in athletic performance induced by amphetamine are very small and several studies have failed to show that amphetamine produces any physical advantage. Some evidence suggests that amphetamine may increase confidence before and during an event, and laboratory studies have shown that it may also reduce fatigue in isometric muscle construction.

The induction of dependence and the increased susceptibility to heat-stroke and cardiac abnormalities seem to suggest that amphetamine taking is of little value as a performance-enhancing drug in the long term.

The fact that amphetamine derivatives of lower potency, such as l-amphetamine, are still present in some OTC medications available in some countries, should serve as a reminder to all those competition athletes seeking medication abroad. A recent mistake cost the UK skier Alain Baxter his Olympic bronze medal in 2002.

Ecstasy

This is an amphetamine derivative and was synthesized as early as 1914, being used initially as an appetite suppressant. It has been a class A illegal substance since 1977 in the UK and a controlled drug in the USA since 1985. Ecstasy has amphetamine-like stimulant properties and is associated with increased stamina and endurance. Its abuse is most commonly associated with social activities such as dancing. However, it is described here because of its *possible* misuse by athletes, though since 1990, no cases of positive ecstasy tests have been reported in the UK.

Ecstasy produces its effects by stimulating the release of the neurotransmitter 5HT (serotonin) from 5HT-releasing neurones in the CNS and can induce the destruction of these neurones. Its most serious physical side-effects are hyperpyrexia, which is the most common cause of death, and seizures. It is addictive.

3.3   Other sympathomimetics – ephedrine, pseudoephedrine and phenylpropanolamine

Ephedrine occurs naturally in the plant genus *Ephedra* and has been a component of ancient Chinese medicine for many centuries. This, and other herbal sources of stimulants, has been reviewed recently by Bucci (2000). Pseudoephedrine and phyenylpropanolamine are synthetic drugs.

This group of drugs are structurally related to amphetamine (Figure 3.2). Each of the drugs exert their effect indirectly on neurones of the sympathetic and central nervous systems, by displacing noradrenaline and possibly other monoamine transmitters from neuronal storage sites. Both drugs also exert direct effects on adrenergic α and β receptors and are weak inhibitors of monoamine uptake. They are also resistant to oxidation by the enzyme monoamine oxidase.

Both phenylpropanolamine and ephedrine are reported to be 5 times less potent than amphetamine. Pseudoephedrine is reported to be 20 times less potent than ephedrine at least in terms of its cardiovascular actions. The CNS effects of phenylpropanolamine and ephedrine are also much less than those of amphetamine. For example a 75 mg/70 kg body weight dose of ephedrine is required before it will cross the blood–brain barrier. This may explain why both drugs produce much less depletion of brain monoamines than amphetamine (Wadler and Hainline, 1989).

The effects of phenylpropanolamine and the ephedrines are produced within 40 minutes after administration and can last up to 3 hours with therapeutic effects being associated with plasma levels of between 60 and 200 mg/ml (Wadler and Hainline, 1989).

Uses

Both phenylpropanolamine and ephedrine were sold in pharmacies in the UK and USA as constituents of 'cold cures' (see Chapter 4), but phenylpropanolamine has now been proscribed by the US authorities.

Adverse effects

At the usual therapeutic doses quoted previously the most common side-effects are tachycardia, hypertension, headache and dizziness. Phenylpropanolamine appears to produce serious hypertensive side-effects at doses sometimes as low as 25 mg (Wadler and Hainline, 1989). These drugs may cause anorexia, insomnia, irritability and nervousness at low to medium doses, whereas high doses are associated with mania and a psychosis similar to that occasionally seen with amphetamine.

Abuse in sport

Abuse of ephedrine, pseudoephedrine and phenylpropanolamine by athletes is nebulous since many of those detected as having taken them have claimed they were using the drugs as 'cold cures'. The first comprehensive study of the possible ergogenic effects of these drugs was carried out by Sidney and Lefcoe (1977). They examined the effect of 25 mg of ephedrine versus placebo in a double-blind crossover study using three separate athletic trials during a 3-week period. In this comprehensive experiment 10 variables were measured including strength, endurance, reaction time, anaerobic capacity and speed of recovery from effort. The results showed that, though exercise heart rate and resting pulse pressure increased and post-exercise recovery rate slowed, none of the physical performance measures improved. It was also interesting that no subjective improvements in performance were noted. Using phenylpropanolamine, Swain *et al.* (1997) found no effect on VO_{2max} or perceived exertion compared with placebo. Further evidence that ephedrine is positively ergogenic is contradictory. In South Africa, Gillies *et al.* (1996) found that 120 mg of pseudoephedrine had no effect on prolonged exercise, i.e. a 40 km time-trial 'ride' on a cycle ergometer, or on skeletal muscle function during the ride. By contrast, Bell's group in Canada (2001) measured the effects of 120 mg of the most potent isomer, ephedrine, on power output (electrically braked ergometer) and oxygen debt and VO_{2max} in 16 healthy volunteers. They found that compared with placebo, ephedrine significantly increased power output during the first 10 seconds of cycle exercise but had no effect after this time. Ephedrine also had no effect on O_2 deficit or accumulated VO_2. Interestingly, caffeine alone had no effect on initial power output but had an additive effect to ephedrine in the first 10 seconds of the test. Ephedrine treatment has been associated with increased plasma glucose levels both before and after exercise and increased plasma lactate and noradrenaline levels after exercise. Using a pseudoephedrine dose of 1 mg/kg, Swain *et al.* (1997) found no effect on VO_{2max} or exertion in 10 subjects exercising on a bicycle ergometer compared with placebo. While Gill *et al.* (2000) found that pseudoephedrine produced minor increases in maximum torque, peak power and lung function in 22 male volunteers undergoing cycle ergometer tests, it had no effect in the same volunteers when they underwent strength-tests. There is evidence that ephedrine and phenylpropanolamine may become abused as anorexic agents by gymnasts (Wadler and Hainline, 1989) and possibly also by body builders.

Adverse effects in athletes

The adverse effects observed in athletes are similar to those seen in the general population. Recent investigations into potential side-effects of phenylpropanolamine and ephedrine in athletes have centred on the cardiovascular system. Swain *et al.* (1997) found that phenylpropanolamine had no effect on systolic or diastolic blood pressure at a dose of 0.33 or 0.66 mg/kg. At a dose of 1 mg/kg psuedoephedrine increased peak systolic but not diastolic blood pressure, while a 2 mg/kg dose had no effect at all. However, a number of investigators have warned of possible interactions between phenylpropanolamine and ephedrine and non-steroidal anti-inflammatory agents (NSAIDs). The pharmacology of these anti-inflammatory drugs is described in Chapter 8 and it will be seen that they inhibit the production of endogenous vasodilators, the prostaglandins. Since many athletes may take these anti-inflammatory drugs, an interaction leading to a larger than expected rise in blood pressure may occur when NSAIDs and phenylpropanolamine and ephedrine are taken together. Another possible dangerous interaction may occur with phenylpropanolamine and ephedrine taken with caffeine.

Can abuse be justified?

The prescription of ephedrine and phenylpropanolamine-like drugs has been criticized (Wadler and Hainline, 1989). In the 1972 Olympics, US swimmer, De Mont, was disqualified because of the presence of ephedrine in his urine, which he admitted originated from a medicine. At Seoul, in 1988, the eventual 100 m silver medallist Linford Christie narrowly escaped disqualification when small traces of 'a cold cure substance' were found in his urine. It has been suggested that phenylpropanolamine and ephedrine may indicate more serious abuse of substances like amphetamine and that their presence is a sign of weaning-off from or a mask for the more powerful drug. Pseudo-ephedrine, phenylpropanolamine and phenylephrine were removed from the prohibited list in 2004 by WADA. They are still monitored for misuse in sport by WADA. Ephedrine remains prohibited by WADA.

3.4   Cocaine

Cocaine first became available commercially in the 1880s. It was an ingredient of the famous Vin Mariani beloved by Pope Leo XIII, which was named 'the wine for athletes'.

Sigmund Freud took the drug to try and cure his own bouts of depression and suggested it as a 'cure all' for others. He exclaimed 'I took for the first time 0.05 gm of cocaine and a few moments later I experienced a sudden exhilaration and a feeling of ease'.

The drug fell out of medical use by the 1920s, and social use ten years later, only to reappear in the 1960s as a major drug of abuse.

Pharmacology

Cocaine affects the brain in a complex way. The most obvious initial effects are a decrease in fatigue, an increase in motor activity and an increase in talkativeness, coupled with a general feeling of euphoria and well-being. These mood changes soon subside and are replaced by a dysphoria (mood lowering). Cocaine is possibly the most addictive agent known.

The mechanism by which cocaine produces these effects is not known fully. Animal studies show that cocaine is a powerful 'reinforcer' and rewarding agent. It stimulates elements of the brain's pleasure and reward 'centres' which are distributed throughout the limbic system of the brain and include the dopamine-rich mesocortical and mesolimbic systems. Much of the reinforcing and rewarding behaviour induced by cocaine in animals, i.e. rats, who will repeatedly administer cocaine to themselves in preference to food, can be reduced by dopamine receptor antagonists. The evidence for the action of cocaine on these systems has been reviewed by Fibiger et al. (1992). Further evidence for the involvement of cocaine with dopamine-releasing neurones comes from studies at the molecular level reviewed by Kuhar

(1992). He has shown that cocaine inhibits the re-uptake of dopamine (DA) into the nerve terminals of dopamine-releasing neurones, and it has a similar though less potent effect on noradrenaline uptake in noradenergic neurones (Zhu *et al.*, 2000). This initially leads to a potentiation of the action of DA at post-synaptic receptor sites. This *acute* effect of cocaine on the dopamine transporter has been demonstrated by many investigations (Chen and Reith, 2000), but it is also exhibited by other drugs, such as methylphenidate, which do not have the same addictive potential as cocaine (Volkow *et al.*, 1999). In chronic cocaine abusers, *in vivo* scanning of behaviourally import-ant areas of the cerebral cortex has shown a significant reduction in dopamine D_2 receptors associated with decreased dopamine metabolism. There are also significant decreases in dopamine release in such abusers and these interrelated actions may be part of a mechanism leading to reduced activ-ities of cerebral 'reward circuits' in cocaine abuse and subsequent addiction (Volkow *et al.*, 1999). However, though dopamine receptor antagonists appear to antagonize all the actions of cocaine in rats, in humans they appear to inhibit cocaine craving, but not the euphoria (Kuhar, 1992). Some investigators have linked the dysphoria and craving following a cocaine dose with an increase in post-synaptic receptor numbers (Wadler and Hainline, 1989), though this is contradicted by the studies of Volkow's group (1999). Tricyclic antidepressants which antagonize these post-administration effects are thought to do so by inducing receptor subsensitivity.

Effective treatments for cocaine abuse are still experimental, though a number of potential new cocaine anti-addiction drugs are being investigated (Howell and Wilcox, 2001). At least two of these have been shown to reduce cocaine self-administration in non-human primates.

Metabolism

Cocaine is mainly metabolized, by plasma and liver cholinesterases, to benzoyl ecgonine and ecgonine methyl ester, which are excreted in the urine.

Pharmacokinetics

Cocaine may be administered by injection, orally, intranasally or by inhala-tion. Oral administration produces peak effects at variable times with behavi-oural changes lasting up to one hour. The most popular route is via nasal 'snorting' which produces peak effects from 5–15 minutes lasting for an hour. Inhalation of 'free-base' cocaine produces peak effects in less than 1 minute, but also a short-lived physiological effect measured in minutes. The route of cocaine administration influences the time course and onset of other actions of cocaine. Effects of the drug such as increases in heart rate and blood pressure are longer lasting via the oral compared with the intra-venous (iv) route (Smith *et al.*, 2001). Smith's group also found that regular cocaine abusers could detect if they were receiving active drug or placebo much quicker via the iv route than the oral and also that iv cocaine is some 10 times more potent than oral cocaine. Inhalation of cocaine results in the most intense cravings compared with other routes of administration (Wadler and Hainline, 1989). The pharmacological basis for this observation has been determined by Volkow *et al.* (2000). They compared levels of dopamine transporter blockade induced by iv, snorted and intranasal cocaine in 32 current cocaine abusers. There was dose-dependent transporter blockade for iv and intranasal delivery but not for smoking. Smoked cocaine produced a self-reported 'high' quicker than the iv route which was quicker than the intranasal route. Differences in the reinforcing effect of cocaine associated with route of administration thus depend not on differences in dopamine transporter blockade but on the speed of entry of cocaine into the brain. The frequency of cocaine administration, at least in rats, also influences the density of brain opioid and dopamine receptors and this needs to be considered in future human research (Unterwald *et al.*, 2001).

Adverse effects

Cocaine is highly addictive (more so than amphetamine) and the abuser may experience acute psychotic symptoms and undertake irrational actions, in addition to the well known adverse effects of euphoria. Chronic symptoms include a paranoid psychosis similar to that induced by amphetamine, coupled with spells of delirium and confusion. Other CNS side-effects include epileptogenesis – that is stimulation of epileptic seizures. This adverse effect is particularly dangerous since animal studies have revealed that the epileptogenic effect increases with frequency of cocaine abuse, a process known as reverse tolerance (Smith and Perry, 1992), which is important when the powerful reinforcing properties of the drug are considered. The epileptogenic effect can be produced even by repeated small doses of the drug (Wadler and Hainline, 1989), which may be more toxic than the same dose given less frequently (Unterwald *et al.*, 2001).

Cocaine abuse is strongly associated with cerebrovascular accidents arising either from the rupture or spasm of cerebral blood vessels. Some of these incidents may be due to pre-existing vascular pathologies, but there are several cases where no predisposing cause has been found at autopsy (Wadler and Hainline, 1989). Cocaine is also responsible for a number of cardiovascular side-effects, those relating directly to exercise are discussed later. A recent review of the literature relating to cocaine-induced coronary disease by Benzaquen *et al.* (2001) reveals that a number of factors may influence the development of cardiovascular pathology in cocaine abusers. Original ideas suggesting a simple mismatch between myocardial oxygen supply and demand caused by cocaine-induced vasoconstriction and the resulting increased myocardial workload are too simplistic. They have argued that a more complex interaction between three key factors: coronary vasoconstriction, intracoronary thrombosis and accelerated atherosclerosis may be involved, as all three can be induced by cocaine abuse. Smith and Perry (1992) have suggested that the increase in cardiovascular and cerebrovascular side-effects seen in recent years is due to the rise in abuse of 'crack' cocaine, which is rapidly absorbed and produces a concentrated effect on cerebral arterioles. A detailed account of cocaine side-effects is given by Wadler and Hainline (1989). A summary of the neuropsychiatric effects of cocaine abuse, including disruption of executive function in prefrontal brain regions is provided by Bolla *et al.* (1998).

Effects in athletes and on exercise

Cocaine was used by South American natives for centuries to increase efficiency, vigour and physical endurance. In 1884, Freud tested the effects of 0.1 g of cocaine hydrochloride, taken intranasally, on hand grip strength and on reaction time. He noted that the positive effect of cocaine was greatest when he was fatigued (Freud, 1885 quoted by Conlee, 1991).

In 1930, Theil and Essing reported that 0.1 g of cocaine administered to subjects before exercising on a cycle ergometer improved work efficiency, as determined by VO_2 measurements per unit work, and that exercise could be maintained for longer. The results were attributed to reduced CNS perception of fatigue. A second study using the same cocaine dose revealed no increase in work efficiency but a more rapid increase in recovery after exercise (Conlee, 1991). In his review of pre-1983 studies of the effects of cocaine on exercise, Conlee (1991) concluded that they were all contradictory and were usually poorly controlled and carried out. Many of the studies reviewed since 1983 have been in animals because of ethical considerations and have involved measurements undertaken in rats trained to run on treadmills connected to ergometers.

Early studies have demonstrated that cocaine had no beneficial effect on running times within a dose range of 0.1–20.0 mg/kg bodyweight and at doses above 12.5 mg/kg the cocaine actually reduced running time. At all doses used, cocaine significantly increases glycogen degradation while increasing plasma lactate concentration without producing consistent changes in plasma catecholamine levels. In 1991 Conlee and co-workers demonstrated in rats exercising voluntarily that cocaine increases glycogen metabolism and enhances the exercise-induced sympathetic responses. None of these studies have explained how cocaine reduces endurance performance. Conlee (1991) suggested three possible mechanisms to explain cocaine's action that could operate in parallel: (1) cocaine releases catecholamines which increase glycogenolysis and lactate production leading to early fatigue; (2) cocaine may induce skeletal muscle vasoconstriction, reducing oxygen delivery, oxidative metabolism, strength and reaction time, and stimulating glycogen breakdown; and (3) cocaine may have a direct effect on muscle glycogen breakdown. Indirect evidence originally suggested that mechanism (2) is less likely since cocaine-induced reduction of myocardial bloodflow is not associated with increased myocardial glycogen breakdown, but in 1994, Braiden *et al.* demonstrated a three-fold increase in muscle lactate accumulation in the white vastus muscle of rats under cocaine–exercise conditions.

These experiments in animals may explain the detrimental effects of cocaine, but do not explain the continued use of the drug and the claims made for it. Perhaps there are other aspects of the action of cocaine which may contribute to the perception that it is ergogenic. Hanna (1970) investigated the effects of male coca leaf chewing on exercise/performance in male habitual coca leaf chewers in the Peruvian Andes. He found that compared with non-chewers there was no significant effect of coca chewing on exercise or recovery rates or blood pressure. A further study (Hanna, 1971) found that coca leaf chewing did not increase work capacity but might increase endurance times. In these studies cocaine blood levels were not measured and the stated 4.5 g 'dose' of leaves was not strictly regulated. A more sophisticated study of the effect of coca leaf has been described by Spielvogel *et al.* (1996). In this experiment, metabolic and hormonal changes in habitual coca chewers were compared with non-coca chewers during incremental exercise to exhaustion. The coca leaf ingestion was controlled at 12 g and this produced a mean cocaine blood concentration of 72 ng/ml. At rest, both habitual and naive coca chewers had similar noradrenaline and adrenaline plasma levels but habitual chewers had higher free fatty acid levels. During exercise, oxygen uptake and work efficiency were similar in both groups, while in incremental exercise habitual chewers demonstrated lower arterial oxygen saturation, which was not due to reduced ventilatory response. Free fatty acid levels were increased during incremental exercise in the coca chewers. This interesting study remains inconclusive as the possible 'benefits' of raised free fatty acid levels could not be determined. There were no simultaneous measurements of changes in carbohydrate metabolism or endurance. Therefore it is unclear whether a carbohydrate-sparing 'mechanism' was activated by coca chewing and since catecholamine (i.e. noradrenaline and adrenaline) plasma levels remained unaltered, the mechanism for the elevation of plasma free fatty acid was unknown.

A similar increase in free fatty acid concentration following coca chewing has been described by Favier *et al.* (1996), though they observed increased adrenaline and free fatty acid levels during exercise, coupled with lower blood glucose concentrations. Their conclusion was that this might be evidence that cocaine might prolong work and postpone fatigue by increasing fat mobilization and sparing glycogen utilization, but it did not increase time to exhaustion. Thus the previous reviews of this topic (George, 1996, 2000; Clarkson and Thompson, 1997) are still correct in stating that cocaine appears to have no established benefit in exercise/athletic performance. Long-term cocaine smoking is associated with reduced maximum exercise performance, which is probably due to poor motivation or altered perception of effort (Marques-Magallanes *et al.*, 1997). In their critique of the research situation up to 1997, Clarkson and Thompson sympathetically (with regard to ethical issues) analysed the current research by questioning the validity of experiments using coca leaves rather than pure cocaine, even where the plasma cocaine concentration has been subsequently determined. The pharmacokinetics of cocaine may be altered by ingesting it via this route and also the coca leaf may contain other naturally occurring ingredients which might (a) influence cocaine metabolism and disposition, (b) influence cocaine action at receptors or transporters, and (c) have metabolic effects of their own. Habitual and naive cocaine/coca users may exhibit different responses, and experiments in rats seem to support this (Conlee *et al.*, 2000). A more detailed analysis of cocaine's effects on exercise in animals has been attempted by Robert Conlee's group since 1995. They demonstrated that cocaine caused an exaggerated rise in the exercise-induced production of lactate and secretion of noradrenaline and adrenaline (Han *et al.*, 1996).

This effect of cocaine on catecholamine secretion could be the basis of the ergolytic effect of cocaine on exercise and *may* be involved in the response to cocaine in athletes. These cocaine effects may not be caused by a vascular action of noradrenaline since blockade of α_1-receptors does not block the action of cocaine on glycogenolysis or lactic acid production (Conlee *et al.*, 2000). Since it is quite likely that athletes abusing cocaine will be chronic abusers, Conlee's group compared cocaine responses in naive and chronic cocaine-administered rats. They found that responses to cocaine in terms of noradrenaline and adrenaline release were greater in rats that had previously received cocaine on a regular basis (Kelly *et al.*, 1995). It may be that cocaine's positive ergogenic effect is manifested only on activities of short duration requiring a burst of high intensity energy output and activities associated with the drug's central stimulatory effect rather than its action on peripheral metabolism. It has been suggested that it is precisely for these central heightened arousal and increased alertness effects, achieved principally at 'low' doses, that cocaine is abused in sport (Wadler and Hainline, 1989).

A 1984 study quotes 17 per cent of 2039 US NCAA athletes admitting to use cocaine in the year preceding the study. Two years later 50 per cent of the respondents in a survey of US National Football League Players revealed that they felt cocaine was 'the number one drug of abuse in the NFL' (Wadler and Hainline, 1989). In Chicago, 2.4 per cent of 1117 male high school athletes admitted to using cocaine in a study conducted by Forman *et al.* (1995). It is not clear from these surveys whether the cocaine was abused for social or athletic performance-enhancing reasons.

Side-effects in athletes

In a previous edition of this book a paper detailing the deaths of two athletes from cocaine abuse was described (George, 1996). These sudden deaths of a basketball player and a US footballer from cocaine-induced coronary occlusion provided the most dramatic evidence of the potential adverse side-effects of cocaine abuse in athletes. In this paper, Cantwell and Rose (1981) describe the recovery of a 21-year-old cocaine and amphetamine abusing athlete from a coronary occlusion. These cases were followed by the cocaine-related deaths of basketball players Bias and Rogers in 1986 (Wadler and Hainline, 1989). The authors have also described the reported experiences of several US baseball players who testify to the mood-enhancing but often performance-inhibiting effects of cocaine. Significantly, baseball players complained of the deleterious central effects of cocaine, i.e. they were most liable to misjudge pitching and hitting. The authors also reported time disorientation in basketball players. New York Yankees' pitcher Steve Howe was arraigned on charges of cocaine abuse in 1991, but escaped a lifetime ban from baseball. The apparent leniency of US Baseball League administrators towards drug transgression has been criticized (Hoffer, 1992).

There have also been reports of athletes combining cocaine abuse with other drugs such as alcohol and anabolic steroids. According to Welder and Melchert (1993), heavy alcohol consumption combined with cocaine abuse enhances cocaine's cardiotoxicity, possibly by the production of a unique metabolite 'cocaethylene'. The existence and structure of cocaethylene, as the ethyl ester of the cocaine metabolite benzoylecgonine, has been established by Farre et al. (1993), and its actions in animals and man have been reviewed and investigated by McCance-Katz et al. (1998). They have detailed the following facts: that cocaine and alcohol taken together have additive deleterious effects, that simultaneous consumption of alcohol and cocaine leads to the formation of cocaethylene, and that though cocaethylene is less potent than cocaine, it is eliminated more slowly and could thus accumulate during or following an alcohol/cocaine binge. Further dangers arise from the possibility that the increased sense of well-being produced by the cocaine/alcohol mixture would lead to further abuse leading to increased toxicity from the drugs plus the toxicity of cocaethylene. Is this relevant to sport? Most certainly it is. This may well have been the ultimate cause of death of the Canadian ice-hockey player John Kordic who abused cocaine, alcohol and anabolic steroids. His downfall has been chronicled in detail by Scher (1992) and included frequent fights on the pitch, with opponents, team-mates and officials.

Conclusion

I concluded earlier (George, 1996) that 'whatever sporting advantage might be gained by cocaine abuse is far outweighed by the serious cardiovascular consequences'. It is quite possible that it is the occasional short-term abuse in sport which is the major problem and athletes think that such an abuse pattern will prevent their experiencing harmful side-effects. However, as with anabolic steroids, the cardiotoxic damage is probably insidious; with any current cardiac damage causing problems in later life. Another aspect is that much of the cocaine abuse in sport may be social, with young, naive individuals, suddenly with massive salaries, able to fund an experimental abuse that leads to addiction.

3.5 Caffeine, theophylline and other methyl xanthines

The three psychoactive drugs most commonly used are alcohols, nicotine and caffeine and all are self-administered! It has been suggested that caffeine has been in use as a stimulant since the Stone Age! Caffeine is a member of the methyl xanthine group of compounds, which also includes theophylline and theobromine. Caffeine occurs naturally in coca, coffee beans and tea leaves. The amount of caffeine obtained from each source depends on the method of extraction and the particle size of the extracts. Caffeine is added to soft drinks such as many types of colas and is also present in a number of 'over-the-counter' medicines (Table 3.1). Caffeine was removed from the prohibited list in 2004 by WADA, however, it is still monitored for its misuse in sport.

Pharmacology

Caffeine usually exerts an effect on the CNS in doses ranging from 85–200 mg and in this dose range it produces a reduction in drowsiness and fatigue, an elevation in mood, improved alertness and productivity, increasing capacity for sustained intellectual effort and a rapid and clearer flow of thought. This dose range of caffeine also causes diuresis, a relaxation of

Table 3.1 Caffeine content of some beverages, drinks and medicines

	Caffeine content (mg)
Coffee (per 5 oz cup)	
Percolated	64–124
Instant	40–108
Filter	110–150
Decaffeinated	2–5
Tea (per 5 oz cup)	
1 minute brew	9–33
5 minute brew	25–50
Soft drinks (per 12 oz serving)	
Pepsi Cola	38.4
Coca-Cola	46
Proprietary medicines	
Anadin tablet	15
Cephos tablet	10
Coldrex cold treatment tablet	25
Phensic tablet	50

smooth muscle, activation of gastric acid secretion and an increase in heart rate, blood pressure and blood vessel diameter. A caffeine dose in excess of 250 mg is considered to be high and may cause headaches, instability and nervousness. The American Psychiatric Association (1994) considers caffeine intoxication as occurring at doses greater than 250 mg.

The pharmacokinetics of caffeine has been comprehensively reviewed by Sawynok and Yaksh (1993). They concluded that caffeine absorption after oral administration is almost 100 per cent and that caffeine can appear in the blood in as little as 5 min after ingestion. An important point is that though peak plasma concentrations usually occur 30–60 min after oral administration, the range can be as wide as 15–20 min because of individual variations in gastric emptying. Using an oral dose of 175 mg, it can be shown that almost 90 per cent of the caffeine dose can be absorbed from the stomach giving rise to plasma concentrations of 5–10 µg/ml. In 17 subjects who consumed coffee and tea, with an average daily consumption of 6.8 mg/kg per day of caffeine, mean 24 h plasma levels of 4.4 µg/ml were observed. The range of concentrations during the 24 h sampling period was 1.2–9.7 µg/ml (Lelo et al., 1986). This information has important consequences for athletes who drink caffeine-containing beverages regularly and who might take additional pure caffeine, as the plasma levels of the two ingestions will be additive. They should also be aware that caffeine is absorbed more slowly from soft drinks such as Coca-Cola than from tea or coffee. Caffeine is water and lipid soluble and is therefore rapidly distributed through all tissues from the plasma and moves into the brain rapidly by simple diffusion. The plasma half-life, that is the time for a given concentration in the plasma to reduce by half, varies from 3–5 hours (Sawynok and Yaksh, 1993).

Five important features governing caffeine disposition relevant to athletes have been discussed by Sawynok and Yaksh (1993). These are age, genetics, exercise, smoking and other drugs. Caffeine, like all methyxanthines, is metabolized by the liver P450 enzyme system to theophylline (4 per cent), theobromine (12 per cent) and paraxanthine (84 per cent). This system also metabolizes the hydrocarbons produced by tobacco smoke, and several common drugs such as the phenobarbitone, the new serotonin-selective re-uptake inhibitor (SSRI) antidepressants and the steroids of oral contraceptives. This has been reviewed recently by Sinclair and Geiger (2000). Several studies have shown that age has very little effect on caffeine metabolism, but there can be marked genetic variabilities in the ability to metabolize it. Moderate exercise appears to increase peak plasma concentrations of caffeine. Smoking increases caffeine removal from the plasma, by increasing the rate at which it is metabolized. Drugs as varied as oral contraceptives, the SSRI antidepressants and alcohol reduce caffeine metabolism, thus raising its plasma levels. Strenuous exercise decreases caffeine elimination more in women than in men.

Some researchers have suggested the optimum ergogenic effect of caffeine occurs 3 hours after ingestion, which correlates with an apparent peak in lipolysis. This theory has been discounted by Graham (2001) as there is no evidence that the increased lipolysis correlates with ergogenicity.

Many athletes are convinced that caffeine improves their performance, while many a student (and this author) have improved their mental concentration by taking drinks containing caffeine. These uses aside, it must be remembered that caffeine consumption (as coffee) has been associated with a number of systemic disorders which include hypertension, myocardial infarction, peptic ulcer and cancers of the gastrointestinal tract and urinary tract.

An interesting study by Graham et al. (1998) showed that caffeine contained in normal coffee was much less effective in improving the endurance of athletes in a 10 km run than equivalent doses of pure caffeine. Later Graham (2001) compared this result with other studies which indicated that coffee was an ergogenic aid. He concluded that coffee may also contain compounds with an anti-ergogenic effect. This should be considered in further studies as should the possible confounding of any results by smoking, since tobacco hydrocarbons alter the activity of enzymes that metabolize caffeine. There have been suggestions that combination of caffeine with carbohydrate supplements enhances the ergogenicity of both substances compared to when either is used alone. Graham (2001) found the evidence for this inconclusive but did conclude that there was no detrimental effect with a combination of caffeine and carbohydrate supplements.

The effects of caffeine

Caffeine causes:

*   increased gastric acid and pepsin secretion plus increased secretion into the small intestine;
*   increased heart rate, stroke volume, cardiac output and blood pressure at rest;
*   tachycardia;
*   increased lipolysis;
*   increased contractility of skeletal muscles;
*   increased oxygen consumption and metabolic rate;
*   increased diuresis;
*   increased anti-nociceptive action of NSAIDs and exerts a mild anti-nociceptive action itself.

Mechanism of action

Caffeine is a powerful inhibitor of the cyclic nucleotide phosphodiesterase group of enzymes, of which there are five distinct types. These enzymes inactivate the so-called intracellular 'second messengers', such as cyclic AMP, which act as one of the links between receptor stimulation and cellular response. When these cellular enzymes are inhibited the action of intracellular messengers such as cyclic AMP is increased. For many years, researchers doubted that this was the main mechanism of action of caffeine since the intracellular concentration of caffeine (0.1–1 mmol) required to achieve significant enzyme inhibition could not be produced by the blood concentrations provided by normal caffeine dosing (Sawynok and Yaksh, 1993). However, phosphodiesterase inhibition as a mechanism of action should not be entirely dismissed. Caffeine also inhibits 5′-nucleotidase enzymes which convert AMP to adenosine, but this has not been thought to be of consequence in the mechanism of action of caffeine. However, recent research by Latini and Perdata (2001) suggests that this action may need to be investigated owing to the possible role of adenosine as a tissue mediator during tissue ischaemia.

It is now widely accepted that the majority of the pharmacological effects of caffeine are mediated by antagonism of adenosine receptors, though some of the cardiac and renal actions may still be brought about by inhibition of phosphodiesterases. In 1983, Daly et al. showed that the central stimulatory activity of caffeine is correlated with its ability to bind to and inhibit adenosine receptors. There are currently four types of adenosine receptor (A_1, A_{2A}, A_{2B} and A_3) and the relative importance of these is still under investigation (Fredholm et al., 1999; Latini and Perdata, 2001). Reviews of current literature by Nyce (1999) and Sinclair and Geiger (2000) illustrate the widespread distribution and complex actions of the adenosine receptor sub-types. Activation of receptors depresses neurotransmission, induces sleep, suppresses pain, causes bronchoconstriction and sodium retention and opposes the action of β receptors. Stimulation of A_2 receptors leads to peripheral and cerebral vasodilatation and inhibition of inflammation, while A_3 receptor stimulation inactivates eosinophil migration. An intriguing insight into the significance of adenosine receptors in metabolism and exercise is revealed by Latini and Perdata (2001). They state that the higher affinity A_1 and A_{2A} adenosine receptors are those involved in 'normal' adenosine neurotransmission. Under conditions of increased metabolic activity or a mismatch between energy supply and demand, adenosine is released from non-neuronal cells (possibly tissue mediators) and this extra adenosine is sufficient to stimulate the less sensitive A_3 receptors. Since caffeine is a weak antagonist of these A_3 receptors, this may be a mechanism by which caffeine produces some of its effects. It is also apparent that caffeine and other methyl xanthines may influence the response to ischaemia during exercise, since adenosine acting on A_1 and A_3 receptors may have a pre-conditioning and protective effect towards ischaemia in cardiac and striated muscle (Fredholm et al., 2001). Since caffeine, theobromine and theophylline are potent antagonists of A_1 and A_2 receptors, and caffeine is a weak antagonist of A_3 receptors, it can be seen that the actions of caffeine on individuals either at rest or during exercise will take some time to evaluate fully.

Central effects

Caffeine is widely accepted as a mild stimulant, though clinical tests often reveal a wide variability in its action. Caffeine increases vigilance, attention and prevents the decrement in performance and information processing that occurs during fatigue or where boring repetitive jobs are being carried out (Weiss and Laties, 1962). Compared with controls, subjects taking caffeine report improved alertness, reaction times and attention span. The common finding of most placebo-controlled studies carried out in the last 30 years is that caffeine produces the most consistent improvements in tests where fatigue or a stressful workload are part of the research protocol (Sawynok and Yaksh, 1993). Investigations into the effects of caffeine on numerical reasoning, verbal fluency, short-term memory or digital skill have produced conflicting results. This may be explained by the effect of differences in personality on the action of caffeine; that is, extroverts may react differently to introverts. The impulsiveness of subjects may also influence their response to caffeine, as may their normal pattern of caffeine consumption.

Many subjects report increased feelings of well-being indicated by improvements in mood, vigour and euphoria. However, some researchers have shown that the response to caffeine is dependent on expectations and that in controlled trials subjects are able to detect caffeine from placebo (Sawynok and Yaksh, 1993). The most favourable improvements in mood seem to occur when doses of up to 100–200 mg are taken. When the dose exceeds 400 mg the major response seems to be dysphoria (lowering of mood) and increased anxiety (Sawynok and Yaksh, 1993). It has been suggested that caffeine may act as a reinforcing agent in that caffeine abstinence for up to 24 h following chronic caffeine consumption leads to a withdrawal state characterized by irritability, insomnia, muscle twitching and headaches. Avoidance of this negative state could therefore act as a reinforcement of caffeine administration. Tolerance to and dependency on caffeine have been described by Strain and Griffins (1997), who state that such dependent individuals exhibit all the symptoms characteristic of substance dependency. Tolerance has been claimed to be associated with an up-regulation of adenosine A_1 or A_2 receptors, but this may not occur in humans.

Caffeine has been shown to be anxiogenic in a number of studies (Sawynok and Yaksh, 1993) and this has led to the description of a clinical syndrome – caffeinism – by Greden (1974). The anxiogenic or alerting effect may be caused by antagonism by caffeine of adenosine action at CNS A_2 receptors, where adenosine has a sedative effect. This 'alerting' action of caffeine may well be coupled to the reduction in 'perceived exertion' measurable in inactive and exercising volunteers whereby athletes feel they have done less work and expended less energy than they actually have (Sinclair and Geiger, 2000).

Adverse reactions

When coffee drinking became fashionable in Great Britain during the seventeenth century the effects of caffeine were immediately noticed and there were suggestions that it should be banned.

The average intake of caffeine in the USA is 206 mg per person per day and 10 per cent of the population consume greater than 1000 mg per day (Conlee, 1991). The major side-effects have been described and categorized as acute, severe and chronic by Wadler and Hainline (1989). Mild effects include nervousness, irritability, insomnia and gastrointestinal distress.

Severe effects include peptic ulcer, delirium, coma, seizures and supraventricular and ventricular arrhythmias, associated with doses greater than 200 mg/kg. Chronic effects mainly involve raised serum cholesterol levels. A particular cluster of side-effects involving anxiety, mood changes, sleep disruption, psychophysiological changes and withdrawal symptoms has been recognized as caffeinism and is described by Greden (1974). The Diagnostic and Statistical Manual of Mental Disorders (DSM IV) of the American Psychiatric Association describes caffeine intoxication as a condition simulating an anxiety attack in which the person experiences nausea, insomnia, restlessness and jitteriness.

Effects in athletes

In 1965 Bellet et al. described the elevation of blood fatty acids that occurred with caffeine ingestion. They concluded that caffeine improved endurance by enhancing fat utilization, thus sparing glycogen stores. Using nine competitive cyclists, Costill et al. (1978) studied the effects of caffeine on their general metabolism. Each cyclist exercised to exhaustion on a cycle ergometer at 50 per cent of their aerobic capacity after ingesting either decaffeinated or normal coffee (containing 330 mg caffeine). The caffeine takers managed to exercise for 19.5 per cent longer than the control group and had significantly higher levels of plasma fatty acids and blood glycerol. In the caffeine group, the respiratory quotient (RQ) was reduced, possibly indicating a shift from carbohydrate to fat utilization. It was suggested that increased lipolysis postponed exhaustion by slowing the rate of glycogen utilization in liver and skeletal muscle. Ivy et al. (1979) found that caffeine increased work production in athletes by 7.4 per cent compared with control conditions and in the same study fat oxidation was elevated by 31 per cent during the last 70 min of the trial. Essig et al. (1980) measured the effect of caffeine on insulin secretion and glycogen utilization in seven untrained male cyclists. Compared with controls, the caffeine group had a 51 per cent increase in lipid oxidation. Muscle biopsies showed a 39 per cent reduction in glycogen utilization. They concluded that caffeine ingestion can increase oxidation of fatty acids and glycerol in muscle. In contrast, Perkins and Williams (1975) could find no effect with 4, 7 or 10 mg of caffeine per kg body weight in 14 male students exercising to exhaustion. They found no significant difference between control and caffeine-taking groups in exercise time to exhaustion, even though there was a caffeine-induced increase in fatty acid level. In the 6 years since the last edition of this book, the glycogen sparing theory has not advanced further. Two studies in 2000 by Laurent et al. (2000) and Graham et al. (2000) failed to demonstrate any glycogen sparing at 60 and 70 per cent VO_{2max}, respectively. Many of these older studies, though often well-controlled, did not measure the substances about which they were speculating! Several studies have indicated a role for lactate in the mechanism of action of caffeine as it has been shown to raise blood lactate levels. Graham et al. (2000) compared the effect of caffeine administration with placebo in individuals where one leg was exercised while the other was static. Arterial lactate levels rose in the caffeine-treated subjects compared with placebo, but lactate exchange was unaltered by caffeine in either the exercising or the non-exercising leg. The role of lactate is thus unclear.

The results of the pioneering studies of the putative ergogenicity of caffeine led me to summarize in the previous editions of this book that 'caffeine has a positive ergogenic effect on large muscles and on short term exercise which requires both strength and power' (George, 1996). Since then a number of studies have been carried out in both animals and humans, some of which support and some of which refute this statement. By the 1990s some reviewers began to have doubts whether caffeine was a true ergogenic aid. In his 1991 review, Conlee listed six crucial factors which he claimed accounted for the variability in the effect of caffeine on athletic performance. These were dose, type of exercise, intensity of exercise, pre-exercise feedings, previous caffeine use and training status. He also identified from his literature survey optimal conditions for the ergogenic effect of caffeine, which are: use of untrained, caffeine-abstaining subjects, caffeine doses of 6–10 mg/kg, abstinence from high carbohydrate diets and an experimental protocol involving prolonged activities at 70–85 per cent VO_{2max}. Some of the questions raised by Conlee (1991) had also been addressed previously by Powers and Dodd (1985), who reviewed the evidence for caffeine ergogenicity prior to 1985 and in particular noted discrepancies between the positive effect of caffeine during graded exercise but its lack of effect on VO_{2max}. Research evidence has been further complicated by the increasing number of animal studies, particularly those involving isolated muscle preparations. A detailed analysis of the conflicting results produced by these various studies was made by Dodd et al. (1993). They examined all the studies of caffeine on exercise performance (1985–1992) and found that they could be divided into three major groups, including short-term high-intensity exercise, graded incremental exercise and prolonged endurance exercise, each group containing both human and animal studies.

During short-term high-intensity exercise, caffeine was shown to enhance muscle force production in isolated muscle preparations while most human studies demonstrate no effect. Caffeine appears to increase peak muscular tension and decrease the time required to achieve peak tension and this is associated with increased release of Ca^{2+} from the sarcoplasmic reticulum. However, in this situation, the muscle Ca^{2+} was also depleted more rapidly resulting in earlier fatigue. Studies in humans, however, have shown that caffeine does not increase force, electromyographic activity or muscular power during either hand grip exercise or short maximal bouts of cycle exercise. Dodd *et al.* (1993) have concluded that the major source of discrepancy between human and *in vitro* animal studies is the dosage of caffeine used. They have calculated that most *in vitro* studies utilize caffeine doses of 200–3500 µmol/l, while human studies have used caffeine doses below 10 mg/kg. In the blood, even assuming the caffeine remained unbound to plasma proteins, the concentration of caffeine would be 60–100 µmol/l. If the allowance is made for 15–17 per cent binding of caffeine to plasma proteins then the amount of caffeine available for cellular action is some 100 µmol *less* than the lowest dosage used in *in vitro* studies. Conversely, to produce a positive ergogenic effect in humans of the same order as that achieved during *in vitro* experiments, it would require caffeine doses which would produce urinary caffeine concentrations well in excess of the then IOC limits of 12 µg/ml urine. It is surprising that so few caffeine studies have involved determinations of blood caffeine levels following administration and during exercise.

More recently, the effects of caffeine on graded incremental exercise have been investigated. Two studies, both of which administered caffeine at 10–15 mg/kg to moderately fit, caffeine-naive subjects, 1–3 hours before exercise testing, demonstrated an improved performance during graded incremental exercise (McNaughton, 1987; Flinn *et al.*, 1990). Performance improvement was identified as an increase in time to exhaustion, and a reduced lactate threshold. The significance of the results is that they were obtained using high doses of caffeine and it is unclear whether they were influenced by any caffeine intolerance of the subjects. However, in 1993, Dodd and co-workers produced evidence to show that the caffeine tolerance within a subject has no effect on performance during exercise of moderate intensity and duration. From these findings it was concluded that the results of the original studies were associated with the high dosage of caffeine used.

The other major area of exercise research involving caffeine concerns prolonged endurance exercise, the subject of the much quoted early research of Costill *et al.* (1978). In the past four years the initial findings have been disputed. Conlee (1991) has stated that the evidence supporting the positive ergogenic effect of caffeine during prolonged exercise is inconclusive. In contrast Dodd *et al.* (1993) have reviewed the studies of caffeine and prolonged exercise since 1978 and have produced a detailed re-analysis of the series of tests. There was a considerable variability in the experimental design used. For example, some studies used caffeine-naive, others caffeine-habituated subjects and dietary control was employed in some subjects but not in others. With the exception of one study that involved a 21 km ski run, all the studies quoted involved cycle ergometer or treadmill measurements. From these, Dodd *et al.* (1993) concluded that moderate to high doses of caffeine are ergogenic during prolonged moderate-intensity exercise in both caffeine-naive and caffeine-habituated subjects. It was argued in their review that the positive ergogenic effect of caffeine on endurance exercise is apparent only when studies of high intensity exercise are omitted from the analysis. Thus, in their table of endurance studies, two of which used continuous low-intensity exercise (50–60 per cent of VO_{2max}) for 2–8 hours followed by exercise to exhaustion at 90 per cent of VO_{2max}, there was no evidence of an ergogenic effect of caffeine. The biochemical and physiological basis of the ergogenic effect of caffeine during endurance exercise is unclear. The possible explanations cited by Ivy *et al.* (1979) and Essig *et al.* (1980) have been added to by Conlee (1991) and now include: (1) a stimulatory effect on the CNS, (2) enhanced release of catecholamines, (3) free fatty acid mobilization from adipose tissue leading to increased β oxidation in muscle and the sparing of glycogen, (4) indirect inhibition of muscle glycogenolysis, thus sparing muscle glycogen, and (5) increased use of muscle triglycerides, also leading to muscle glycogen sparing.

Studies where caffeine effects on glycogen depletion have been investigated simultaneously with prolonged exercise (Essig *et al.*, 1980; Erickson *et al.*, 1987; Spriet *et al.*, 1992) all show that caffeine brings about glycogen sparing, thus confirming the original hypothesis of Bellet *et al.* (1965) quoted earlier. Research by Essig *et al.* (1980) suggesting that fat metabolism, fuelled by increased lipolysis, is enhanced following caffeine ingestion has not been unequivocally supported by recent research. Dodd *et al.* (1993) quote the results of seven experiments, five of which demonstrate an increase in plasma free fatty acid levels during exercise following caffeine ingestion which, however, was not accompanied in any study by a rise in the respiratory quotient. Thus caffeine may well antagonize adenosine-mediated inhibition of lipolysis, but the consequent increased availability of free fatty acids does not appear to influence energy production. The anomalous results obtained with caffeine on free fatty acids and the respiratory quotient may be explained by the observation that caffeine ingestion raises plasma catecholamine levels. This may lead to a pre-exercise increase in free fatty acid utilization, which masks any effect of caffeine during the exercise period (Conlee, 1991). However, French *et al.* (1991) showed that caffeine ingestion immediately prior to exercise to exhaustion improved the distance that was run by six trained athletes. In this experiment blood lactate was raised only at the end of the study and blood triglycerides were elevated by caffeine only after 45 min of exercise. This, then, is the position up to the mid-1990s.

In recent years, research into the effects of caffeine has been more intensive, but though we have much further evidence that caffeine *is* ergogenic, the nature, mechanism and circumstances of its effects in exercise are hardly any clearer. Research has been clouded by investigations into whether the IOC limit of 12 µg/ml urinary concentration was acceptable and also by experiments involving the addition of caffeine to other ergogenic agents and the effects of caffeine added to so-called power supplements. Spriet (1995) is adamant that caffeine does have a measurable ergogenic effect on endurance exercise at doses which did not contravene the IOC urinary concentration limit.

Many of the effects of stimulants on exercise are subtle and may only be revealed using the most accurate ergometers and timing devices currently available. There is also confusion about which environment is best to research and observe the effects of caffeine: the controlled laboratory situation or the semi-controlled competitive arena. Terry Graham (2001) has attempted to organize the current state of our knowledge about caffeine (up to April 2001) in a comprehensive review. He has divided caffeine effects into five major categories:

- endurance in long-term exercise;
- speed and power in long-term exercise;
- endurance in short-term intensive exercise;
- power in short-term intensive exercise; and
- strength activity.

Comparing results over the past 6 years and back to 1981, he found 13 studies which examined the effect of caffeine on endurance exercise (half an hour to 1 hour fatigue) and only two failed to find a positive ergogenic effect for caffeine. In these experiments, power was kept constant or controlled so that the only 'athletic' variable being measured was endurance time. His review concludes that whether this is a true increase of the competition situation is debatable but that, even so, such an effect of caffeine might be useful in training.

The earlier studies on speed and power have often been criticized for the small numbers of subjects involved and the lack of vigour in the protocol design. Power and speed studies tend to be more equivocal but still seem, on balance, to support an ergogenic effect of caffeine. In contrast to the highly positive effect of caffeine on speed in cross-country skiers, Cole *et al.* (1996) showed that caffeine ingestion did not benefit one athlete in a 21 km road run. Caffeine reduced the 1.5 km time by 23 seconds in a group of 12 swimmers (Mackintosh and Wright, 1995). In a well-controlled study by Kovacs *et al.* (1998) caffeine enhanced the power output by 20 cyclists in a 1 hour time-trial, but this study was complicated by the co-administration of a power/electrolyte drink: the effects of caffeine being additive.

Short-term endurance and internal exercise

Collomp and his group (1990) found no effect of caffeine on exercise duration at VO_{2max} compared with placebo, while Jackman's group (1996) found there was a statistically significant effect of caffeine on endurance under these conditions. Analysis of five studies of caffeine in progressive exercise regimes has shown that in four of these, caffeine or theophylline has a positive effect, or at least 'a non-significant improvement in exercise time' (Graham, 2001). Pasman et al. (1995) found that though incremental doses of caffeine enhanced endurance performance time in cyclists exercising to exhaustion on an ergometer, there was no dose–response relationship between caffeine and performance or blood glycerol concentration.

During short-term intensive exercise the effects of caffeine seem to be more equivocal. We now seem to be in a position to overturn the perceived wisdom that caffeine has no effects on power output in these conditions. Whereas Wiles' group in 1992 showed that caffeine improved running speed in non-elite athletes, the degree of improvement did not correlate with caffeine intake. Collomp's group (1990) of four trained swimmers improved their 100 m sprint times while taking caffeine, whereas a group of untrained swimmers noted no improvement.

Thus, caffeine does seem to have an ergogenic effect in at least four categories of exercise evaluation. How is this achieved? Early experiments (described under Effects in athletes, above) rely heavily on the so-called 'glycogen-sparing theory': caffeine stimulates adrenaline secretion resulting in increased lipolysis and plasma free fatty acid (FFA) concentration, increased fat oxidation and a reduction in the utilization of carbohydrate. Graham (2001) has stated that there is now much less support for this hypothesis, particularly since caffeine has now been shown to enhance aspects of short-term and/or intense activity exercise in which the influence of fatty acids is negligible. Also, van Baak and Saris (2000) have demonstrated that FFAs are not elevated in the blood during endurance performance exercise regimes. He has revised the theory: caffeine stimulates FFA release by antagonizing A_1 adenosine receptors on adipocytes, increased FFA concentration is taken up by the liver, which oxidizes them or converts them to triglycerides. Excess FFAs are partially oxidized to keto acids (ketone bodies), which can be used as an energy source by muscle, heart and other tissues. Central to the older hypotheses is the concept of glycogen sparing. The work of Ivy et al. (1979), mentioned previously, was supported by other contemporary studies but has not found support since then. Chesley et al. (1998) found no difference in the glycogen content of exercising muscle either 3 or 15 minutes into an exercise regime at 85 per cent of VO_{2max} and Greer et al. (2000) have shown that theophylline and caffeine increased endurance time, but did not change muscle glycogen depletion. Further work needs to be done to investigate these conflicts, possibly re-evaluating and re-running the earlier experiments.

Graham (2001) has cited six reports of caffeine-induced increases in blood glucose but states that generally it has little or no effect. To add to the confusion surrounding caffeine action, it has frequently been demonstrated in the past that it increases blood lactate levels during exercise. However, this increase in lactate does not originate from the muscle, as demonstrated recently by Graham's team (Graham *et al.*, 2000), and they were able to demonstrate no effect of caffeine or theophylline on fat or carbohydrate metabolism during exercise. Recent work by Chesley *et al.* (1998) has concluded that caffeine may reduce phosphocreatine degradation and reduce the formation of ADP in exercising muscle, but this was carried out in a small sample of volunteers. Caffeine increases plasma adrenaline levels, but this increase does not seem to be related to caffeine-induced improvements in endurance, power output or speed during exercise. One recent study (Graham *et al.*, 2000) has demonstrated a caffeine-induced increase in noradrenaline release in exercising muscle and this needs to be investigated in relation to different exercise programmes in a concentration- and dose-dependent manner. So, if we have destroyed the fashionable glycogen/lactate/FFA theories; what remains? Other possibilities for caffeine mechanisms of action include: actions on ion balance, blood flow and the striated muscle excitation–contraction coupling mechanism. The role of adenosine and, therefore, the action of adenosine receptor antagonism in these processes needs to be examined. Another neglected area of caffeine/methyl xanthine research includes the CNS. Each of the adenosine receptor types found in the brain and the full implications for the inhibitor of these receptors on behaviour needs to be investigated. In 1996, Cole *et al.* showed that caffeine may alter the perception by an athlete of how much exercise they had actually performed. The basis of this may well be simiar to the observations of Plaskett and Cafarelli (2001), who showed that alterations in muscle proprioception may be involved in the caffeine-enhanced ability to endure repeated isometric quadriceps contractions. Anselme *et al.* (1992) noted that caffeine enhanced maximum power in 6-second sprints but failed to do so in a 30-second Wingate test. Graham (2001) concluded from this limited evidence that 'caffeine can be ergogenic in exercise lasting as long as 60 seconds'. In this review, Graham (2001) notes the many anecdotal reports of caffeine use in strength athletes and suggests that the use could be related to perceived improvements in strength, power or fatigue. His review of the small number of experiments on the direct effects of caffeine on muscle contractility and the spinal reflex also suggests that caffeine may have direct actions on muscle strength, which are disassociated from its assumed metabolic actions. Some support for this theory comes from a small study by Tarnopolsky and Cupido (2000). They found that caffeine potentiates low frequency (20 Hz) muscle force but has no effect at 40 Hz. This study involved only six volunteers in each of a habitual and non-habitual caffeine group. It may indicate that some of the ergogenic effect of caffeine is produced by a direct effect on muscle.

Another largely unresearched area, surprisingly, is in team sports. Paton *et al.* (2001) examined the effect of caffeine on mean sprint performance and fatigue over 10 sprints and found that the effect of caffeine was negligible, and further doses of caffeine worsened the time taken to complete the final sprint compared with placebo.

Caffeine combinations

Caffeine appears to have an additive effect on performance when combined with stimulants such as ephedrine. Bell's group in Toronto, Canada (1998), have examined the effects of caffeine and ephedrine together in a number of exercise situations. They found that combined caffeine and ephedrine significantly improved performance in the so-called 'harrier test' and resulted in improved run times and increased heart-rate (Bell and Jacobs, 1999). Using an anaerobic exercise programme, Bell *et al.* (2001) found that ephedrine increased power output during the early phase of the test but caffeine increased time to exhaustion. They explained their result on the basis of central stimulation by ephedrine and muscle stimulation by caffeine.

I observed in 1996 that future research might be devoted to understanding the underlying psychological processes that influence the abuse of central stimulants by athletes and possibly those mental factors that contribute to success or failure in sport. Begel in 1992 reviewed the psychodynamic factors influencing the development of the athlete and the maintenance of his/her performance. Several sport scientists have attempted to devise models and measurement techniques for the evaluation of mental and psychological influences on sport. John Raglin's recent review (2001) of the MHM (Mental Health Model) revealed that successful athletes enjoyed better mental health than their less successful colleagues and that successful athletes were less likely to be introverted. He also admitted that mental health in the unsuccessful athletes was still normal when compared with the rest of the population and that introversion has been shown to be advantageous in sports involving extreme manual skill such as shooting. Mood state in many of the studies reviewed by Raglin was closely related to training levels and in particular to overtraining. There may be a connection, then, between reduced performance, overtraining and lowered mood. Possibly, athletes particularly resort to central stimulants when coaches fail to identify or help to rectify problems in the athletes' approach and technique or fail to counsel them adequately when their performance drops. It would also be interesting to know, as Begel concluded, what particular personalities are associated with central stimulant abuse in sportspersons and whether psychiatric disorders contribute to abuse of stimulants by them. Could there be a biochemical–psychopharmacological connection? The authors of two reviews on the influence of CNS neurotransmission systems on mental and physical performance suggest this is possible. Strüder and Weicker (2001a) argue that exhaustive, intensive exercise may lead to disruption of normal neurotransmission patterns in the brain, particularly those involving the neurotransmitter 5HT (serotonin). Their second proposition (Strüder and Weicker, 2001b) is that the mental symptoms experienced by many over-training athletes are not caused by systemic metabolic changes but by 'central, exhaustive exercise stress'. It may be too simplistic to link stimulant abuse in sport to tenuous changes in CNS neurotransmission, but since many of the drugs of abuse discussed in this chapter cause profound changes in these processes, it is a subject worthy of further investigation.

It is interesting that both voluntary running and cocaine administration have similar effects on certain brain 'reward' centres in rats' brains (Werme et al., 2000). Perhaps scanning studies will reveal similar findings in the human brain.

3.6   Conclusions and the future

The effect of stimulants on sporting performance is proving to be more subtle than was originally forecast. Not only are we to revise our concepts of what aspects of performance are enhanced by these drugs but we are having to revisit long-held theories about modes of action. Many of the current anomalies in the results obtained with stimulant drugs could be resolved by more carefully standardized and controlled experiments. For example, we need to differentiate studies on endurance from speed, power from work and to include analysis of subtle central actions like the perception of work done. It is also obvious that we must control for the subjects' athletic prowess and state of training because this has confounded investigations into anabolic steroids for many years (see Chapter 5). Studies also illustrate differences in responses between naive and habitual 'users' of a drug in both animal and human studies and this also must be incorporated into experimental design. Finally, we must learn to be more thorough and rigorous in the overall design of our experiments. Good studies should measure the plasma/blood concentration of any drug being administered together with physiological and physical measures of its effect. Also a full and detailed analysis of the impact of the drug under investigation over time in several exercise paradigms should be undertaken as the maximum effect of ephedrine, for example, seems to occur after only 10 seconds of exercise.

3.7   References

American Psychiatric Association (1994) *Diagnostic and Statistical Manual of Mental Disorders*, 4th edn revised (DSM IV).

Anselme, F., Collomp, K. and Mercier, B. (1992) Caffeine increases maximal aerobic power and blood lactate concentration. *Eur. J. Appl. Physiol.*, **65**, 188–191.

Begel, D. (1992) An overview of Sport Psychiatry. *Am. J. Psychiat.*, **149**, 606–614.

Bell, D.G. and Jacobs, I. (1999) Combined caffeine and ephedrine ingestion improves run times of Canadian Forces Warrior Test. *Aviat. Space Environ. Med.*, **70**, 325–329.

Bell, D.G., Jacobs, I. and Zamecoik, J. (1998) Effects of caffeine, ephedrine and their combination on time to exhaustion during high-intensity exercise. *Eur. J. Appl. Physiol.*, **77**, 427–433.

Bell, D.G., Jacobs, I. and Ellerington, K. (2001) Effect of caffeine and ephedrine ingestion on anaerobic exercise performance. *Med. Sci. Sport Exerc.*, **33**, 1399–1403.

Bellet, S., Kershbaum, A. and Aspe, J. (1965) The effect of caffeine on free fatty acids. *Arch. Int. Med.*, **116**, 750–752.

Benzaquen, B.S., Cohen, V. and Eisenberg, M.J. (2001) Effects of cocaine on the coronary arteries. *Am. Heart J.*, **142**, 402–410.

Bolla, K.I., Cadet, J.L. and London, E.D. (1998) The neuropsychiatry of chronic cocaine abuse. *J. Neuropsychiat. Clin. Neurosci.*, **10**, 280–289.

Braiden, R.W., Fellingham, G.W. and Conlee, R.K. (1994) *Med. Sci. Sports Exerc.*, **26**, 695–700.

Brookes, L.G. (1985) Central Nervous System Stimulants. In *Psychopharmacology: Recent Advances and Future Prospects*, (ed.) S.D. Iverson, Oxford, Oxford University Press, pp. 264–277.

Bucci, L.R. (2000) Selected herbals and human performance. *Am. J. Clin. Nutr.*, **72**, 624S–636S.

Cantwell, J.D. and Rose, F.D. (1981) Cocaine and cardiovascular events. *Phys. Sports Med.*, **14**, 77–82.

Chandler, J.V. and Blair, S.N. (1980) The effect of amphetamines on selected physiological components related to athletic success. *Med. Sci. Sports Exerc.*, **12**, 65–69.

Chen, N. and Reith, M.E.A. (2000) Structure and function of the dopamine transporter. *Eur. J. Pharmacol.*, **405**, 329–339.

Chesley, A., Howlett, R.A., Heignehauser, G.J. *et al.* (1998) Regulation of muscle glycogenolytic flux during intense aerobic exercise after caffeine. *Am. J. Physiol.*, **275**, 596–603.

Clarkson, P.M. and Thompson, H.S. (1997) Drugs and sport – research findings and limitations. *Sports Med.*, **24**, 366–384.

Cole, K.J., Costill, D.L., Starling, R.D. *et al.* (1996) Effect of caffeine ingestion on perception of effort and subsequent work production. *Int. J. Sport Nutr.*, **4**, 14–23.

Collomp, K., Caillaud, C. and Audran, M. (1990) Influence de la prise aigue ou chronique de caffeine sur la performance et les catecholamines au cours d'un exercice maximal. *C.R.Seances Soc. Biol. Fil.*, **184**, 87–92.

Comer, S.D., Hart, C.L., Ward, A.S. *et al.* (2001) Effects of repeated oral methamphetamine administration in humans. *Psychopharmacology*, **155**, 397–401.

Conlee, R.K. (1991) Amphetamine, caffeine and cocaine. In *Perspectives in Exercise Science and Sports Medicine 4*, (ed.) Lamb, D.R. and Williams, M.H. New York, Brown and Benchmark, pp. 285–328.

Conlee, R.K., Han, D.H., Kelly, K.P. *et al.* (1991) Effects of cocaine on plasma catecholamine and muscle glycogen concentrations during exercise in the rat. *J. Appl. Physiol.*, **70**, 1323–1327.

Conlee, R.K., Kelly, K.P., Ojuka, E.O. and Hammer, R.L. (2000) Cocaine and exercise: alpha-1 receptor blockade does not alter muscle glycogenolysis or blood lactacidosis. *J. Appl. Physiol.*, **88**, 77–81.

Connell, P.H. (1958) *Amphetamine psychosis*. London, Chapman and Hall.

Costill, D.L., Dalsky, G.P. and Fink, W.J. (1978) Effects of caffeine ingestion on metabolism and exercise performance. *Med. Sci. Sports Exerc.*, **10**, 155–158.

Daly, J.W., Butts-Lamb, P. and Padgett, W. (1983) Sub-classes of adenosine receptors in the central nervous system interaction with caffeine and related methyl xanthines. *Cell. Mol. Neurobiol.*, **3**, 69–80.

Dodd, S.L., Herb, R.A. and Powers, S.K. (1993) Caffeine and exercise performance – an up date. *Sports. Med.*, **15**, 14–23.

Erickson, M.A., Schwarkopf, R.J. and McKenzie, R.D. (1987) Effects of caffeine, fructose, and glucose ingestion on muscle glycogen utilisation during exercise. *Med. Sci. Sport Exerc.*, **19**, 579–583.

Essig, D., Costill, D.L. and Van Handel, P.J. (1980) Effects of caffeine ingestion on utilisation of muscle glycogen and lipid during leg ergometer cycling. *Int. J. Sports Med.*, **1**, 86–90.

Farre, M., De La Tour, R., Llorente, M. *et al.* (1993) Alcohol and cocaine interactions in humans. *J. Pharmacol. Exp. Ther.*, **266**, 1364–1373.

Favier, R., Caceres, E. and Koubi, H. (1996) Effects of coca chewing on metabolic and hormonal changes during prolonged submaximal exercise. *J. Appl. Physiol.*, **80**, 650–655.

Fibiger, H.C., Phillips, A.G. and Brown, E.E. (1992) The neurobiology of cocaine-induced reinforcement. In *Cocaine: scientific and social dimensions. Ciba Foundation Symposium 166*, (ed.) Wolstenholme, G.E.W., Chichester, John Wiley, pp. 96–124.

Flinn, S., Gregory, J., McNaughton, L.R. *et al.* (1990) Caffeine ingestion prior to incremental cycling to exhaustion in recreational cyclists. *Int. J. Sports Med.*, **11**, 188–193.

Forman, E.S., Dekker, A.H., Javors, J.R. *et al.* (1995) High risk behaviour in teen-age male athletes. *Clin. J. Sport. Med.*, **5**, 36–47.

Fredholm, B.B., Battig, K., Holman, J. *et al.* (1999) Actions of caffeine in the brain with special reference to factors that contribute to its widespread use. *Pharmacol. Rev.*, **51**, 83–133.

Fredholm, B.B., Izerman, A.P., Jacobson, K.A., Klotz, K-N. and Linden, J. (2001) International Union of Pharmacology. XXV. Nomenclature and classification of adenosine receptors. *Pharmacol. Rev.*, **53**, 527–552.

French, C., McNaughton, L., Davies, P. *et al.* (1991) Caffeine ingestion during exercise to exhaustion in elite distance runners. *J. Sport Med. Phys. Fitness*, **31**, 425–432.

George, A.J. (1996) CNS Stimulants. In *Drugs in Sport*, 2nd edn, (ed.) Mottram, D.R., London, E and F.N. Spon, pp. 86–112.

George, A.J. (2000) Central nervous system stimulants. *Ballière's Clin. Endocrinol. Metab.*, **14**, 79–88.

Gill, N.D., Shield, A., Blazevich, A.J. *et al.* (2000) Muscular and cardiorespiratory effects of pseudo ephedrine in human athletes. *Br. J. Clin. Pharmacol.*, **50**, 205–213.

Gillies, H., Derman, W.E., Noakes, T.D. *et al.* (1996) Pseudoephedrine is without ergogenic effects during prolonged exercise. *J. Appl. Physiol.*, **81**, 2611–2617.

Golding, L.A. (1981) Drugs and hormones. In *Ergogenic Aids and Muscular Performance*, (ed.) Morgan, W.P. New York: Academic Press, pp. 368–397.

Golding, L.A. and Barnard, J.P. (1963) The effect of D-amphetamine sulphate on physical performance. *J. Sports Med.*, **3**, 221–224.

Graham, T.E. (2001) Caffeine and exercise – metabolism, endurance and performance. *Sports Med.*, **31**, 785–807.

Graham, T.E., Hibbert, E. and Sathasivam, P. (1998) Metabolic and exercise endurance effects of coffee and caffeine ingestion. *J. Appl. Physiol.*, **85**, 883–889.

Graham, T.E., Helge, J.W., MacLean, D.A. *et al.* (2000) Caffeine ingestion does not alter carbohydrate or fat metabolism in human skeletal muscle during exercise. *J. Physiol.*, **529**, 837–847.

Greden, J.F. (1974) Anxiety of caffeinism: a diagnostic dilemma. *Am. J. Psychiat.*, **131**, 1089–1092.

Greer, F., McLean, C. and Graham, T.E. (1998) Caffeine, performance, and metabolism during repeated Wingate exercise tests. *J. Appl. Physiol.*, **85**, 1502–1508.

Greer, F., Friars, D. and Graham, T.E. (2000) Comparison of caffeine and theophylline ingestion: exercise metabolism and endurance. *J. Appl. Physiol.*, **89**, 1837–1844.

Haldi, J. and Wynn, W. (1959) Action of drugs on efficiency of swimmers. *Res. Q.*, **31**, 449–553.

Han, D.H., Kelly, K.P., Fellingham, G.W. *et al.* (1996) Cocaine and exercise: temporal changes in plasma levels of lactate, glucose and cocaine. *Ann. J. Physiol.*, **270**, 438–445.

Hanna, J.M. (1970) The effects of coca chewing on exercise in the Quechua of Peru. *Hum. Biol.*, **42**, 1–11.

Hanna, J.M. (1971) Further studies on the effects of coca chewing on exercise. *Hum. Biol.*, **43**, 200–209.

Hart, C.L., Ward, A.S., Harvey, M. *et al.* (2001) Methamphetamine self-administration by humans. *Psychopharmacology*, **57**, 75–81.

Hoffer, R. (1992) A career of living dangerously. *Sports Illustr.*, **76**, 38–41.

Howell, L.L. and Wilcox, K.M. (2001) The dopamine transporter and cocaine medication development: Drug self-administration in non-human primates. *J. Pharmacl. Exp. Ther.*, **298**, 1–6.

Ivy, J.L., Costill, D.L. and Fink, W.J. (1979) Influence of caffeine and carbohydrate feedings on endurance performance. *Med. Sci. Sports*, **11**, 6–11.

Jackman, M., Wendling, P., Friars, D. *et al.* (1996) Metabolic catecholamine, and endurance responses to caffeine during intense exercise. *J. Appl. Physiol.*, **81**, 1658–1663.

Kelly, K.P., Han, D.H., Fellingham, G.W., Winder, W.W. and Conlee, R.K. (1995) Cocaine and exercise: physiological responses of cocaine-conditioned rats. *Med. Sci. Sports Exerc.*, **27**, 65–72.

Kennedy, L. (1974) *Pursuit, The chase and sinking of the Bismarck*. London, Collins.

Knuepfer, M.M. and Miller, P.J. (1999) Review of evidence for a novel model of cocaine-induced cardiovascular toxicity. *Pharmacol. Biochem. Behav.*, **63**, 489–500.

Kovacs, E.M.R., Stegen, J.H.C.H. and Brouns, F. (1998) Effect of caffeinated drinks on substrate metabolism, caffeine excretion, and performance. *J. Appl. Physiol.*, **85**, 709–715.

Kuhar, M.J. (1992) Molecular pharmacology of cocaine: a dopamine hypothesis and its implications. In *Cocaine: scientific and social dimensions. Ciba Foundation*

Symposium 166, (ed.) Wolstenholme, G.E.W. Chichester, John Wiley, pp. 81–95.

Laties, V.G. and Weiss, B. (1981) The amphetamine margin in sports. *Fed. Proc.*, **40**, 2689–2692.

Latini, S. and Perdata, F. (2001) Adenosine in the central nervous system: release mechanisms and extracellular concentrations. *J. Neurochem.*, **79**, 463–484.

Laurent, D., Scheider, K.E., Prusaczyk, W.K. *et al.* (2000) Effects of caffeine on muscle glycogen utilisation and the neuroendocrine axis during exercise. *J. Clin. Endocrinol. Metab.*, **85**, 2170–2175.

Lelo, A., Miners, J.O., Robson, R. *et al.* (1986) Assessment of caffeine exposure: caffeine content of beverages, caffeine intake and plasma concentrations of methylxanthines. *Clin. Pharm. Ther.*, **39**, 54–59.

Mackintosh, B.R. and Wright, B.M. (1995) Caffeine ingestion and performance of a 1500 m swim. *Can. J. Appl. Physiol.*, **20**, 168–170.

Mandell, A.J. (1979) The Sunday Syndrome: A unique pattern of amphetamine abuse indigenous to American Professional Football. *Clin. Toxicol.*, **15**, 225–232.

Mandell, A.J., Stewart, K.D. and Russo, P.V. (1981) The Sunday Syndrome from Kinetics to altered consciousness. *Fed. Proc.*, **40**, 2693–2696.

Marques-Magallanes, J.A., Koyal, S.N., Cooper, C.B., Kleenip, E.C. and Tashkin, D.P. (1997) Impact of habitual cocaine smoking on the physiological response to maximum exercise. *Chest*, **112**, 1008–1016.

McCance-Katz, E.F., Kosten, T.R. and Jatlow, P. (1998) Concurrent use of cocaine and alcohol is more potent and potentially more toxic than use of either alone – a multi-dose study. *Bio. Psychiat.*, **44**, 250–259.

McNaughton, L. (1987) Two levels of caffeine ingestion on blood lactate and free fatty acid response during incremental exercise. *Res. Q. Exerc. Sport*, **58**, 255–259.

Nyce, J.W. (1999) Insight into adenosine receptor function using anti-sense and gene knockout approaches. *Trends Pharmacol. Sci.*, **20**, 79–83.

Pasman, W.J., van Burak, M.A., Jeukendup, A.C. and Dehaan, A. (1995) Effect of different dosages of caffeine on endurance performance time. *Int. J. Sports Med.*, **16**, 225–230.

Paton, C.D., Hopkins, W.G. and Vollebregt, L. (2001) Little effect of caffeine ingestion on repeated sprints in team sports athletes. *Med. Sci. Sports Exerc.*, **33**, 822–825.

Perkins, R. and Williams, M.H. (1975) Effects of caffeine upon maximal muscular endurance of females. *Med. Sci. Sports*, **7**, 221–224.

Plaskett, C.H. and Cafarelli, E. (2001) Caffeine increases endurance and alternates force sensations during submaximal isometric contractions. *J. Appl. Physiol.*, **91**, 1535–1544.

Powers, S.K. and Dodd, S. (1985). Caffeine and endurance performance. *Sports Med.*, **2**, 165–174.

Raglin, J.S. (2001) Psychological factors in sport performance. *Sports Med.*, **31**, 875–890.

Sawynok, J. and Yaksh, T.L. (1993) Caffeine as an analgesic adjuvant. A review of pharmacology and mechanisms of action. *Pharmacol. Rev.*, **45**, 43–85.

Scher, J. (1992) Death of a goon. *Sports Illustr.*, **76**, 112–116.

Seiden, L.S., Sabol, K.E. and Ricaurte, G.A. (1993) Amphetamine: effects on catecholamine systems and behaviour. *Annu. Rev. Pharmacol. Toxicol.*, **32**, 639–677.

Sidney, K.H. and Lefcoe, W.M. (1977) The effects of ephedrine on the physiological and psychological responses to submaximal and maximal exercises in man. *Med. Sci. Sports*, **9**, 95–99.

Silverstone, T. and Goodall, E. (1985) How amphetamine works. In *Psychopharmacology: Recent Advances, Future Prospects*, (ed.) Iversen, S.D., Oxford, Oxford University Press, pp. 315–325.

Sinclair, C.J.D. and Geiger, J.D. (2000) Caffeine use in sports. *J. Sports Med. Phys. Fitness*, **40**, 71–79.

Smith, B.J., Jones, H.E. and Griffiths, R.R. (2001) Physiological, subjective and reinforcing effects of oral and intravenous cocaine in humans. *Psychopharmacology*, **156**, 435–444.

Smith, D.A. and Perry, P.J. (1992) The efficacy of ergogenic agents in athletic competition, Part II: Other performance-enhancing agents. *Ann. Pharmacother.*, **26**, 653–659.

Smith, G.M. and Beecher, H.G. (1959) Amphetamine sulphate and athletic performance. *J. Am. Med. Assoc.*, **170**, 542–551.

Spielvogel, H., Caceres, E., Karbritt, B. *et al.* (1996) Effects of coca chewing on metabolic and hormonal changes during graded incremental exercise to maximum. *J. Appl. Physiol.*, **80**, 643–649.

Spriet, L.L. (1995) Caffeine and performance. *Int. J. Sport Nutr.*, **5**, 84–99.

Spriet, L., MacLean, D., Dyck, D. *et al.* (1992) Effects of caffeine on muscle glycogenolysis and acetyl group metabolism during prolonged exercise in humans. *Am. J. Physiol.*, **262**, 891–898.

Strain, E.C. and Griffins, R.R. (1997) Caffeine use disorders. In *Psychiatry*, vol 1, (eds) Tasman, A., Kay, J. and Lieberman, J.A., Philadelphia (PA), W.B. Saunders Co., 779–794.

Strüder, H.K. and Weicker, H. (2001a) Physiology and pathophysiology of the serotonergic system and its implications on mental and physical performance. Part 1. *Int. J. Sports Med.*, **22**, 467–481.

Strüder, H.K. and Weicker, H. (2001b) Physiology and pathophysiology of the serotonergic system and its implications on mental and physical performance. Part 2. *Int. J. Sports Med.*, **22**, 482–497.

Swain, R.A., Harsha, D.M., Baenziger, J. *et al.* (1997) Do pseudo ephedrine or phenylpropanolamine improve maximum oxygen uptake and time to exhaustion. *Clin. J. Sport. Med.*, **7**, 168–173.

Tarnopolsky, M. and Cupido, C. (2000) Caffeine potentiates lower frequency skeletal muscle force in habitual and non-habitual caffeine consumers. *J. Appl. Physiol.*, **89**, 1719–1724.

Theil, D. and Essing, B. (1930) Cocaine und muskelarbeit I. Der einfluss auf leistung und gastoffwechsel. *Arbeitsphysiologie*, **3**, 287–297.

Unterwald, E.M., Kreek, M.J. and Cuntapay, M. (2001) The frequency of cocaine administration impacts cocaine-induced receptor alteration. *Brain Res.*, **900**, 103–109.

Van Baak, M.A. and Saris, W.H.M. (2000) The effect of caffeine on endurance performance after non-selective beta-adrenergic blockade. *Med. Sci. Sport Exerc.*, **32**, 499–503.

Volkow, N.D., Fowler, J.S. and Wang, G.J. (1999) Imaging studies on the role of dopamine in cocaine reinforcement and addiction in humans. *J. Psychopharmacol.*, **13**, 337–343.

Volkow, N.D., Wang, G.J., Fischman, M.W. *et al.* (2000) *Life Sci.*, **67**, 1507–1515.

Wadler, G.A. and Hainline, B. (1989) *Drugs and the Athlete*. Philadelphia, F.A. Davies Company.

Weiss, B. and Laties, V.G. (1962) Enhancement of human performance by caffeine and the amphetamines. *Pharmacol. Rev.*, **14**, 1–36.

Welder, A.A. and Melchert, R.B. (1993) Cardiotoxic effects of cocaine and anabolic-androgenic steroids in the athlete. *J. Pharmacol. Toxicol. Meth.*, **29**, 61–68.

Werme, M., Thoren, P., Olson, L. and Brene S. (2000) Running and cocaine both upregulate dynorphin mRNA in medial caudate putamen. *Eur. J. Neurosci.*, **12**, 2967–2974.

Wiles, J.D., Bird, S.R. and Hopkins, J.R. (1992) Effect of caffeinated coffee on running speed, respiratory factors, blood lactate and perceived exertion during 1500 m treadmill running. *Br. J. Sports Med.*, **26**, 116–120.

Wyndham, G.H., Rogers, G.G., Benade, A.J.S. *et al.* (1971) Physiological effects of the amphetamines during exercise. *S. Afr. Med. J.*, **45**, 247–252.

Zhu, M.Y., Shamburger, S., Li, J. *et al.* (2000) Regulation of human dopamine transporter by cocaine and amphetamine. *J. Pharmacol. Exp. Ther.*, **295**, 951–959.

Chapter 4

WADA regulations in relation to drugs used in the treatment of respiratory tract disorders

David. J. Armstrong and Neil Chester

4.1 Introduction

Maximum performance in aerobic events, at whatever level of competition, is only achievable if respiratory function is optimal. Participants will always be concerned about respiratory problems, be they major disease such as asthma or minor ailment such as the common cold. Their recourse to medications either to control or to alleviate symptoms of these conditions has brought many sportspersons into conflict with their national federations and Olympic committees. Thus in the XXVII Olympiad in Sydney (2000), there were 31 positive drug tests reported to the Chairman of the IOC Medical Commission by the head of the Australian Sport Drug Testing Laboratory. Of those 31, 6 were quality control samples. Of the remaining 25 positive results, 14 were for drugs used to treat asthma and 1 was for treatment of the common cold (IOC Medical Commission, 2000b). No further action was taken against the users of the anti-asthma medications because they were permitted drugs, the quantity used fell within the stipulated urine concentration and prior notification had been provided. However, the drug used to treat the common cold resulted in the loss of a gold medal for the individual concerned. It would appear from those figures that drugs used to treat respiratory problems are still of concern to both participants and those responsible for drug testing. This chapter will describe the pathophysiology of asthma, exercise-induced asthma and of coughs and colds. It will discuss the treatments of those conditions with reference to current British Thoracic Society (BTS) guidelines and to the IOC and World Anti-Doping Agency (WADA) Regulations. It will also provide some historical background to the problems encountered by sportspersons as counsel to those who have used or might anticipate using these drugs, albeit inadvertently.

4.2 Asthma and its treatment

Definition

Asthma is a chronic inflammatory disorder of the airways. In susceptible individuals this inflammation causes recurrent episodes of coughing, wheezing, chest tightness and dyspnoea. Inflammation makes the airways sensitive to stimuli such as allergens, chemical irritants, tobacco smoke, cold air or exercise. When exposed to these stimuli, the airways may become swollen, constricted, filled with mucus and hyper-responsive to stimuli. The resulting airflow limitation is reversible (but not completely so in some patients), either spontaneously or with treatment. When asthma therapy is adequate, inflammation can be reduced over the long term, symptoms can usually be controlled and most asthma-related problems prevented (Global Initiative for Asthma, 2001).

Epidemiology

Asthma is one of the commonest chronic conditions. It affects children more commonly than adults. It is estimated that 1 in 7 children (ages 2–15) and 1 in 25 adults (aged 16 and over) in the UK has asthma symptoms currently requiring treatment. That is equivalent to 1.5 million children and 1.9 million adults (National Asthma Audit, 1999/2000). The global incidence of asthma is estimated to be 100 million (Global Initiative for Asthma, 2001).

Pathophysiology

An asthma attack always consists of an early phase and frequently contains a late phase. The early phase occurs within minutes of exposure to the trigger factor, reaches a maximum in 15–20 minutes and normally resolves within an hour. It is caused by bronchoconstriction. The late phase occurs 2–4 hours after exposure to the trigger factor and reaches a maximum after 6–8 hours. It is caused by inflammation of the airways.

Historically, it was thought that airway obstruction and hence difficulty of breathing in asthma were caused by contraction of airway smooth muscle, i.e. bronchoconstriction. However, post-mortem findings in asthma have revealed the cardinal features of inflammation. There is disruption of the airway epithelium (desquamation) and exposure of subepithelial tissue. The subepithelium demonstrates increased blood flow (hyperaemia), oedema (caused by increased vascular permeability), hypertrophy of airway smooth muscle and accumulations of pro-inflammatory cells (particularly eosinophils and mononuclear cells). The molecular mechanisms of the inflammation are extremely complex and not fully understood. The putative mediators of asthma parallel the chronology of the discovery of inflammatory mediators. Thus they have changed from histamine to the cyclo-oxygenase-mediated metabolites of arachidonic acid, to platelet-activating factor and currently to the lipoxygenase-mediated metabolites of arachidonic acid (namely the leukotrienes). It is unlikely that the inflammatory processes in asthma can be attributed to either a single mediator or a family of mediators. Nevertheless, appreciation of the change of emphasis from bronchoconstriction to inflammation as the cause of airway obstruction has underpinned the change in approach to the management of asthma as defined by organizations such as the British Thoracic Society (1997).

Trigger factors

There are numerous factors which can trigger an asthma attack. The commonest are allergens. These can be either inhaled, such as pollens and/or animal danders (hairs and feathers), or ingested, such as dairy produce or strawberries. Viral, but not bacterial, infection of the upper respiratory tract can trigger asthma. Indeed, the initial presenting feature of asthma may be a persistent wheeze after a self-limiting, upper respiratory tract, viral infection. Occupational pollution can cause asthma. It is difficult to estimate the number of people suffering from this form of asthma. Government figures suggest some 500–600 new cases per annum in the UK. The National Asthma Campaign suggests that the true figure may be nearer 1500–2000 new cases per annum. Asthma attacks can be precipitated by emotional factors. This should not be misinterpreted as an indication that asthma is psychosomatic. Rather it is a reflection of neuroendocrine changes which, as yet, are poorly understood. Certain drugs may precipitate an asthma attack. Beta blockers and non-steroidal anti-inflammatory drugs (NSAIDs), particularly aspirin, can evoke a potentially fatal asthmatic attack. Beta blockers cause bronchoconstriction by blocking the bronchodilating β_2-receptors on airway smooth muscle. They should not be administered to asthmatics. The mechanism by which NSAIDs evoke bronchospasm is hypothetical but may involve a shift in balance between bronchodilating and bronchoconstricting metabolites of arachidonic acid. Approximately 10 per cent of asthmatics are aspirin sensitive and will develop bronchoconstriction if given the drug. For this reason, aspirin and other NSAIDs should be used with caution in asthmatics. Finally, and most importantly in the context of sport, exercise can cause bronchoconstriction, in which case exercise-induced asthma (EIA) is diagnosed. An asthmatic may be sensitive to a variety of trigger factors or to just one.

4.3   Management of asthma

Non-drug treatment of asthma involves avoidance of known trigger factors. Drug treatment of asthma is now directed at arresting and reversing the inflammatory process. The emphasis has shifted from the excessive and inappropriate use of β_2-agonist bronchodilator therapy towards the early use of anti-inflammatory drugs. β_2-Agonists merely relieve the symptoms of asthma without addressing the underlying inflammation. This has been likened to 'painting over rust'. Guidelines for treatment of chronic asthma have been prepared in several countries including Britain and the United States. They constitute a systematic approach to the treatment of increasing severity of symptoms. It must be remembered that the treatment of asthma can also be stepped down if the severity of the symptoms declines. The following is a resumé of guidelines published by the British Thoracic Society in 2004.

Step 1

Mild intermittent asthma

Inhaled short-acting β_2-agonists should be prescribed as short-term reliever therapy for all patients with symptomatic asthma. Unless individual patients are shown to benefit from regular use of inhaled short-acting β_2-agonists, then as required use is recommended.

Using two or more canisters of β_2-agonists per month or > 10–12 puffs per day is a marker of poorly controlled asthma.

Step 2

Regular preventer therapy

Inhaled steroids are the recommended preventer drug for adults and children for achieving overall treatment goals. They should be considered for patients with any of the following:

- exacerbations of asthma in the last two years;
- using inhaled β_2-agonists three times a week or more;
- symptomatic three times a week or more, or waking one night a week.

Inhaled steroids should be initiated twice daily. The dose should be titrated to the lowest at which effective control of asthma is maintained.

Step 3

Add-on therapy

Before initiating a new drug therapy, practitioners should recheck compliance, inhaler technique and eliminate trigger factors.

A trial of other treatments should be undertaken before increasing the inhaled steroid dose beyond 800 µg/day in adults.

The first choice would be the addition of an inhaled long-acting β_2-agonist (LABA) which have been shown to improve lung function and symptoms, and decrease exacerbations. If asthma control remains sub-optimal after the addition of an inhaled long-acting β_2-agoinst, then the dose of inhaled steroids should be increased to 800 µg/day in adults.

If control is still inadequate after a trial of LABA and after increasing the dose of inhaled steroid, consider a sequential trial of one of the following add-on therapies:

- leukotriene receptor antagonists provide improvement in lung function and symptoms, and a decrease in exacerbations;
- theophyllines improve lung function and symptoms, but side-effects occur more commonly;
- slow release β_2-agonist tablets also improve lung function and symptoms, but side-effects occur more commonly.

Step 4

Persistent poor control on moderate dose inhaled steroid + add-on therapy: addition of fourth drug

If control remains inadequate on 800 µg/day inhaled steroid plus a long-acting β_2-agonist, the following interventions should be considered:

- increasing inhaled steroids to 2000 µg/day;
- leukotriene receptor antagonists;
- theophyllines;
- slow release β_2-agonist tablets, though caution needs to be used in patients on long-acting β_2-agonist.

Step 5

Continuous or frequent use of oral steroids

Prednisolone is the most widely used steroid tablet for maintenance therapy in chronic asthma. There is no evidence that any other formulation is more advantageous.

Patients on long-term steroid tablets (e.g. longer than three months) or requiring frequent courses of steroid tablets (e.g. three to four per year) will be at risk of systemic side-effects:

- blood pressure should be monitored;
- diabetes mellitus may occur;
- reduction in bone density occurs and should be monitored.

In adults, the recommended method of eliminating or reducing the dose of steroid tablets is inhaled steroids, at doses of up to 2000 µg/day.

Stepping down

Stepping down therapy once asthma is controlled is recommended. It has been demonstrated that it is reasonable to attempt to halve the dose of inhaled steroid every month in patients who are stable.

Regular review of patients as treatment is stepped down is important. When deciding which drug to step down first and at what rate, the following should be taken into account:

- the severity of asthma;
- the side-effects of treatment;
- the beneficial effect achieved;
- the patient's preference.

4.4   Pharmacology of anti-asthma drugs

Anti-inflammatory drugs

There are three groups of drugs which are used prophylactically, i.e. to prevent an asthma attack from occurring. They do not dilate a constricted airway and should not be used for symptomatic relief during an acute asthma attack. They are referred to colloquially as 'preventers'.

Sodium cromoglycate (SCG)

Administration is by inhalation of dry powder, by aerosol or nebulizer. SCG is better tolerated than inhaled corticosteroids but less effective. Side-effects are rare. Infrequently, a slight cough, bronchospasm or throat irritation can be caused by inhalation of the dry powder. This can be circumvented either by using an aerosol or more simply by drinking a little water after administration of the drug. Alternatively, a short-acting β_2-agonist can be inhaled shortly before SCG (BNF, 2004). SCG is effective in 40–50 per cent of children but relatively ineffective in adults. The mode of action is controversial. The classical explanation is that SCG stabilizes the membrane of mast cells and prevents the release of the mediators of inflammation and bronchoconstriction. However, other mast cell stabilizers have been ineffective in the treatment of asthma. There is an increasing volume of evidence which suggests that the anti-inflammatory activity of SCG may be attributable to inhibition of airway sensory receptors and hence of neurogenic inflammation of the airways. It must be emphasized to the patient that SCG prevents airway inflammation but does not dilate constricted airways. Consequently, it will not relieve the symptoms of an attack. Hence, SCG should be used regularly to prevent attacks and not to relieve symptoms of an established attack. If this is not explained to the patient then they may dismiss the drug as being ineffective. The duration of action is 2–4 hours.

Nedocromil sodium, a derivative of SCG, has a similar profile of activity but a longer duration of action (6–12 hours). SCG has no effect on the cardiovascular system and is of no ergogenic value. It should be used from Step 2 onwards of the British Thoracic Society guidelines (1997) for the treatment of asthma. Its use is permitted by WADA.

Corticosteroids

Glucocorticosteroids (GCS) are the mainstay of the treatment of chronic asthma in both children and adults. They are also a quintessential component of the emergency treatment of acute severe asthma in both children and adults. At the molecular level they increase the synthesis of anti-inflammatory mediators. Therapeutically, they decrease the swelling and oedema of the inflamed bronchial mucosa, reduce mucus secretion and airway hypersensitivity, whilst increasing the sensitivity to β_2-agonists. Steroids may be administered by inhalation, orally, or by injection. Inhaled steroids are the anti-inflammatory drugs of choice for the prophylaxis of chronic asthma. It is estimated that 3 per cent of the total population in the UK is currently taking an inhaled steroid. Moreover, approximately one-fifth of these patients or 333 000 are using doses in excess of 1000 µg a day (Walsh, LJ in Tattersfield, 1997). The dose that is used should be the minimum that is commensurate with satisfactory control of symptoms. Because budesonide and fluticasone have a longer duration of action than beclomethasone, they need only be administered twice daily, whereas beclomethasone may be administered up to a maximum of 4 times daily. Together with β_2-agonists (see below), inhaled corticosteroids account for almost 90 per cent of UK prescriptions for asthma (Tattersfield, 1997). The glucocorticoid group of steroid hormones do not have an anabolic effect. Glucocorticosteroids are included on the WADA prohibited list. Apart from dermatological preparations, which are not prohibited, administration of glucocorticosteroids is subject to Therapeutic Use Exemption (TUE). Athletes may therefore use glucocorticosteroids to treat asthma having obtained a TUE and in the case of inhaled glucocorticosteroids, the most common route of administration, the athlete can apply for an Abbreviated TUE.

Leukotriene antagonists

Leukotrienes (LTs) are a family of lipid mediators derived from arachidonic acid by the action, initially, of the enzyme 5-lipoxygenase. LTs are released from pro-inflammatory cells in response to a variety of stimuli and can evoke many of the cardinal features of asthma, such as increased mucus production, airway wall oedema, eosinophil accumulation and activation, and bronchoconstriction. Leukotriene antagonists selectively block the receptors for a sub-group of LTs, the cysteinyl leukotrienes (Jones and

Rodger, 1999). There are currently two drugs licensed in the UK, montelukast and zafirlukast. When they were licensed in 1998 they were the first novel treatment for asthma in 25 years. They are orally active, which is an advantage over existing inhaled medications because it is more convenient and may help patient compliance with therapy. However, they should be considered as add-on therapy for those patients with mild to moderate asthma that is not controlled with an inhaled corticosteroid and a short-acting β_2-agonist. In the UK, the Committee on Safety of Medicines (CSM) has advised that LT antagonists should not be used to relieve an attack of acute severe asthma and that their use does not necessarily allow a reduction in existing corticosteroid treatment (BNF, 2004). Their use is permitted by WADA.

Bronchodilator drugs

There are three groups of drugs which are used to relax the constricted airways of the asthmatic during an attack. These drugs are used to treat the symptoms of asthma, rather than to prevent an attack from occurring. They are referred to colloquially as 'relievers'.

Selective β_2-adrenoceptor agonists

The first β-agonist to be used in the treatment of asthma was isoprenaline. The increase in asthma mortality which paralleled the introduction of isoprenaline prompted the development of a new generation of selective β_2-agonists for use as bronchodilators. There are currently six selective β_2-agonists licensed in the UK for the treatment of asthma (Table 4.1).

All the selective β_2-agonists are potent bronchodilators. They differ in their time to onset and duration of action. Salbutamol and terbutaline are short acting and the most frequently used β_2-agonists in the UK. There are many formulations of salbutamol and terbutaline including tablets, slow-release tablets, elixirs, aerosols and dry powder, solutions for injection and inhalation from a nebulizer. Inhalation is the route of choice because it is the most rapidly effective (1–2 minutes) and is associated with the fewest side-effects. Tremor is the only common side-effect after inhalation. The side-effects after oral administration include: fine tremor (usually of the

Table 4.1 Selective β_2-adrenoceptor agonists

Salbutamol (Ventolin™)
Terbutaline (Bricanyl™)
Bambuterol (Bambec™)
Fenoterol (Berotec™)
Formoterol/Eformoterol (Foradil™/Oxis™)
Salmeterol (Serevent™)

hands), nervous tension and headache. Tachycardia, peripheral vasodilation and hypokalaemia may occur after oral dosing but are commoner after intravenous injection. Tachycardia is most common after nebulization. The duration of action of salbutamol and terbutaline after aerosol administration is approximately 4 hours. Formoterol (eformoterol) and salmeterol are the most frequently prescribed long-acting β_2-agonists with a duration of action of approximately 12 hours.

The properties of different β_2-agonists determine their use in the treatment of asthma. Rapid-onset, short-acting β_2-agonists are used to give immediate and/or emergency relief from symptoms. There are differences between the time to onset of action for formoterol and salmeterol. The former begins to take effect within 1–3 minutes whilst the latter takes 10–20 minutes. Nevertheless, long-acting β_2-agonists should not be used for immediate relief of symptoms. Instead, they should be used in addition to inhaled corticosteroids to treat troublesome nocturnal symptoms and to prevent exercise-induced asthma (see below) when their longer duration of action confers a definite advantage. What is more, their respective role in the management of asthma is still evolving. It was thought that short-acting β_2-agonists should be used to a maximum of 4 times a day. However, this provides no clear clinical benefit when compared with their use 'as required'. Indeed, a recent clinical trial has shown greater efficacy of formoterol compared with terbutaline when used 'as required' in terms of improved lung function, symptoms and quality of life (Tattersfield *et al.*, 2001). This has considerable cost implications since long-acting β_2-agonists are considerably more expensive than short-acting β_2-agonists.

The use of β_2-agonists is governed by WADA Regulations. Historically, controversy over the use of sympathomimetics has centred upon the potential ergogenic value of the cardiovascular and central nervous system side-effects that these drugs can evoke. Thus, some α-agonists, non-selective α/β-agonists and non-selective β-agonists are included in Class S6 (stimulants) of the WADA Prohibited Substances and Methods. The 1992 Olympics in Barcelona turned the spotlight on to a new controversy surrounding selective β_2-agonists, namely the putative anabolic effects of β_2-agonists, in general, and clenbuterol in particular. Two British weightlifters were withdrawn from the Olympic Games that year when they tested positive for clenbuterol. A USA competitor and a German athlete also tested positive and were banned for using clenbuterol. In July 1992, the IOC classification of selective β_2-agonists was changed radically. Only salbutamol and terbutaline were permitted and then only by inhalation and following written notification to the relevant medical authority by the team physician (IOC, 1992). All β_2-agonists, except salbutamol and terbutaline, were re-classified into sub-group 2 (other anabolic agents) of Doping Class C Anabolic Agents. This sub-group included only β_2-agonists and specified clenbuterol as the example. Since 1992 there have been several positive tests for clenbuterol. In

1997, Djamolidin Abduzhaparov tested positive in the Tour de France and was withdrawn. Clenbuterol was one of the frequently used drugs cited by Willy Voet in his account of the notorious 'Festina Affair' in the 1998 Tour de France (Voet, 2001). In 1999, two Chinese swimmers received 3-year bans after testing positive for the second time (*Irish Times*, 1999). In the 2000 Olympic games in Sydney, there was one positive test upon which no action was taken because there had been prior notification of use (IOC, 2000b).

Clenbuterol is a long-acting β_2-agonist which is licensed for the treatment of asthma in several countries including Germany, Italy and Spain. The drug is available in a variety of formulations including syrup, aerosol, injectable solutions and granules. It is not licensed for human use in either the UK or the USA. It is licensed for veterinary use (Ventopulmin®, Boehringer Ingelheim) in horses for the treatment of bronchoconstriction caused by several equine respiratory diseases. The therapeutic dose for the treatment of asthma is 20–30 μg per day. It is misused in humans as an anabolic agent when doses of 100–140 μg per day are commonly employed. It is widely available on the Internet and the 'black market'. The maximum effective dose is limited by availability of β_2-receptors. One of the advantages of clenbuterol is that it is not a steroid and therefore does not cause steroid-related side-effects. However, it is a β_2-agonist and has side-effects which are typical of this group of drugs, i.e. tremor, restlessness, agitation, headache, increased blood pressure and palpitations. These side-effects are dose-related and purported to decrease after 8–10 days. This is due to a decrease, i.e. down-regulation, of β_2-receptors, a consequence of which is also a decrease in the anabolic effect of the drug. This has resulted in various dose-cycle regimens being adopted by abusers, details of which are readily available on the Internet. The 'off' periods are often associated with withdrawal symptoms (referred to colloquially as 'crash') as the CNS stimulant effects decline. There is anecdotal evidence that a variety of sympathomimetic drugs have been used to attenuate the severity of the withdrawal symptoms.

The molecular mechanism of the anabolic effect is complex and discussed in detail in Chapter 5. Colloquially, clenbuterol is described as either a 'fat burner' or a 'repartitioning agent'. In the high doses at which the drug is abused, it is reported to increase non-shivering thermogenesis by increasing metabolism in brown fat. A 1° increase of body temperature will increase basal calorific utilization by 5 per cent. Because of the effect upon metabolic rate, clenbuterol is contraindicated in people with hyperthyroidism. In addition β_3-agonists activate lipolysis in fat cells (Katzung, 2001). The evidence for the anabolic effect of clenbuterol in animals is considerable. It increases muscle mass by causing hypertrophy but not hyperplasia. It inhibits muscle protein catabolism, which is why it is reported to be abused in humans after discontinuation of steroids to reduce the catabolic phase (Prather *et al.*,

1995). The combination of an increase in lipolysis and an increase in muscle mass results in an increase in lean body mass, hence the description of 'a repartitioning agent'.

The current regulations regarding the use of β_2-agonists are explained in the World Anti-Doping Agency (WADA) Code (January 2005). The only β_2-agonists that are permitted within Class S3 are formoterol, salbutamol, salmeterol and terbutaline subject to TUE. The use of these drugs is restricted to inhaler only to prevent and/or treat asthma and exercise-induced asthma. TUE is requested from the relevant medical authority, by a respiratory or team physician, of asthma and/or exercise-induced asthma is necessary prior to competition. At the Olympic Games, athletes who required an inhaled β_2-agonist to treat asthma and/or exercise-induced bronchoconstriction (exercise-induced 'asthma') were required to submit to the IOC-MC clinical and laboratory (including respiratory function tests) evidence that justified such treatment. This had to be received by the IOC-MC at least 1 week prior to the athlete's first competition. A panel of scientific and medical experts reviewed the submitted information. In doubtful cases, the panel had the authority to perform appropriate scientifically validated tests. All other β_2-agonists are also prohibited under Class S1 Anabolic Agents. The definition of a positive test for salbutamol as a stimulant is a urine concentration greater than 100 nanograms/ml and as an anabolic agent, 1000 ng/ml ($1 \text{ ng} = 10^{-9}\text{g}$).

Methyl xanthines

Both theophylline and aminophylline (the soluble ethylenediamine-derivative of theophylline) are related to caffeine. They are classed as additional bronchodilators and should be confined to Stages 3, 4 and 5 of the BTS Guidelines (1997). They constitute the second line of bronchodilator therapy. They must be given orally or intravenously and the risk of side-effects is much greater than with selective β_2-agonists. The dose should be adjusted to provide a therapeutic plasma theophylline concentration of 10–20 µg/ml. Although the absolute threshold varies between individuals, both the frequency and severity of side-effects increases with the plasma concentration. Thus 15 µg/ml is associated with nausea, vomiting, abdominal pains, headache, nervousness and muscle tremor. Plasma concentrations between 20 and 40 µg/ml can cause convulsions and ventricular arrhythmias increasing in severity from tachycardia to fibrillation and ultimately cardiac arrest. Sustained-release tablets are now the formulation of choice because they have reduced the fluctuations in plasma concentrations of theophylline and hence have reduced the incidence of side-effects. Cardiovascular side-effects are associated more with theophylline and central nervous system side-effects with caffeine.

Their mode of action is contentious. The classical explanation is that they inhibit phosphodiesterase, the enzyme responsible for the inactivation of cAMP. However, the plasma concentration required to achieve this inhibition *in vivo* is a factor of 10 times the accepted upper limit of therapeutic plasma concentrations. Alternatively, there is evidence that methyl xanthines antagonize adenosine receptors. Theophylline and aminophylline also down-regulate the activity of pro-inflammatory cells. Whatever the mode of action, these drugs have a place in treatment of both chronic and acute severe asthma. The methyl xanthines are permitted by WADA.

Anticholinergic drugs

The parasympathetic nervous system causes contraction of bronchial smooth muscle by the effect of acetylcholine upon muscarinic cholinergic receptors. Theoretically, therefore, anticholinergic drugs should be of benefit in the treatment of asthma. In practice, they have a greater bronchodilator effect in chronic bronchitics than in asthmatics. Inhaled ipratropium bromide, which is a quaternary derivative of atropine, is a useful alternative for individuals who cannot tolerate or respond to β_2-agonists. It is classed as an additional bronchodilator and should be used in Stage 4 or 5 of the BTS Guidelines (1997). It has a slow onset time (30–60 min) and is active for 3–4 hours and hence should be taken four times per day. Oxitropium bromide, a derivative of ipratropium, has a longer duration of action and need only be taken twice daily. Neither drug will give rapid relief of symptoms. The side-effects of antagonism of the parasympathetic nervous system are dry mouth, urinary retention and constipation. However, ipratropium bromide is poorly absorbed and is not associated with significant side-effects when standard doses are administered by inhalation. WADA permits the use of ipratropium bromide for the treatment of asthma.

4.5   Exercise and asthma

Asthma presents a twofold problem to elite sportspersons. First, it can impair performance if not treated correctly. However, many athletes compete successfully at the highest level despite asthma, for example Paula Radcliffe who captained the British female athletes at the Sydney Olympics and who is the 2002 Commonwealth 5000 m, European 10 000 m and long-course, World cross-country champion. Second and perhaps of greater concern, treatment can expose the sportsperson to drugs which are contained in the WADA lists of Prohibited Classes of Substances. The incidence of asthma is reported to be more common in elite athletes than in the general population. In 1984, it was reported that 11.2 per cent of US athletes competing in the Los Angeles Olympics had exercise-induced asthma (Voy, 1986). A second study was undertaken of 699 athletes prior to the 1996 Summer Olympics in Atlanta: 16.7 per cent had a history of asthma, took anti-asthma medications or both; 10.4 per cent had active asthma (Weiler *et al.*,

1998). This compares with 3–7 per cent of the general population in the USA.

Exercise may be one of a number of trigger factors for an individual's asthma or it may be the only trigger factor. This led to the concept of exercise-induced asthma (EIA) as a syndrome discrete from asthma. Thus, EIA has been defined in terms of the trigger factor, i.e. as reversible airway obstruction that occurs during or after exertion. The initial response to exercise in both non-asthmatics and asthmatics is bronchodilation. However, in the asthmatic, initial bronchodilation is not sustained and bronchoconstriction develops, most dramatically once the exercise has been terminated. The maximum decrease in peak expiratory flow rate (PEFR) and forced expiratory volume in the first second (FEV_1) normally occur between 3 and 15 minutes after the exercise has been completed (Rupp, 1996). The ventilatory changes in EIA are identical to those observed during a spontaneous asthma attack, i.e. decreased V_t (tidal volume), PEFR, FEV_1, FVC (forced vital capacity) and increased residual volume (RV) leading to hyperventilation and dyspnoea. The symptoms include coughing, wheezing, excessive sputum production, dyspnoea and/or chest tightness (Lacroix, 1999). All of these changes are observed in asthma induced by factors other than exercise. In the laboratory, the exercise needs to be of 6–8 minutes duration at greater than 80 per cent of predicted maximal heart rate (Lacroix, 1999), although in their sport, the early phase may take longer to develop. The maximum decrease in lung function occurs after 15 minutes and returns towards normal function after approximately one hour. This is known as the early phase of EIA. EIA may consist of just an early phase or, in approximately 30 per cent of EIA patients, may also develop a late phase after 6–8 hours (Lacroix, 1999). In 50 per cent of individuals affected by EIA, a second period of exercise within 2 hours of the initial period evokes a weaker bronchoconstrictor response (less than 50 per cent of the original response). The period during which the response is less is referred to as the refractory period. Advantage can be taken of the refractory period for both training and competition. Exercise-induced asthma occurs in up to 90 per cent of people with chronic asthma and 40 per cent of people with allergic rhinitis (Rupp, 1996; Lacroix, 1999). A 23 per cent incidence of exercise-induced asthma was found among 1998 US Winter Olympians. Random testing of asymptomatic children found that 7 per cent had EIA (Nastasi et al., 1995).

The pathophysiology of EIA is only partially understood. It is accepted that the severity of EIA is dependent upon the level of ventilation and the temperature and humidity of the inspired air. Cold dry air is more asthmogenic than warm humid air. This challenges the homeostatic regulation of airway temperature and water loss. Water loss from the airway epithelial cells decreases the cell volume and increases the viscosity of mucus. The latter can obstruct airflow and stimulate the cough reflex. After the challenge has subsided, the airways must be re-warmed and the intracellular fluid that was lost must be replaced. This can cause reactive hyperaemia (increased blood flow to the airway wall) and rebound increase in cell volume. This may be the key event that causes release of mediators and triggers bronchoconstriction and inflammatory changes in the airway wall. It may also explain the time course of the changes in lung function. Moreover, cycling may be the most asthmogenic sport because both training and competition involve longer periods of challenge to the respiratory tract. Typical cycling road races can last in excess of 4 hours whereas marathons last 2.5 hours and football matches last 1.5 hours. Finally, the environment in which the exercise takes place is important. Thus cross-country skiing, which is conducted in cold dry air environments, has one of the highest incidences of reported EIA (Larsson *et al.*, 1993).

4.6   Treatment of exercise-induced asthma (EIA)

The management of EIA consists of both non-drug and drug interventions and is directed at two goals: optimal control of base-line symptoms and prevention of an asthmatic attack following exercise. Relief of symptoms of EIA should be considered as an indication that the first two goals have not been achieved satisfactorily.

Non-drug treatment

Aerobic fitness

Fitness does not prevent EIA as indicated by the number of Olympians who suffer from the syndrome. However, aerobic fitness does improve lung function, retards deterioration in lung function with age (in non-asthmatics) and enables asthmatics to exercise with less EIA. It also facilitates social interactions and improves self-esteem of asthmatics. There is no evidence to suggest that aerobic training is deleterious to asthmatics provided that their treatment is optimal and that they have a satisfactory management plan which includes access to appropriate bronchodilator therapy, if required. The only contraindication for strenuous aerobic activity in an asthmatic would be if they demonstrated significant arterial desaturation upon exercise-testing during laboratory investigations.

Minimize cooling and drying of the airways

This can be achieved in several ways. First, if possible, select a physical activity such as walking and swimming which are less likely to evoke bronchoconstriction. Second, utilize nasal breathing whenever possible. Third, seek to avoid exercising in a cold, dry environment. If this is unavoidable then a face mask may reduce cooling and drying of the airways.

Warm-up

This can help to maximize the benefit of the training session and, if possible, should take cognizance of the refractory period that many asthmatics experience after an initial episode of EIA. The warm-up should be of 15 minutes' duration. It is debatable whether this should involve high intensity bursts to increase ventilation rapidly or moderate sustained activity. It is also advisable to cool down gradually after the exercise to minimize rebound warming of the airways.

Monitoring of PEFR

This will provide objective assessment of the current status of base-line control of asthma. Inadequate base-line control requires revision of maintenance therapy. Concurrent conditions such as hay fever and allergic rhinitis should also be satisfactorily controlled. If possible, training and participation should not be undertaken on days when symptoms are poorly controlled.

Drug treatment

The treatment of EIA focuses upon prevention rather than relief of symptoms. β_2-Agonists and mast cell stabilizers are the most effective and proven therapies for the prevention of EIA.

β_2-Agonists

These drugs are the most effective prophylactic treatment of EIA. Salbutamol, terbutaline, formoterol and salmeterol are the only β_2-agonists which are permitted by WADA subject to TUE. Short-acting β_2-agonists (i.e. salbutamol, formoterol or terbutaline) should be administered 15 (Rupp, 1996) to 30 minutes (Lacroix, 1999) before commencing exercise. They induce bronchodilation within 5 minutes and afford protection against EIA for approximately 3–6 hours (Rupp, 1996; Lacroix, 1999). They prevent asthma symptoms in 90 per cent of patients (Lacroix, 1999). They should be available to the athlete for rapid relief of symptoms should they develop despite pre-exercise treatment. Salmeterol, a long-acting β_2-agonist, should be taken 30 minutes before exercise and is effective for up to 9 hours (Hansen-Flaschen and Schotland, 1998). It is licensed in the UK for the treatment of troublesome nocturnal symptoms and exercise-induced asthma (BNF, 2004; BTS Guidelines, 1997). Its long duration of action makes it suitable for children who require prophylaxis against EIA throughout the school day. Because of its slower onset of action, salmeterol should not be used as a rescue medication to relieve symptoms of an asthma attack. Salbutamol or terbutaline should be used instead. There is controversy about the relative merits of the long-term prophylactic use of short- and long-acting β_2-agonists.

Tachyphylaxis to salmeterol has been shown to develop after 4 weeks of regular use (Nelson *et al.*, 1998). Alternatives to regular use of salmeterol are either short-acting β_2-agonists before exercise and 'on-demand' for relief of symptoms or leukotriene antagonists before exercise (see below).

Mast cell stabilizers

Sodium cromoglycate (SCG) and nedocromil sodium are the next most effective and most frequently used drugs for the treatment of EIA. It should be remembered that neither SCG nor nedocromil sodium is a bronchodilator. They are anti-inflammatories and are used prophylactically to prevent EIA. Neither drug is as effective as short-acting β_2-agonists which also prevent EIA, but by causing bronchodilation. They should be administered 10–15 minutes before the start of exercise and will provide up to two hours' protection against bronchoconstriction (Morton and Fitch, 1992). They prevent asthma symptoms in 70–85 per cent of patients with EIA (Smith and LaBotz, 1998). SCG is often extremely effective when combined with a short-acting β_2-agonist in those patients for whom monotherapy is ineffective (Rupp, 1996). Neither SCG nor nedocromil sodium is included in the WADA lists of Prohibited Substances and Prohibited Methods. It should be noted that sodium cromoglycate is available as a compound formulation with salbutamol. This preparation is not recommended because it may be used inappropriately to relieve symptoms, whereas it should be used prophylactically (BNF, 2004).

Methyl xanthines

Theophylline is administered orally either as a rapid-release or a sustained-release formulation. The rapid-release formulation must be administered 1–2 hours before exercise. The narrow therapeutic window of theophylline coupled with the many factors that can affect plasma concentrations and either increase toxicity or decrease efficacy of the drug mean that it is impracticable to administer a single dose as a prophylactic against EIA. The sustained-release formulation is used prophylactically in order to maintain better base-line control of asthma in accordance with BTS Guidelines (1997). The aforementioned factors, together with the greater risk of cardiovascular and CNS side-effects from theophylline, compared with either inhaled short-acting β_2-agonists or mast cell stabilizers, relegates theophylline to the third line of therapy for EIA. Theophylline is not included in the WADA lists of Prohibited Substances and Prohibited Methods.

Corticosteroids

The time to onset of anti-inflammatory effects of inhaled steroids is 8–12 hours. Hence, single doses of inhaled steroids immediately prior to exercise do not afford protection against EIA. A 4-week trial of inhaled betamethasone valerate produced a significant improvement in EIA, but this was probably related to better base-line control of asthma (Hartley *et al.*, 1977). Inhaled budesonide twice a day for 4 weeks produced a significant improvement in resting pulmonary function and in the benefit derived from pre-exercise terbutaline (Henriksen and Dahl, 1983). The role of inhaled steroids in the treatment of EIA is now considered to be in the establishment of satisfactory base-line control of symptoms (BTS Guidelines, 1997).

Anticholinergics

These drugs are of minor importance in the treatment of EIA. Bronchodilatation produced by inhalation of 0.5 mg of ipratropium bromide was equal to that of a β_2-agonist, but was not effective against EIA (Bundgaard *et al.*, 1980). Two studies have demonstrated a synergistic effect between SCG and ipratropium bromide in the treatment of EIA (Bundgaard *et al.*, 1980). However, ipratropium bromide alone does not compare with β_2-agonists in either the prevention or the reversal of EIA. Neither ipratropium nor its longer-acting derivative, oxitropium, is included in the WADA lists of Prohibited Substances and Prohibited Methods.

Leukotriene antagonists

In the UK, montelukast and zafirlukast are licensed for the prophylaxis of asthma. In the USA, an inhibitor of LT synthesis, zileuton, is also marketed. For this reason, in the USA, the group of drugs is referred to as LT modifiers rather than simply as the LT antagonists. It is suggested that LT antagonists may be of benefit in preventing exercise-induced asthma and in those asthmatics who are aspirin sensitive (BNF, 2004). An 8-week, multicentre, randomized, double-blind comparison of oral, once daily, montelukast (10 mg) with inhaled, twice daily (50 µg) salmeterol showed that montelukast provided consistent long-term protection against EIA without tachyphylaxis (Edelman *et al.*, 2000). A significant loss of protection was seen over the 8-week period with salmeterol (Edelman *et al.*, 2000). Montelukast offers several advantages over other prophylactic therapies. First, it is available as a once daily, oral medication. In those who respond, it is effective for up to 20–24 hours. It is permitted by WADA. However, there are two potential disadvantages. First, not all patients will respond and the figure may be as high as 75 per cent (Hansen-Flaschen and Schotland, 1998). Second, Churg–Strauss syndrome has been reported, albeit rarely, in association with the use of LT antagonists. Whilst a causal relationship may not have been established and the possibility exists that the syndrome may be caused by reduction or withdrawal of corticosteroids, the CSM advises that patients be informed and alerted to the possible risks (BNF, 2004).

4.7   Treatment of coughs and colds

Cough is a protective reflex that is initiated by either mechanical or chemical stimulation of the oral pharynx, larynx, trachea or bronchi. Its purpose is to remove mucus and irritants from the upper respiratory tract (URT). Most commonly it is a symptom of a self-limiting URT infection that will normally resolve, without treatment, within 3–4 days. Antibiotics are of no value because the infection is normally viral and not bacterial. There is evidence to support a causal link between intense exercise and the incidence of URT infection (Nieman *et al.*, 1990; Heath *et al.*, 1991). In the case of male endurance runners, there appears to be a dose-related effect of exercise training on the risk of URT infection (Peters and Bateman, 1983; Nieman *et al.*, 1990; Heath *et al.*, 1991). This relationship is highlighted by the 'J' curve model proposed by Nieman *et al.* (1993) whereby the risk of URT infection is reduced below that of sedentary individuals when engaged in mild to moderate intensity exercise training and increased when engaged in high intensity exercise training. However, a direct link between infection and disturbed immune function in athletes has not been fully established.

Less frequently, cough is a symptom of serious disease of the respiratory tract (e.g. chronic obstructive pulmonary disease, tuberculosis and bronchial carcinoma), but this is unlikely to be relevant to an individual who is participating in top level competitive sport. However, this was most certainly not the case with Lance Armstrong, seven times winner of the Tour de France, whose cough was a symptom of pulmonary metastases secondary to testicular cancer.

The important therapeutic distinction is between productive and nonproductive coughs. A productive cough should not be suppressed but should be facilitated by adequate fluid intake and, possibly, with the use of an expectorant. A non-productive cough may be suppressed or perhaps converted into a productive cough by increased fluid intake and the use of either an expectorant or, in exceptional circumstances, a mucolytic.

The number of OTC (over-the-counter or non-prescription) medications available for the treatment of coughs and colds is enormous. The global market for 1999 was valued at $6.5 bn (Anon, 2000). There are approximately 500 OTC cough and cold preparations available in the USA. There are approximately 160 OTC cough and cold preparations in the UK with a market value of £337.4 million in 1999 (Proprietary Association of Great Britain, personal communication, 2001). The majority of these preparations contain more than one active ingredient, some of which are banned by WADA, for example sympathomimetics and narcotic analgesics. Therefore, great care must be taken by the sportsperson when purchasing a cough or cold remedy for consumption at a time when they may be subject to testing under WADA regulations.

The major classes of drugs which are contained in cough and cold preparations are: cough suppressants, sympathomimetics, expectorants, demulcents, and xanthines.

Cough suppressants

There are two groups of centrally active cough suppressants: narcotic analgesics and antihistamines.

Centrally acting cough suppressants reduce coughing by inhibiting the cough centre in the medulla oblongata in the brainstem. The three main drugs in this category are the opioid derivatives, codeine, pholcodine and dextromethorphan. They can each cause drowsiness, respiratory depression and constipation. Codeine is a narcotic analgesic which can cause both physical and psychological dependence and hence potentially is a drug of abuse. However, the antitussive dose (normally 15–30 mg, 3–4 times a day) is less than that required for analgesia and the risk of unwitting addiction is merely theoretical. Pholcodine has less potential for addiction and causes less respiratory depression and constipation than codeine. For these reasons, it is preferable to codeine as a cough suppressant. The recommended daily dose is 5–10 mg, 3–4 times a day. Dextromethorphan was introduced in 1958 and is essentially free of analgesic and addictive properties and causes less respiratory depression and constipation than either codeine or pholcodine. It is available in many OTC cough and cold preparations and is the safest of the three cough suppressants. The recommended daily dose is 10–30 mg, 3–4 times a day. The use of all three centrally acting cough suppressants (codeine, pholcodine and dextromethorphan) is permitted by WADA. However, although these drugs are widely available for cough suppression and are permitted by WADA, there is scant justification for their use by a sportsperson. First, there is little conclusive evidence that they completely suppress a cough. Second, they can cause drowsiness and constipation. Third, it should be remembered that they should only be used to suppress a non-productive cough when a demulcent may be more appropriate and have fewer adverse side-effects.

Antihistamines are of potential value in the treatment of nasal allergies, particularly hay fever, and may reduce rhinorrhoea and sneezing. They are less effective than sympathomimetics in reducing nasal congestion associated with the common cold. They are present in many cough and cold remedies. Antihistamines reduce coughing by two mechanisms. First, they have a central suppressant action that is non-narcotic but which does suppress the cough reflex. Second, their anticholinergic action reduces the rate of mucus secretion. This can increase the viscosity of mucus, which is why antihistamines should be used with caution in asthmatics. The overall decrease in mucus production complements the effects of sympathomimetics, which is why the two groups of drugs are commonly combined in cough and cold preparations. The older antihistamines, such as brompheniramine and chlorpheniramine, have greater sedative activity than the newer antihistamines, such as acrivastine and cetirizine. However, the former are most commonly contained in OTC cough and cold preparations whilst the latter are only contained in POMs (prescription-only medicines) for the treatment of hay fever and other allergies. The use of antihistamines is permitted by WADA.

Sympathomimetic amines

Drugs which mimic the effects of the endogenous mediators of the sympathetic nervous system (i.e. adrenaline and noradrenaline) are referred to as sympathomimetic amines. Sympathomimetic amines work through the stimulation of adrenoceptors. The response of any cell or organ to sympathomimetic amines is directly related to the density and proportion of α- and β-adrenoceptors present.

According to Hoffman and Lefkowitz (1990) the actions of sympathomimetic amines can be classified into the following types: (1) peripheral excitatory action on vascular smooth muscle in blood vessels supplying the skin, kidneys and mucous membranes and glandular smooth muscle in salivary and sweat glands; (2) peripheral inhibitory action on the smooth muscle of the gut wall, the bronchioles and the blood vessels supplying the skeletal muscles; (3) cardiac excitatory action, inducing increased heart rate and force of contraction; (4) metabolic actions, including increased rate of glycogenolysis in the liver and muscles and mobilization of free fatty acids from adipose tissue; (5) endocrine actions, including regulation of the secretion of insulin, renin and pituitary hormones; (6) CNS actions, including respiratory stimulation, increased wakefulness, psychomotor activity and reduction in appetite; and (7) presynaptic actions resulting in the inhibition or facilitation of release of neurotransmitters such as acetylcholine and noradrenaline. Not all sympathomimetic amines display all of the actions mentioned to the same degree, and many of the differences in their effects are only quantitative.

The profile of effects of each sympathomimetic amine is determined by its relative affinity for the sub-groups of adrenoceptors and forms the basis for their classification (Table 4.2).

β_2-Receptors are located on airway smooth muscle and cause bronchodilation when stimulated. α_1-Receptors are located on arterial smooth muscle and cause vasoconstriction when stimulated. Consequently, β_2-agonists (e.g. salbutamol) are used as bronchodilators to treat asthma whilst α_1-agonists (e.g. ephedrine) are used as vasoconstrictors to treat coughs and colds. The primary role of sympathomimetic amines in the treatment of coughs and colds is to act as a decongestant. When the mucous membrane lining the nose is irritated by infection (e.g. in the common cold) or allergy (e.g. in

Table 4.2 Sympathomimetic amines categorized according to the principal adrenoceptors that they stimulate

Sympathomimetic amine	Principal adrenoceptor stimulated
Salbutamol	β_2
Terbutaline	β_2
Clenbuterol	β_2
Ephedrine	α_1
Phenylephrine	α_1
Phenylpropanolamine	α_1
Pseudoephedrine	α_1

seasonal allergic rhinitis), the blood vessels supplying the membrane become enlarged. This leads to fluid accumulation in the surrounding tissue and encourages the production of larger than normal amounts of mucus. As well as affecting the nasal passages, congestion can also occur in the sinuses resulting in sinusitis. α_1-Agonists cause constriction of the blood vessels, so reducing the swelling in the lining of the nose and sinuses and acting as decongestants. The most widely available α_1-agonists present in OTC medications are referred to collectively as the ephedrines. Ephedrines can be defined as those compounds that are either isomers or stereoisomers of ephedrine and include pseudoephedrine, norephedrine (phenylpropanolamine) and norpseudoephedrine (cathine). Phenylephrine, also a sympathomimetic, is also commonly found in OTC formulations. The ephedrines and phenylephrine pose several potential problems for the sportsperson. First, they can cause significant side-effects. Second, the use of some α_1-sympathomimetics is prohibited by WADA. Third, they are of doubtful ergogenic value. Finally, the choice is enormous and even the names of the proprietary preparations can be misleading. There are many opportunities to make a costly mistake. Even though these prohibited OTC substances appear on WADA's specified substances list, thereby allowing reduced sanctions, it remains the athlete's responsibility to establish that the use of such specified substances was not intended to enhance performance.

Potential side-effects of sympathomimetic amines

The decongestants, although widely available in OTC preparations, are potent vasoconstrictors as evinced by their licensed indications. In the UK, ephedrine is licensed for the treatment of hypotension caused by spinal or epidural anaesthesia. It should be used with caution in hypotensive patients. Phenylephrine is licensed for the treatment of acute hypotension and is contraindicated in hypertensive patients. Pseudoephedrine is available in OTC cough and cold preparations and in tablet form as a systemic decongestant.

Table 4.3 Recommended maximal therapeutic doses of the four commonest decongestants in OTC decongestant preparations

Sympathomimetic	Single dose (mg/4 hours)	Daily dose (mg)
Ephedrine	25	100
Phenylephrine	10	40
Phenylpropanolamine	25	100
Pseudoephedrine	60	240

It has few sympathomimetic side-effects. Phenylpropanolamine (PPA), on the other hand, is the most controversial of the sympathomimetics available in OTC cough and cold preparations. Its use has been linked with hypertensive reactions, cerebral haemorrhage and psychosis (Gibson and Warrell, 1972; Norvenius *et al.*, 1979; Berstein and Diskant, 1982; Johnson *et al.*, 1983). It does not have a licensed indication within the BNF but is widely available in OTC cough and cold preparations. In the USA, it is also marketed as an appetite suppressor. A recent study has demonstrated an odds ratio for association between haemorrhagic stroke and the use of PPA of 1.23 for cough and cold preparations and 15.92 for appetite suppressants (Yale Hemorrhagic Stroke Project, Horwitz *et al.*, 2000). This has led to the United States Food and Drugs Administration (FDA) taking steps to remove PPA from all drug products (FDA, 2000). It is considered that although the risk is small, it cannot be justified for treatment of minor ailments. The Committee on Safety of Medicines in the UK has not recommended a ban on PPA for two reasons (CSM, 2000). First, the drug is not marketed in appetite suppressants in the UK. Second, the maximum approved daily OTC dose in the UK is 100 mg compared with 150 mg in the USA.

It is obvious, therefore, from clinical data that, when taken orally, α_1-agonist sympathomimetic amines can evoke profound systemic cardiovascular side-effects. Moreover, these effects are both drug-specific and dose-dependent. The current recommended oral doses for the four commonest decongestants are shown in Table 4.3.

There have been numerous reports of the effects upon cardiovascular parameters of those sympathomimetic amines which are contained in OTC medicines. Thomas *et al.* (1991) reported significant increases in heart rate and both systolic and diastolic blood pressure following administration of two proprietary cold cure preparations containing the equivalent of double the therapeutic dose of phenylpropanolamine. Increases in diastolic blood pressure to 100 mmHg or more were reported in 12 out of 37 subjects taking preparations containing 85 mg of phenylpropanolamine (Horowitz *et al.*, 1980). However, only 4 out of 34 subjects reached 100 mmHg diastolic blood pressure following treatment with a lower dose of 50 mg of phenylpropanolamine. Doses equivalent to over three to four times the recommended therapeutic dose of pseudoephedrine raised diastolic pressure above 90 mmHg (Drew *et al.*, 1978). These results were in accord with two other studies. Bye *et al.* (1974) reported significant increases in heart rate and systolic blood pressure following relatively high doses (180 and 120 mg) of pseudoephedrine. Empey *et al.* (1980) found doses of 120 and 180 mg produced statistically significant increases in both pulse and systolic blood pressure. However, the increases were deemed to be clinically unimportant as they were quantitatively considerably less than might be expected to occur with either emotion or mild exercise.

Whilst several studies have reported increased cardiovascular stimulation following ingestion of ephedrines, it is evident that doses used were at least twice the recommended single therapeutic dose. The reports of the effects of ingestion of ephedrines in single therapeutic doses have been conflicting. Thus Bye *et al.* (1974) found that a single dose of ephedrine (25 mg) significantly elevated both heart rate and systolic blood pressure. In the same study, a single dose of pseudoephedrine (60 mg) significantly elevated only systolic arterial blood pressure. Bright *et al.* (1981) found only a non-significant rise in resting heart rate following a single therapeutic dose of pseudoephedrine. Empey *et al.* (1980) reported that ingestion of pseudoephedrine in a therapeutic dose of 60 mg provided maximal nasal decongestion without any cardiovascular or other side-effects.

Few researchers have examined the effects of multiple dosing regimes on cardiovascular parameters. Chester *et al.* (2003b) found significant increases in blood pressure following multiple, therapeutic dosing regimen for pseudoephedrine (i.e. six 60 mg doses over a 36-hour period) and phenylpropanolamine (i.e. six 25 mg doses over a 36-hour period). Bye *et al.* (1975) reported significant increases in heart rate but not systolic arterial blood pressure after three different dose regimes, one involving two different sustained-release formulations. Prolonged administration of a sustained-release formulation of pseudoephedrine (180 mg twice daily for 2 weeks) increased heart rate and decreased systolic arterial blood pressure. The authors could only speculate at the possible explanations for these results and the variance from those in the earlier study. Other studies that have addressed prolonged usage of ephedrines have been conflicting. Goodman *et al.* (1986) found no significant increase in blood pressure following daily administration of a 75-mg controlled release preparation of phenylpropanolamine for a period of 7 days. In an extensive study by Noble (1982), more than 400 obese patients were administered 50 mg of phenylpropanolamine three times a daily over a 12-week period. Results showed no significant increase in blood pressure when compared with placebo.

The bronchodilator effects of ephedrines have been less well documented than the cardiovascular effects as might be expected from their receptor affinities. Ephedrines exert their effect principally on the α_1-receptors on

Table 4.4 Urinary concentrations above which a WADA accredited laboratory must report results

Drug	Urinary concentration
Salbutamol	> 100 ng/ml
Cathine	> 5 μg/ml
Ephedrine	> 10 μg/ml
Methylephedrine	> 10 μg/ml

vascular smooth muscle with minimal effect on β_2-receptors in the bronchial smooth muscle. There have been no published reports on the stimulatory effects of phenylpropanolamine; however, some brochodilation has been claimed following administration of supratherapeutic doses of ephedrine (60 mg) and pseudoephedrine (210 mg) (Drew *et al.*, 1978).

In terms of action on the CNS, most evidence suggests that ephedrines have no stimulatory effect in the relatively low doses used (Bye *et al.*, 1975; Kuitunen *et al.*, 1984). Bye *et al.* (1974) found that whilst pseudoephedrine lacked any stimulatory effect even at supratherapeutic doses (180 mg), ephedrine possessed a stimulatory effect at therapeutic doses. Nevertheless, according to Wadler and Hainline (1989), ephedrines exhibit less central stimulatory effects than amphetamines because they are less lipid soluble. Differences in central stimulation are related to differences of lipid solubility within the biological membranes and hence penetration of the blood–brain barrier determines the ease with which these compounds gain access to central receptors (Lanciault and Wolf, 1965).

WADA regulations and sympathomimetic amines

The use of sympathomimetic amines is restricted by WADA. A WADA accredited laboratory must report results in excess of those shown in Table 4.4. This constitutes a doping offence.

Data reveals a total of 205 cases of stimulant detection from the UK Sport's testing programme of which a high proportion were sympathomimetics (UK Sport, 2000) (Figure 4.1).

Indeed, just over 50 per cent of cases were for ephedrines found commonly in OTC formulations. There have been numerous instances of positive tests for ephedrine. In the 1972 Munich Olympics, there was a positive test in ice hockey, but the more famous case from those Games was that of Rick Demont who lost his gold medal in the 400 m freestyle. Demont claimed that he had taken Marax for his asthma and had not been told that it contained ephedrine. In 1988, eight US athletes tested positive for ephedrine prior to the Seoul Olympics. They were let off having claimed that it was contained within Ma Huang which they had taken inadvertently (Nichols,

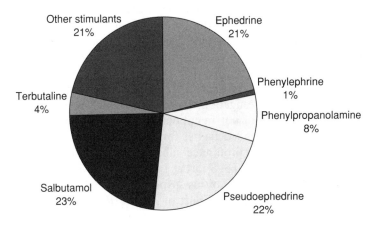

Figure 4.1 Results from UK Sport's testing programme between 1995 and 2000 regarding the detection of stimulants.

2001). In 1994, Diego Maradona was banished from the World Cup after testing positive for a cocktail of ephedrine and ephedrine-related substances. In 2000, the Russian synchronized swimmer, Maria Kisseleva, was stripped of her European duet title after testing positive. She claimed that it had been given to her by a team doctor to help her lose weight. She was only given a 1-month ban and subsequently won gold in Sydney. There have also been high profile cases that have involved positive tests for pseudoephedrine. In 1988 at the Seoul Olympics, the UK and subsequent Olympic 100 m champion, Linford Christie tested positive for pseudoephedrine. He was exonerated as he was believed to have taken the drug inadvertently as an ingredient of the Chinese health supplement, ginseng. What is more, although he had finished in the bronze medal position, he received the silver medal because Ben Johnson was stripped of his gold medal for using stanozolol. More recently the IOC have shown less leniency as Andreea Raducan, the Romanian gymnast was stripped of her individual gold medal at the Sydney Olympic Games after testing positive for pseudoephedrine, contained in a cold cure prescribed by the team doctor. There was an unsuccessful appeal by Raducan. Although she lost her gold medal she did not receive a ban. The doctor was less fortunate in that respect and was banned from the next two Olympiads by the IOC. The most recent example of a positive test for a respiratory drug was that of Alain Baxter at the 2002 Winter Olympics in Salt Lake City. Alain Baxter won a bronze medal in the men's slalom but subsequently tested positive for methamphetamine. The IOC stripped Baxter of his medal. Baxter contested that he had taken the methamphetamine inadvertently by using a nasal decongestant, Vicks Inhaler (Proctor & Gamble). The medicine sold over-the-counter in the UK contains menthol as the active ingredient whilst that sold in the US contains methamphetamine. What is of greater significance is that the methamphetamine in the Vicks Inhaler is the l-isomer (i.e. l-methamphetamine). It is the d-isomer (d-methamphetamine) which is known colloquially as 'speed' and which has greater abuse potential because it is a central nervous system stimulant. However, the IOC test does not distinguish between the two isomers. The British Olympic Association asked the IOC to carry out the differential test but IOC President, Jacques Rogge, refused to re-open the investigation. The International Ski Federation (FIS), who ruled that Baxter had not intentionally sought to enhance his performance, subsequently suspended Baxter for three months for the first offence of unintentionally using a prohibited substance. Baxter successfully appealed to the Court of Arbitration in Sport at Lausanne (16 August 2002), who brought forward the termination of his suspension from 15 December 2002 to 18 August 2002. However, the Court of Arbitration in Sport later rejected his appeal against disqualification by the IOC and his bronze medal was not returned (16 October 2002). On 27 September 2002, the IOC issued a revised Prohibited List of Substances and Prohibited Methods for implementation, effective from 1 January 2003 (IOC, 2002). Included explicitly amongst several revisions were both the L- and D- isomers of the prohibited substances referred to in both Class 1.A.a. and Class 1.A.b. stimulants. There have been two less high profile cases of positive tests for ephedrines in the Olympics. There were positive tests for norephedrine (phenylpropanolamine) in yachting in Montreal (1976) followed by one in athletics in Barcelona (1992) (IOC, 2000a).

In an attempt to reduce the number of positive cases and limit those athletes using sympathomimetics for legitimate reasons, the IOC introduced quantitative levels below which drug detection would not be deemed to be a positive case (Table 4.4). It is evident that such measures are futile since pharmacokinetic data suggests that such levels are exceeded following normal therapeutic dosing (Lefebvre et al., 1992; Chester et al., 2003a). Data from a study by Chester et al. (2003a) showed urine drug levels to remain above the IOC limits, in operation at the time, for both pseudoephedrine and phenylpropanolamine following multiple therapeutic dosing (i.e. six 60-mg doses of pseudoephedrine and six 25-mg doses of phenylpropanolamine over a 36-hour period) (Figures 4.2 and 4.3). Drug urine concentrations were found to remain above IOC limits for a minimum of 16 hours following final administration of pseudoephedrine and a minimum of 6 hours following final administration of phenylpropanolamine.

According to the IOC, following the detection of both norpseudoephedrine and the parent compound pseudoephedrine in urine, concentrations are added in order to gain an indication of drug misuse.

It is apparent that no clear relationship exists between the amount of drug ingested and a single urine drug concentration. Indeed, drug elimination and thus urinary drug concentration are affected by several factors, including diet and activity level, all of which have an effect on urine pH and urine

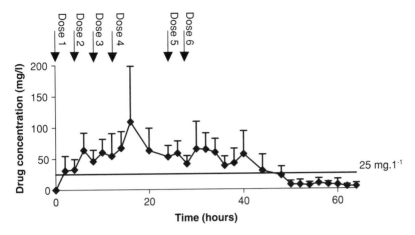

Figure 4.2 Mean urine pseudoephedrine concentrations (± SD) following multiple dosing of immediate-release capsules (D).

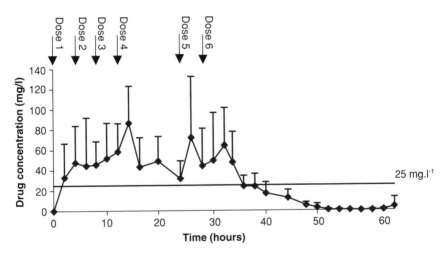

Figure 4.3 Mean urine phenylpropanolamine concentrations (± SD) following multiple dosing of immediate-release capsules (D).

flow rate (Brater *et al.*, 1980). Noakes and Gillies (1994) found significant increases in urinary pseudoephedrine concentration following endurance exercise and concluded that exercise had a large but variable effect on drug elimination. The elimination of such drugs is significantly influenced by the pH of urine (Wilkinson and Beckett, 1968) because basic drugs, such as sympathomimetic amines, are excreted more rapidly if urinary pH is acidic and retained in the body for longer if the urinary pH is more alkaline.

Information regarding the pharmacokinetics of particular drugs is therefore essential if drug testing is to be successful in differentiating between deliberate and inadvertent drug use. In 2004, WADA removed pseudoephedrine, phenylpropanolamine and phenylephrine from the prohibited list. However, the misuse of these substances is still under review through WADA's monitoring programme.

Reputed ergogenic effects

The sympathetic response involves a myriad of reactions that heighten the capacity of the body to respond to stressful situations. Such responses include increased cardiac activity, bronchodilation, increased oxygen uptake and ventilation, redistribution of blood flow to the working muscles and increased glycogenolysis and free fatty acid mobilization. Stimulation of the central nervous system also results in an elevation in mood, an increased alertness and decreased fatigue. These actions enable an individual to perform physical activity and relate to an increased potential in terms of sports performance.

Amphetamines are structurally related to the OTC sympathomimetics and are possibly the most well known of stimulants banned by WADA. Enhanced performance following amphetamine administration may be explained by the fact that amphetamines appear to mask the body's symptoms of fatigue. Recent data show that amphetamines are a relatively minor drug of abuse in sport these days (UK Sport, 2000). Ephedrines, which are much more frequently abused, are banned by WADA because of their chemical similarity to amphetamines. Therefore, it is assumed that they, like amphetamine, have ergogenic properties. However, the literature regarding the effects of ephedrines on sports performance is limited.

Studies of the effects of sympathomimetics during exercise can be divided into two distinct areas: those that have investigated their effects either during sub-maximal exercise (Bright et al., 1981) or during maximal exercise (De Meersman et al., 1987; Clemons and Crosby, 1993; Gillies et al., 1996; Voelz et al., 1996; Swain et al., 1997).

Few studies have examined the effects of OTC stimulants on steady-state exercise. Bright et al. (1981) investigated the effects of pseudoephedrine on sub-maximal treadmill exercise. They concluded that pseudoephedrine in single or double therapeutic doses failed to cause significant cardiovascular and metabolic adjustments in healthy subjects during sub-maximal exercise. It was likely that any sympathoadrenergic effects which occurred as a result of drug administration were masked during exercise.

Most research that has attempted to elucidate the effects of such drugs on exercise has focused on performance parameters (De Meersman et al., 1987; Clemons and Crosby, 1993; Gillies et al., 1996; Swain et al., 1997). One of the most appropriate physiological indicators of physical endurance capacity is maximal oxygen consumption (VO_{2max}). An increase in this parameter following drug administration may indicate increased aerobic power and the potential to enhance aerobic exercise performance. Swain *et al.* (1997) reported no effect of pseudoephedrine and phenylpropanolamine on maximal aerobic capacity following the administration of single or double the therapeutic dose. Similarly, Sidney and Lefcoe (1977) found no effect of a therapeutic dose of ephedrine on VO_{2max}. Clemons and Crosby (1993) examined the effect of a single 60-mg dose of pseudoephedrine prior to performance of a graded exercise test and found no difference in total exercise time to exhaustion. Gillies *et al.* (1996) administered double the therapeutic dose of pseudoephedrine to male cyclists prior to both a 40-km time trial performed on a cycle ergometer and to a knee extension exercise. No significant effect was found either to cycling performance time or to knee extension strength. Voelz *et al.* (1996) investigated the effects of supratherapeutic doses of ephedrine on high intensity treadmill exercise. There was no effect on time to exhaustion, suggesting ephedrine has no ergogenic effect even at high doses on endurance exercise. Of those studies addressing the performance effects of ephedrines, very few have used highly trained individuals or attempted to simulate competitive events.

Conduction of simple motor tasks is also an important contributing factor in athletic performance. Despite no reported ergogenic effects of OTC sympathomimetic amines upon complex exercise performance, it is possible that effects may be evident upon less complex athletic parameters such as isometric muscle strength and reaction time. However, Sidney and Lefcoe (1977) found no effect of a single therapeutic dose of ephedrine on grip strength or endurance, muscle power, anaerobic capacity or reaction time. Following multiple therapeutic doses of pseudoephedrine (i.e. six 60-mg doses over a 36-hour period) and phenylpropanolamine (six 25-mg doses over a 36-hour period) Chester *et al.* (2003b) found no effect on isometric grip, leg and back strength or reaction time.

Danger during endurance exercise has been associated with impaired thermoregulation as a result of the use of sympathomimetic amines. Indeed, the deaths of several cyclists during major competition, most notably that of Tom Simpson on Mont Ventoux in the 1967 Tour de France, have been attributed to hyperthermia related to the use of amphetamine (Williams, 1974). It is likely that hyperthermia is a consequence of increased motor activity and impaired thermoregulation. Although published studies have identified increased thermogenesis (Dulloo and Miller, 1986) and a reduction in the drop in core temperature during exposure to low temperature (Vallerand, 1993) following administration of ephedrine, no studies have assessed body temperature at comfortable ambient temperatures following the administration of ephedrines.

The use of ephedrines in sport has sometimes been associated with simultaneous use of caffeine. Bell and colleagues (1998) investigated the time to exhaustion during high intensity cycling exercise following ingestion of such a combination of drugs (5 mg/kg body weight caffeine and 1 mg/kg body weight ephedrine). Results showed a significant increase in time to exhaustion when compared with trials following placebo ingestion and ingestion of caffeine and ephedrine alone. These results were attributed to increased central nervous system stimulation. Caffeine, *per se*, is suspected of widespread abuse in sport. Caffeine was prohibited if the urine concentration exceeds 12 µg/ml. There was a single positive test for caffeine in the modern pentathlon in the Seoul Olympics (1988). There is strong anecdotal evidence of caffeine abuse in cycling (Kimmage, 1998; Orr and Stannard, 1999). In response to a questionnaire, all 12 'A' grade cyclists in a National series race in Australia reported taking caffeine before the race. Six reported taking caffeine both before and during the race. All caffeine ingested during the race was taken within 35–50 km of the finish (Orr and Stannard, 1999). The most outrageous example of simultaneous use of caffeine and other stimulants is the legendary 'pot belge'. This is a concoction purportedly used in the not-too-distant past by some cyclists and which is alleged to contain amphetamines, caffeine, cocaine, heroin, painkillers and, sometimes, corticosteroids (Voet, 2001). At least the corticosteroids are not used all the time!

The proposal that ingestion of sympathomimetic drugs can promote weight loss by increasing energy expenditure and reducing food intake through appetite suppression has resulted in considerable interest by researchers. In an animal study performed by Ramsey *et al.* (1998), it was reported that energy expenditure was increased and, in some animals, food intake was reduced following the administration of ephedrine and caffeine. Consequently it was concluded that ephedrine and caffeine treatment could promote weight loss. It appears that ephedrine is effective in increasing thermogenesis and has the potential for body weight loss in obese individuals (Bukowiecki *et al.*, 1982), especially when combined with caffeine or aspirin (Astrup and Toubro, 1993). However, there have been no studies that have focused on sympathomimetic drug use and non-obese, athletic populations to promote leanness.

The number of OTC preparations which contain banned sympathomimetics is extremely high. In the USA there are over 120 formulations that contain prohibited decongestants, 36 of which contain PPA. In the UK there are over 40 formulations that contain prohibited decongestants, 11 of which contain PPA. Moreover, even the names of products can confuse the purchaser. Thus the name Sudafed™ is associated with pseudoephedrine. But Sudafed™ tablets contain pseudoephedrine whilst Sudafed™ Nasal Spray contains oxymetazoline.

Expectorants

These are intended to increase the volume and decrease the viscosity of respiratory mucus. They are emetics, i.e. they cause vomiting at high concentrations. At sub-emetic doses they are thought to irritate the gastric mucosa, which in turn stimulates secretion of respiratory mucus by a vagal reflex, though there is little evidence to support this theory. Moreover, there is little evidence to suggest that OTC expectorants are effective. Consequently, they are frequently dismissed as little more than harmless placebos. Guaiphenesin (guaifenesin) is the only expectorant listed by the FDA as having scientific evidence of safety and efficacy. Thick tenacious mucus that cannot be cleared by coughing is normally a feature of a bacterial infection of the lower respiratory tract rather than of a self-limiting, viral infection of the upper respiratory tract. As such, this condition may require antibiotic therapy. An alternative approach is to decrease the viscosity of mucus with a mucolytic. Steam is an excellent expectorant and mucolytic. It is permitted by WADA and is a most acceptable alternative to the aforementioned expectorants.

Demulcents

Demulcents substitute for the natural function of the mucus, i.e. a physical and chemical barrier which coats and protects the epithelium of the respiratory tract. Viral infections of the URT damage the epithelial lining of the respiratory tract. This reduces the production of mucus, decreases the ciliated cells which transport the mucus and reduces the protective barrier above the inflamed mucosa. A persistent, non-productive cough exacerbates the removal of cells from the respiratory epithelium and should be prevented. Demulcents are often effective in preventing dry, non-productive coughs merely by coating the inflamed tissue and protecting the exposed sensory nerve endings which initiate the cough reflex. Throat lozenges which contain a local anaesthetic (benzocaine) may be advantageous in these circumstances. Alternatively, simple linctus, syrups and lozenges containing glycerin (glycerol), honey and lemon are widely available. Note that demulcents and local anaesthetics are only effective in those areas of the URT that they can reach, i.e. the oral pharynx and larynx. However, they are often all that is needed to treat a dry, non-productive cough caused by a self-limiting viral infection and they have no side-effects. In that respect, they are preferable to centrally acting cough suppressants. Their use is permitted by WADA.

Xanthines

Caffeine and theophylline are methylxanthines. In the UK, seven OTC cough and cold preparations contain caffeine and three contain theophylline. One preparation even contains ephedrine in addition to both caffeine and theophylline. Theophylline is a bronchodilator which is used in Step 4 of the BTS Guidelines for the treatment of chronic asthma in adults. Caffeine is a central nervous stimulant with weak diuretic activity and little or no bronchodilator activity. Bronchodilators are of no relevance to the treatment of a congested nasal cavity, pharynx, larynx or trachea. Bronchodilators would only be appropriate for lower respiratory tract infections where there is bronchoconstriction or a wheeze. However, in these circumstances, the presence of a cough may well be a symptom of poorly controlled asthma when the use of an OTC preparation containing a xanthine would be entirely inappropriate. There can be no justification, whatsoever, for recommending a preparation containing a xanthine to a sportsperson.

4.8   Recommendations for treatment of coughs and colds

In view of the myriad of problems facing the sportsperson who seeks a short-term remedy for the symptoms of a cough or cold, the following recommendations are offered:

1.   Hydration. This will prevent dehydration when there is copious secretion and will aid expectoration when a cough is non-productive.
2.   Since a cough is designed to remove mucus, a productive cough should **never** be suppressed. A cough should only be suppressed when it is dry and non-productive (often a prelude to a viral infection of the upper respiratory tract). However, demulcents are preferable to cough suppressants if the cause is an inflamed throat because they have no side-effects and they are not banned by WADA.
3.   A purulent secretion requires antibiotic therapy from a medical practitioner.
4.   Many cough and cold remedies cannot be recommended because they contain irrational combinations of either cough suppressants and expectorants, expectorants and antihistamines, decongestants and expectorants. Some compound preparations contain sub-therapeutic concentrations of the active ingredients. Many of the active constituents are banned by WADA. Therefore, always attempt to purchase a product with a single active constituent. Moreover, it is cheaper to purchase an analgesic and a decongestant separately than to purchase them together in a cough and cold preparation.
5.   If a decongestant is desired, then caution must be applied. A topical nasal spray is always preferable as it is targeted at the desired site of action and will not have systemic side-effects. Oxymetazoline and xylometazoline are long-acting decongestants which are available as topical formulations. They need only be administered 2 and 3 times a day, respectively. Oxymetazoline, xylometazoline and phenylephrine (when administered topically) are permitted by WADA.
6.   Finally, always check the list of active drugs in the pharmaceutical preparation against the list of banned drugs that is readily available. If

in doubt about either the mode of action or the type of drug and whether it is likely to be banned, ask a pharmacist and then your coach.

Sportspersons should heed the following emboldened warning from the IOC (August 1993) *'Thus no product for use in colds, flu or hay fever purchased by a competitor or given to him/her should be used without first checking with a doctor or pharmacist that the product does not contain a drug of the banned stimulant class'.*

4.9 Summary

Historically, the treatment of asthma and the common cold has resulted in positive drug tests and personal tragedies in the lives of elite sportspersons from Rick Demont to Andreea Raducan. As the lack of action taken against the positive tests for salbutamol and terbutaline showed in the 2000 Summer Olympiad in Sydney, it is possible to be treated for asthma and to remain within the proscribed limits set by WADA. However, this is manifestly not the case with ephedrines when used to treat the common cold. Whilst this might deny a sportsperson the legitimate use of an OTC medication for a minor ailment, they would be well advised to avoid all such medications until such time as WADA reviews the acceptable urinary concentrations of these sympathomimetics. Even allowing for the fact that certain OTC drugs appear in WADA's specified substances list, it is beholden on the athlete to establish that the use of such a substance was not intended to enhance performance. This does not mean that all treatments are denied them; rather, that individual medicines such as a permitted analgesic, e.g. paracetamol, and a topical decongestant, e.g. oxymetazoline, constitute a much wiser course of action and one that is not likely to end in tragedy after many years of preparation and sacrifice.

4.10 References

Anon (2000) Editorial: OTC sales top $40bn. *Pharm. J.*, **265**, 225.

Astrup, A. and Toubro, S. (1993) Thermogenic, metabolic and cardiovascular responses to ephedrine and caffeine in man. *Int. J. Obes.*, **17**, S41–S43.

Bell, D.G., Jacobs, I. and Zamecnik, J. (1998) Effects of caffeine, ephedrine and their combination on time to exhaustion during high-intensity exercise. *Eur. J. Appl. Physiol. Occup. Physiol.*, **77**, 427–433.

Berstein, E. and Diskant, B.M. (1982) Phenylpropanolamine: A potentially hazardous drug. *Ann. Emerg. Med.*, **11**, 311–315.

BNF (2004) *British National Formulary.* Number 47 (September, 2004). British Medical Association and Royal Pharmaceutical Society of Great Britain, London.

Brater, D.C., Kaojarern, S., Benet, L.Z. *et al.* (1980) Renal excretion of pseudoephedrine. *Clin. Pharmacol. Ther.*, **28**, 690–694.

Bright, T.P., Sandage, B.W. and Fletcher, H.P. (1981) Selected cardiac and metabolic responses to pseudoephedrine with exercise. *J. Clin. Pharmacol.*, **21**, 488–492.

British Thoracic Society (1997) The British Guidelines on Asthma Management. *Thorax*, **52**, Suppl. 1.

Bukowiecki, L., Jahjah, L. and Follea, N. (1982) Ephedrine, a potential slimming drug, directly stimulates thermogenesis in brown adipocytes via β-adrenoreceptors. *Int. J. Obes.*, **6**, 343–350.

Bundgaard, A., Rasmussen, F.V. and Madsen, L. (1980) Pretreatment of exercise-induced asthma in adults with aerosols and pulverized aerosol. *Allergy*, **35**, 639–645.

Bye, C., Dewsbury, D. and Peck, A.W. (1974) Effects on the human central nervous system of two isomers of ephedrine and triprolidine and their interaction. *Br. J. Clin. Pharmacol.*, **1**, 71–78.

Bye, C., Hill, H.M., Hughes, D.T.D. and Peck, A.W. (1975) A comparison of plasma levels of L(+)pseudoephedrine following different formulations, and their relation to cardiovascular and subjective effects in man. *Eur. J. Clin. Pharmacol.*, **8**, 47–53.

Chester, N., Mottram, D.R., Reilly, T. and Powell, M. (2003a) Elimination of ephedrines in urine following multiple dosing: the consequencies for athletes, in relation to doping control. *Br. J. Clin. Pharmacol.*, **71**, 62–67.

Chester, N., Reilly, T. and Mottram, D.R. (2003b) Physiological, subjective and performance effects of pseudoephedrine and phenylpropanolamine during endurance running exercise. *Int. J. Sports Med.*, **24**, 3–8.

Clemons, J.M. and Crosby, S.L. (1993) Cardiopulmonary and subjective effects of a 60 mg dose of pseudoephedrine on graded treadmill exercise. *J. Sports Med. Phys. Fit.*, **33**, 405–412.

Committee on Safety of Medicines (2000) PAGB Statement on DoH Position re Phenylpropanolamine (PPA). http://www.pagb.co.uk/Media_Services/Industry_Positions/ip_01121.htm (accessed 03/05/2001).

De Meersman, R., Getty, D. and Schaefer, D.C. (1987) Sympathomimetics and exercise enhancement: all in the mind? *Pharmacol. Biochem. Behav.*, **28**, 361–365.

Drew, C.D.M., Knight, G.T., Hughes, D.T.D. and Bush, M. (1978) Comparison of the effects of D-(–)-ephedrine and L-(+)-pseudoephedrine on the cardiovascular and respiratory systems in man. *Br. J. Clin. Pharmacol.*, **6**, 221–225.

Dulloo, A.G. and Miller, D.S. (1986) The thermogenic properties of ephedrine methylxanthine mixtures – human studies. *Int. J. Obes.*, **10**, 467–481.

Edelman, J.M., Turpin, J.A., Bronsky, E.A. *et al.* (2000) Oral montelukast compared with inhaled salmeterol to prevent exercise-induced bronchoconstriction – a randomised, double-blind trial. *Ann. Int. Med.*, **132**, 97–104.

Empey, D.W., Young, G.A., Letley, E. *et al.* (1980) Dose–response of the nasal decongestant and cardiovascular effects of pseudoephedrine. *Br. J. Clin. Pharmacol.*, **9**, 351–358.

FDA (2000) Phenylpropanolamine (PPA): Information page. US Food and Drug Administration. http://www.fda.gov/cder/drug/infopage/ppa/default.htm (accessed 06/08/2001).

Gibson, G.J. and Warrell, D.A. (1972) Hypertensive crisis and phenylpropanolamine. *Lancet*, **ii**, 492.

Gillies, H., Derman, W.E., Noakes, T.D., Smith, P., Evans, A. and Gabriels, G. (1996) Pseudoephedrine is without ergogenic effects during prolonged exercise. *J. Appl. Physiol.*, **81**, 2611–2617.

Global Initiative for Asthma. http://www.ginasthma.com/ (accessed 28/09/2001).

Goodman, R.P., Wright, J.T., Barlascini, C.O., McKenny, J.M. and Lambert, C.M. (1986) The effect of phenylpropanolamine on ambulatory blood pressure. *Clin. Pharmacol. Ther.*, **40**, 144–147.

Hansen-Flaschen, J. and Schotland, H. (1998) Editorial: New treatments for exercise-induced asthma. *N. Engl. J. Med.*, **339**, 192–193.

Hartley, J.P.R., Charles, T.J. and Seaton, A. (1977) Betamethasone valerate inhalation and exercise-induced asthma in adults. *Br. J. Dis. Chest*, **71**, 253–258.

Heath, G.W., Ford, E.S., Craven, T.E., Macera, C.A., Jackson, K.L. and Pate, R.R. (1991) Exercise and the incidence of upper respiratory tract infections. *Med. Sci. Sports Exerc.*, **23**, 152–157.

Henriksen, J.M. and Dahl, R. (1983) Effects of inhaled budesonide alone and in combination with low-dose terbutaline in children with exercise-induced asthma. *Am. Rev. Respir. Dis.*, **128**(6), 993–997.

Hoffman, B.B. and Lefkowitz, R.J. (1990) Catecholamines, sympathomimetic drugs, and adrenergic receptor antagonists. In J.G. Hardman, A.G. Gilman and L.E. Limbird (Ed.) *Goodman and Gilman's The Pharmacological Basis of Therapeutics*, 9th edn, pp. 199–249. McGraw-Hill, New York.

Horowitz, J.D., Lang, W.J., Howes, L.G., Fennessy, M.R., Christophidis, N., Rand, M.J. and Louis, W.J. (1980) Hypertensive responses induced by phenylpropanolamine in anorectic and decongestant preparations. *Lancet*, **i**, 60–61.

Horwitz, R.I., Brass, L.M., Kernan, W.M. and Viscoli, C.M. (2000) Phenylpropanolamine and risk of hemorrahagic stroke: Final Report of The Yale Hemorrhagic Stroke Project, 46 pp.

IOC Medical Commission (1992) *Prohibited Classes of Substances and Prohibited Methods*, July 1992.

IOC Medical Commission (1999) *Olympic Movement Anti-doping Code.*

IOC Medical Commission (2001) *Prohibited Classes of Substances and Prohibited Methods*, 1st September 2001.

IOC (2000a) 30 Years of fight against doping. Doping cases. http://www.nodoping.olympic.org/ (accessed 14/03/2001).

IOC Medical Commission (2000b) *Post-Olympic Public Report on doping controls at the Games of the XXVII Olympiad in Sydney (Australia)*. Lausanne, 14 December 2000.

Irish Times (1999). Seven international athletes test positive. *Irish Times*, 10th August 1999.

Johnson, D.A., Etter, H.S. and Reeves, D.M. (1983) Stroke and phenylpropanolamine use. *Lancet*, **ii**, 970.

Jones, T.R. and Rodger, I.W. (1999) Role of leukotrienes and leukotriene receptor antagonists in asthma. *Pulm. Pharmacol. Ther.*, **12**, 107–110.

Katzung, B.G. (2001) *Basic and Clinical Pharmacology*, 8th edn. Appleton and Lange, Stamford, Connecticut.

Kimmage, P. (1998) *Rough Ride*. Yellow Jersey Press, London.

Kuitunen, T., Karkkainen, S. and Ylitalo, P. (1984) Comparison of the acute physical and mental effects of ephedrine, fenfluramine, phentermine and prolitane. *Meth. Find. Exptl. Clin. Pharmacol.*, **6**, 265–270.

Lacroix, V.J. (1999) Exercise-induced asthma. *Phys. Sports Med.*, **27**(12), 75–92.

Lanciault, G. and Wolf, H.H. (1965) Some neuropharmacological properties of the ephedrine isomers. *J. Pharm. Sci.*, **54**, 841–844.

Larsson, K., Ohlsen, P., Larsson, L. *et al.* (1993) High prevalence of asthma in cross-country skiers. *Br. Med. J.*, **307**, 1326–1329.

Lefebvre, R.A., Surmont, F., Bouckaert, J. and Moerman, E. (1992) Urinary excretion of ephedrine after nasal application in healthy volunteers. *J. Pharm. Pharmacol.*, **44**, 672–675.

Morton, A.R. and Fitch, K.D. (1992) Asthmatic drugs and competitive sport: an update. *Sports Med.*, **14**(4), 228–242.

Nastasi, K.J., Heinly, T.L. and Blaiss, M.S. (1995) Exercise-induced asthma and the athlete. *J. Asthma*, **32**(4), 249–257.

National Asthma Audit (1999/2000). http://www.asthma.org.uk/infofa18.html (accessed 13/03/2001).

Nelson, J.A., Strauss, L., Skowronski, M., Ciufo, R. Novak, R. and McFadden, E.R. Jnr. (1998) Effect of long-term salmeterol treatment on exercise-induced asthma. *N. Engl. J. Med.*, **339**, 141–146.

Nichols, P. (2001) Not necessarily guilty: how other ephedrine cases were resolved. *Guardian*, 16 June 2001.

Nieman, D.C., Johanssen, L.M., Lee, J.W. and Arabatzis, K. (1990) Infectious episodes in runners before and after the Los Angeles Marathon. *J. Sports Med. Phys. Fitness*, **30**, 316–328.

Nieman, D.C., Henson, D.A. and Gusewitch, G. (1993) Physical activity and immune function in elderly women. *Med. Sci. Sports Exerc.*, **25**, 823–831.

Noakes, T.D. and Gillies, H. (1994) Drugs in sport. *S. Afr. Med. J.*, **84**, 364.

Noble, R.E. (1982) Phenylpropanolamine and blood pressure. *Lancet*, **i**, 1419.

Norvenius, G., Widerlov, E. and Lönnerhölm, G. (1979) Phenylpropanolamine and mental disturbance. *Lancet*, **ii**, 1367–1368.

Orr, R. and Stannard, S. (1999) Caffeine ingestion in competitive road cyclists in Australia. 5th IOC World Congress on Sport Sciences. http://www.ausport.gov.au/fulltext/1999/iocwc/abs109.htm (accessed 09/08/2001).

Peters, E.M. and Bateman, E.D. (1983) Ultramarathon running and upper respiratory tract infections. *S. Afr. Med. J.*, **64**, 582–584.

Prather, I.D., Brown, D.E., North, P. and Wilson, J.R. (1995) Clenbuterol: a substitute for anabolic steroids? *Med. Sci. Sports Exerc.*, **27**, 1118–1121.

Proprietary Association of Great Britain (2002) Personal Communication.

Ramsey, J.J., Colman, R.J., Swick, A.G. and Kemnitz, J.W. (1998) Energy expenditure, body composition and glucose metabolism in lean and obese rhesus monkeys treated with ephedrine and caffeine. *Am. J. Clin. Nutr.*, **68**, 42–51.

Rupp, N.T. (1996) Diagnosis and management of exercise-induced asthma. *Phys. Sports Med.*, **24**(1), 77–87.

Sidney, K.H. and Lefcoe, N.M. (1977) The effects of ephedrine on the physiological and psychological responses to submaximal and maximal exercise in man. *Med. Sci. Sports*, **9**, 95–99.

Smith, B.W. and LaBotz, M. (1998) Pharmacological treatment of exercise-induced asthma. *Clin. Sports Med.*, **17**(2), 343–363.

Swain, R.A., Harsha, D.M., Baenziger, J. and Saywell, R.M. (1997) Do pseudoephedrine or phenylpropanolamine improve maximum oxygen uptake and time to exhaustion? *Clin. J. Sport Med.*, **7**, 168–173.

Tattersfield, A.E. (1997) Limitations of current therapy. *Lancet*, **350**, Suppl. II, 2427.

Tattersfield, A.E., Lofdahl, C-G., Postma, D.S. *et al.* (2001) Comparison of formoterol and terbutaline for as-needed treatment of asthma. *Lancet*, **357**, 257–261.

Thomas, S.H.L., Clark, K.L., Allen, R. and Smith, S.E. (1991) A comparison of the cardiovascular effects of phenylpropanolamine and phenylephrine containing proprietary cold remedies. *Br. J. Clin. Pharmacol.*, **32**, 705–711.

UK Sport (2000) *The year in detail: UK Sport's 1999–2000 anti-doping programme.*

Vallerand, A.L. (1993) Effects of ephedrine/xanthines on thermogenesis and cold tolerance. *Int. J. Obes.*, **17**, S53–S56.

Voelz, J., Dolgener, F. and Kolkhorst, F. (1996) The effect of high-dose ephedrine HCl on high intensity treadmill performance. *Med. Sci. Sport Exerc.*, **28**, Suppl. S35 (Abstract).

Voet, W. (2001) *Breaking the chain.* Yellow Jersey Press, London.

Voy, R. (1986) The US Olympic Committee experience with exercise-induced bronchospasm 1984. *Med. Sci. Sports Exerc.*, **18**, 328–330.

Wadler, G.I. and Hainline, B. (1989) *Drugs and the Athlete.* F.A. Davis Company, Philadelphia.

Weiler, J.M., Layton, T. and Hunt, M. (1998) Asthma in United States Olympic athletes who participated in the 1996 Summer Games. *J. Allergy Clin. Immunol.*, **102**, 722–726.

Wilkinson, G.R. and Beckett, A.H. (1968) Absorption, metabolism and excretion of the ephedrines in man I. The influence of urinary pH and urine volume output. *J. Pharmacol. Exp. Ther.*, **162**, 139–147.

Williams, M.H. (1974) *Drugs and Athletic Performance.* Charles C. Thomas Publisher, Springfield, Illinois.

Chapter 5

Androgenic anabolic steroids

Alan J. George

5.1 Summary

The conclusions reached in surveying anabolic steroid use in male and female athletes are that anabolic steroids do increase muscle bulk and body weight in all anabolic steroid takers but that increases in strength are certain to occur at low doses only in those undertaking regular training exercise. The long-term side-effects of anabolic steroids may be severe and will depend on dosage and duration. In particular, early death from cardiovascular disease, sterility in men and, in women, masculinization and possible fetal effects constitute the most serious hazards. More recently, studies have suggested that psychological and behavioural changes and addiction may result from chronic anabolic steroid abuse, but methodological inconsistencies still make evaluation of these side-effects very difficult. There is evidence of increased abuse of steroids for cosmetic reasons, and among college and school students and that intensive education programmes have had little effect on steroid abuse so far.

5.2 Introduction

Gliding, racialism, Jesse Owens, anabolic steroids – which is the odd one out? Well, the first three were present at the infamous Berlin Olympics of 1936, and the last one almost certainly wasn't (Yesalis *et al.*, 2000). So when did they first make their appearance in sport? It is suggested that the Helsinki Olympics of 1952 was the debut for anabolic steroids and steroid-filled Russians then swept to numerous golds in the 1954 Vienna Weightlifting Championships. The worried US team doctor, John Ziegler, identified anabolic steroids as the source of Russian success. Armed with the new wonder drugs, the coaches, like Goethe's Sorcerer's Apprentice, wreaked a spell on their athletes, but the Sorcerer is yet to return.

For centuries, it was popularly believed that symptoms of ageing in men were caused by testicular failure. This stimulated a search for an active principle of the testicles which, when isolated, would restore sexual and mental vigour to ageing men. The testicular principle, we now know, is the male sex hormone testosterone, which was first synthesized in 1935.

Experimental studies in both animals and humans soon showed that testosterone possessed both *anabolic* and *androgenic* actions. The androgenic actions of testosterone are those actions involving the development and maintenance of primary and secondary sexual characteristics while the anabolic actions consist of the positive effects of testosterone in inhibiting urinary nitrogen loss and stimulating protein synthesis, particularly in skeletal muscle.

5.3   The testosterone family

Testosterone is a so-called C-19 steroid hormone. The steroid hormones are derived in the body from the substance cholesterol. The structure of testosterone is closely related to the steroid substance androstane and the structure of androstane is used as a reference when naming most of the compounds related to or derived from testosterone (see Figure 5.1). The apparently identical structures of testosterone and epitestosterone can be differentiated by the orientation of the hydrogen atom at the 17 position. When two chemical compounds have the same atomic composition, but different orientations of the constituent atoms, they are known as isomers. Hence epitestosterone is an isomer of testosterone.

Biosynthesis

In humans, the immediate precursor of testosterone in the biosynthetic sequence from cholesterol is androstenedione which is converted to testosterone by the action of the enzyme 17β-hydroxysteroid dehydrogenase (Figure 5.2). This enzyme will also act on other steroids with similar structures, such as 19 nor-androstenedione, to produce 19 nor-testosterone (nandrolone) (Figure 5.2) (Mottram and George, 2000; Wright *et al.*, 2000).

The biochemistry and physiology of testosterone

Testosterone, the most important naturally occurring compound with androgen and anabolic activity is formed in the Leydig cells of the testis but also in the adrenal cortex. Adrenocortical testosterone is important in women, as it is responsible for some secondary sexual characteristics such as pubic and axillary hair growth and in some cases for its influence on sexuality (Greenblatt *et al.*, 1985). Mean testosterone production in men is approximately 8 mg per day of which 90–95 per cent is produced by the testis and the remainder by the adrenal cortex. When testosterone is synthesized in the body, its isomer epitestosterone is also formed. Epitestosterone has exactly the same number of atoms as testosterone but the –H and –OH groups at C-17

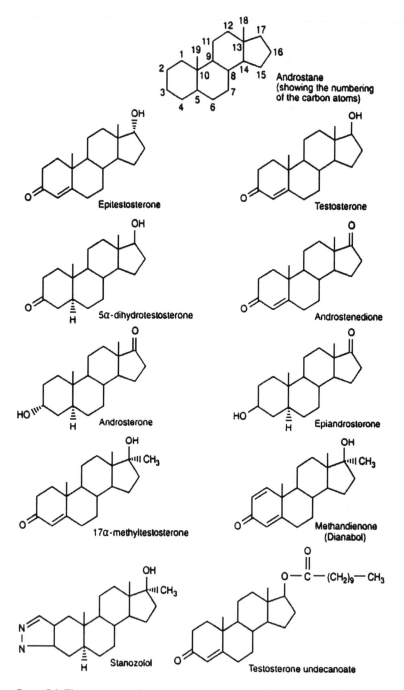

Figure 5.1 The structure of testosterone and some of its derivatives (from George, 1996).

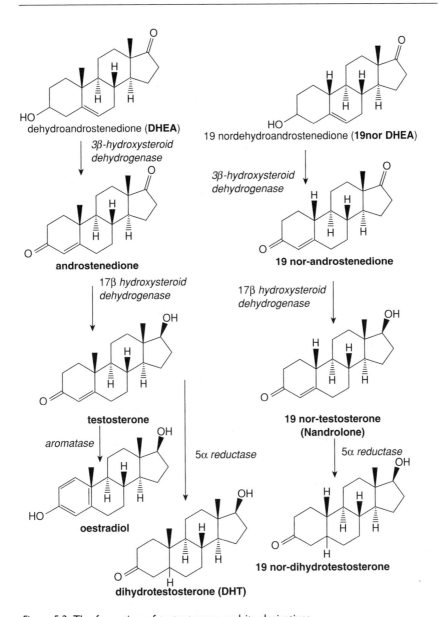

Figure 5.2 The formation of testosterone and its derivatives.

are orientated differently (Figure 5.1). The ratio of testosterone to epitestosterone concentrations in the plasma of normal males is 12:1. (Kicman *et al.*, 1999). The testis also produces 5α-dihydrotestosterone, which is approximately equal in androgenic and anabolic activity to testosterone, and also two compounds with much weaker biological activity: androstenedione and dehydroepiandrosterone. After puberty, plasma testosterone levels are approximately 0.6 mg/dl in males and 0.03 mg/dl in women; 95 per cent of testosterone in the blood is bound to protein, mainly sex hormone-binding globulin (SHBG); 2–3 per cent of testosterone remains free, i.e. unbound, while the remainder is bound to serum albumin.

Mode of action of testosterone

Like most other steroid hormones testosterone produces its principal effect on tissues by altering cellular biochemistry via an interaction with the cell nucleus. Testosterone diffuses into the cell, as it is lipid soluble and thus readily crosses cell membranes. It combines with a testosterone-binding protein which transports it to the cell nucleus. Here the testosterone interacts on a particular chromosome with one or more specific binding sites called hormone receptor elements and activates the synthesis of one or more proteins which may be either enzymes or structural proteins. However, the possibility that testosterone and/or anabolic steroids may produce pharmacological effects via a cell surface receptor should not be ruled out. In some mammalian tissues such cell surface receptors are known to exist for the glucocorticoid hormones, which also possess a similar steroid structure to testosterone. In some tissues testosterone is first converted to 5α-dihydrotestosterone (DHT), also called androstanolone, by the enzyme 5α-reductase (Figure 5.2). The DHT is then transported to the nucleus and produces similar biochemical changes to those of testosterone. In many testosterone-sensitive tissues it is now thought that the anabolic effects of testosterone are mainly produced by the action of DHT. DHT can be formed from testosterone in the testes, liver, brain, prostate gland and external genitalia, but there is little 5α-reductase activity and therefore little *direct* formation of DHT in human skeletal muscle. Generally in the liver, and locally in brain areas such as the hypothalamus, testosterone can be converted by the aromatase enzyme system to oestradiol (Figure 5.2).

The 'aromatization' of testosterone to oestradiol is essential for sexual differentiation of the brain, bone mass consolidation and for epiphyseal fusion of the long bones at the end of puberty (Wu, 1997). DHT is primarily androgenic while oestradiol antagonizes some androgenic actions while enhancing others. The full details of testosterone synthesis and metabolism have been expertly reviewed by Wilson (1988), Lukas (1993), Wu (1997), and Ueki and Okana (1999).

Metabolism

Apart from conversion to DHT in various tissues, testosterone is metabolized in the liver mainly to DHT, androstenedione and then via the 3-keto reductive enzymes to either androsterone or one of its two isomers,

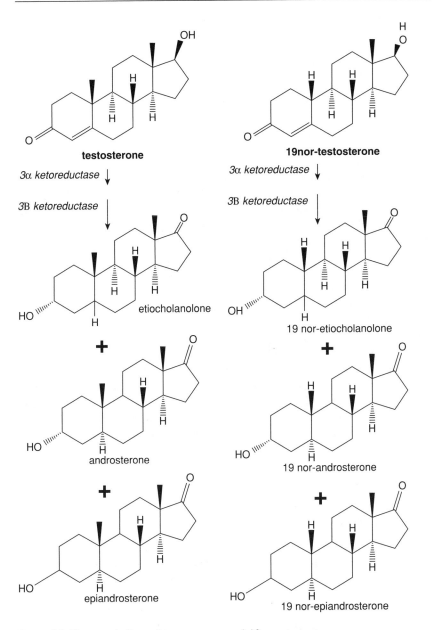

Figure 5.3 The metabolism of testosterone and 19 nor-testosterone.

epiandrosterone or etiocholanolone (Figure 5.3). This has been reviewed recently by Ueki and Okana (1999) and Wright *et al.* (2000). All four metabolites are present in plasma and urine. Androsterone and epiandrosterone have weak androgenic activity, while etiocholanone has none. Some testosterone is converted in the testis to oestradiol. Significant amounts of oestradiol are also thought to be formed from testosterone in the brain.

The physiological role of testosterone

Testosterone and its structurally related analogues possess androgenic and anabolic activity.

Androgenic effects

Testosterone is responsible for the development of primary sexual characteristics in males. Normally in a genetically male fetus, i.e. one with the XY sex chromosome configuration, the embryonic testis begins to differentiate, under the influence of H-Y antigen, the production of which is directed by the Y chromosome. As the male gonad differentiates, Leydig cells are formed which begin to secrete testosterone. Testosterone and a polypeptide factor Müllerian regression factor (MRF) together stimulate the formation of the internal male genitalia, *in utero*. The external genitalia and prostate develop mainly under the influence of DHT (Wu, 1997). From birth until puberty the Leydig cells which secrete testosterone produce small amounts of testosterone providing a plasma testosterone concentration of up to 2 nmol/l. From the age of approximately 10 years, in males, increased testosterone secretion occurs principally from the testicular Leydig cells. The pubertal changes induced by this increase in testosterone are the secondary sexual characteristics which include musculoskeletal configuration, genital size, psychic changes and induction of sperm production. Adult secondary hair growth is stimulated by DHT. The chronology of male puberty and adolescence has been described in detail by Tanner (1962) and the Tanner Index provides a useful guide for the assessment of the progress of puberty, and the attainment of maturity.

Anabolic effects

The anabolic effects of testosterone and anabolic steroids are usually considered to be those promoting protein synthesis and muscle growth, but they also include effects such as stimulation and eventually inhibition of skeletal growth in the young. Attempts to produce purely anabolic, synthetic, testosterone derivatives have been unsuccessful. It should be remembered that though the anabolic action of anabolic steroids may be much greater than testosterone, all anabolic steroids also possess some androgenic activity. There will also be discrete variations in the ratio of androgenic to anabolic activity amongst the family of testosterone derivatives, anabolic steroids and their various metabolites. For example, it has been suggested that, in females, the androgenic effect of the nandrolone metabolite

19 nor-dihydro-testosterone (Figure 5.2) (19 nor-DHT) is less than either DHT or testosterone.

5.4 Structural analogues of testosterone – the anabolic steroids

To the dismay of clinical scientists, it was soon discovered that when the newly isolated testosterone was given orally or injected into patients it was ineffective. When taken by mouth, testosterone is absorbed from the small intestine and passes via the portal vein to the liver where it is rapidly metabolized, mostly to inactive compounds. Injected testosterone also passes rapidly into the blood and then to the liver where it is inactivated. In the late 1940s medicinal chemists began to develop analogues of testosterone which might be degraded less easily by the body. Forty years of intensive research have yielded three major types of testosterone modification, each of which gives rise to a class of anabolic steroids (Figure 5.4). Addition of an alkyl group at position 17 renders the structure orally inactive (B). A type (A) modification makes the compound suitable for 'depot' injection, while type (C) modifications allow oral dosing and sometimes increased potency. A detailed account of the medicinal chemistry of anabolic steroids is provided by Wilson (1988) while a brief introduction to the topic is provided by George (1994).

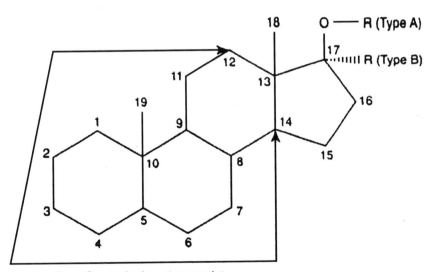

Figure 5.4 The three major types of testosterone modification (after Wilson, 1988).

Clinical uses of androgens/anabolic steroids

Replacement therapy in men

Anabolic steroids may be given to stimulate sexual development in cases of delayed puberty. The therapy is then withdrawn gradually once full sexual maturity is reached. They may also be given in cases where the testicles have been surgically removed either because of physical injury or because of a testicular tumour. In this case the replacement therapy must be continuous for life.

Replacement therapy in women

Testosterone production is necessary in women as well as men. In the rare condition known as sexual infantilism a young female fails to secrete oestradiol, progesterone and testosterone. As a consequence she suffers from amenorrhea, a lack of libido and absence of pubic and axillary hair. Only when she is treated with testosterone does libido appear. Some postmenopausal women suffer from loss of libido. In both these cases administration of testosterone restores sex drive and sexual characteristics (Greenblatt *et al.*, 1985).

Gynaecological disorders

Anabolic steroids are occasionally used to treat gynaecological conditions in women, though long-term usage produces severe side-effects such as erratic menstruation and the appearance of male secondary characteristics. In the USA, they have sometimes been used to repress lactation, after childbirth. They are also sometimes used to combat breast tumours in premenopausal women.

Protein anabolism

The initial use of anabolic steroids in the early 1940s was to inhibit the loss of protein and aid muscle regeneration after major surgery, and to stimulate muscle regeneration in debilitating disorders such as muscular dystrophy and diabetes. Many concentration camp survivors owe their early recovery from debilitation to the skilled use of dietary measures coupled with anabolic steroids. Recently, a number of clinical studies have indicated that nandrolone, oxandrolone and oxy-methalone may be able to attenuate and, in some cases, reverse muscle loss and decline of lean body mass in AIDS patients (Mulligan *et al.*, 1999).

Anaemia

Anabolic steroids are sometimes used in large doses to treat anaemias which have proved resistant to other therapies – this therapy is not recommended in women because of masculinizing side-effects.

Osteoporosis

There is some evidence that combined oestrogen/androgen therapy is able to inhibit bone degeneration in this disorder.

Growth stimulation

Anabolic steroids may be used to increase growth in prepubertal boys who have failed to reach their expected height for their age. The treatment must be carried out under carefully controlled conditions so that early fusion of the epiphyses does not occur.

Side-effects of androgens

Principally in women

These include acne, growth of facial hair, hoarsening or deepening of the voice and reduction in body fat. If the dose given is sufficient to suppress gonadotrophin secretion then menstrual irregularities will occur. Chronic, i.e. long-term treatment with androgens, as for example in mammary carcinoma, may produce the following side-effects – male pattern baldness, prominent musculature and veins, clitoral hypertrophy. A detailed review of this subject has been provided by Elliott and Goldberg (2000). A case of gender identify confusion coupled with pseudohermaphroditism has been reported recently (Choi, 1998).

In children

Administration of androgens can cause stunting of growth, a side-effect directly related to disturbance of normal bone growth and development. The enhancement of epiphyseal closure is a particularly persistent side-effect which can be present up to 3 months after androgen withdrawal.

In males

Spermatogenesis is reduced by testosterone treatment with as little as 25 mg of testosterone per day over a 6-week period. Anabolic steroids will produce the same effect, since they will suppress natural testosterone secretion. The inhibition of spermatogenesis may persist for many months after anabolic steroid withdrawal.

General side-effects

OEDEMA

Oedema or water retention, related to the increased retention of sodium and chloride is a frequent side-effect of short-term androgen administration.

This may be the major contribution to the initial weight gain seen in athletes taking these drugs (see later). Water and electrolyte gain is an unwanted side-effect in all normal individuals but is particularly unhealthy in people with circulatory disorders or in those with a family background of such disorders.

BLOOD VOLUME

Significant increases in steroid-induced water retention are likely to produce an increase in the blood volume. It should be noted that any expansion of the blood volume is likely to be a result of the simultaneous increase in water retention plus the increased erythropoiesis caused by anabolic steroid administration (Rockhold, 1993).

JAUNDICE

Jaundice is a frequent side-effect of anabolic steroid therapy and is caused mainly by reduced flow and retention of bile in the biliary capillaries of the hepatic lobules. Hepatic cell damage is not usually present. Those anabolic steroids with a 17α-methyl group are most likely to cause jaundice.

HEPATIC CARCINOMA

Patients who have received androgens and/or anabolic steroids for pro-longed periods may develop hepatic carcinoma. This is also particularly prevalent in people who have taken 17α-methyl testosterone derivatives.

5.5 Anabolic steroids and sport

The desire to increase sporting performance and athletic prowess by means other than physical training has been experienced for at least 2000 years. Ryan (1981) quotes the observation of the Greeks that a high protein diet was essential for bodybuilding and athletic achievement. The Greeks, of course, knew nothing of protein structure or biosynthesis but they felt that by eating the flesh of a strong animal such as the ox, the athlete would gain strength himself. We have seen previously that one of the first therapeutic uses of anabolic steroids was in treating the protein loss and muscle wasting suffered by concentration camp victims. Following the publication of the results of these treatments it was natural that anabolic steroids should be used in an attempt to increase muscle strength in athletes. Many early studies on the effect of anabolic steroids often involved self-administration and were necessarily anecdotal with no attempt at scientific or controlled investigation of the effect of the steroid drugs. Several studies relied on subjective feelings and lacked any objective measure of increased strength or stamina. Also, side-effects were never admitted to or were simply omitted from the results.

Subsequent studies, many of which were carried out in the late 1960s and early 1970s, were more scientifically based but often entirely contradictory in their results. In this chapter we will discuss what any physician, student or lay person would wish to know about the use of an anabolic steroid: where are they obtained?; how are they used?; does it work?; does it confer any advantage over normal training practices?; what are the side-effects?; what are the long- and short-term consequences? In addition the athlete needs to know whether the practice is ethical and the sports administrator how to discover whether anabolic steroids are being taken. Finally we will consider future trends.

Sources, supply and control

The increased usage of anabolic steroids by athletes and the spread of usage from sport to the general population has prompted governmental intervention in several countries and stimulated investigation into the illicit supply of anabolic steroids and the control of their abuse.

In Great Britain, anabolic steroids are licensed by the Department of Health's Medicine Control Agency (MCA) as prescription-only medicines (POMs) within the meaning of the Medicines Act 1968. This means that it is illegal for a doctor or pharmacist to *supply* them other than by a doctor's prescription and there are recorded cases of individual prosecution for illegal supply. The UK government has legislated to classify anabolic steroids as controlled drugs under the Misuse of Drugs Act (1971). This makes export, import, and supply without prescription illegal. Under UK law, *possession* of anabolic steroids is not illegal unless it is 'with intent to supply' whether for profit or not (Tucker, 1997). This attitude has been contested by many experts on addiction and those closely associated with counselling and treating anabolic problems in gyms and sports clubs (Dawson, 2001). Denmark has recently raised anabolic steroids to 'controlled' status and has made possession a criminal offence punishable by two years in jail.

In the USA anabolic steroids were added to Schedule III of the Controlled Substances Act of 1994, making supply and possession of the drugs a federal offence. However, the American Medical Association opposed this legislation because they contend that most of the illicitly used anabolic steroids are illegally smuggled in or manufactured, and such legislation, when enacted for cocaine led to an *increase* in its illegal supply (Daigle, 1990).

There are numerous sources of anabolic steroids, which vary between nations. In the USA, the major external sources appear to be Panama and Mexico, while illegal synthesis by 'street traders' is another major source. Both these internal and external sources provide drugs which are untested, unstandardized, contain potentially toxic impurities and have not been produced in the stringently hygienic conditions of the modern pharmaceutical industry. Musshoff *et al.* (1997) analysed 42 illicit 'anabolic' substances seized by the police and customs officials in Germany. Fifteen of these contained counterfeit ingredients such as 'cheaper' anabolic steroids substituted for more expensive products, for example metenolone gestagen (a progestogen) substituted for nandrolone. In two cases tocopherole (an anabolically inactive compound) was substituted for the steroid trenbolone. There are anecdotal tales of body builders taking 'anabolic steroids' which were actually stilboestrol, an *oestrogen* used in Europe for improving the muscle mass of chickens. Perry *et al.* (1992) described the supply of Equipoise, an equine anabolic steroid, to gym users in Glamorgan. Catlin *et al.* (2000) examined seven brands of androstenedione available 'over the counter' in US health shops and only one contained the pure compound; the others consisted of adulterated product, impurities such as testosterone and in one sample no drug at all. Surveys show that the majority of steroid abusers in the USA are supplied by the black market (Lamb, 1991) with the remaining supplies coming from physicians and pharmacists. In their survey of college student athletes, Green *et al.* (2001) found that 32 per cent of anabolic steroid abusers in the USA obtained their drugs from a physician not associated with the college team!

All these criminal activities are insignificant in terms of organization and scale compared with the sponsored and managed promotion and supply of anabolic steroids by the government of the former German Democratic Republic (GDR). Release of State documents following the GDR's collapse indicates the extent of the systematic, programmed dosing of thousands of GDR athletes in the period 1970–1990. A full account of this governmental network of drug supply and administration in the cause of athletic abuse has been provided by Franke and Berendonk (1997). There is every reason to suppose that the practice has occurred elsewhere and is continuing.

Patterns of administration and use

No two groups of athletes who abuse anabolic steroids seem to use the same pattern of drug administration. It is this observation that above all confounds attempts to make scientific comparisons between various studies of anabolic steroid efficacy (see below). There are a number of administration regimes in use (Wilson, 1988; Rogol and Yesalis, 1992), though each has its variations and often combinations of regimes may be used concurrently.

Cycling

A period of administration followed by a similar period of abstinence before the administration is recommenced. Typical cycling patterns are short: 6–8 weeks on drug, 6–8 weeks' abstinence; or long: 6–18 weeks on drug with up to 12 months' abstinence. The rationale here is that the periods of abstinence may reduce the incidence of side-effects. This regime is preferred by body builders.

Pyramiding

A variation of cycling in which the dose is gradually built up in the cycle to a peak and then gradually reduced again towards the end of the cycle. This regime is said to cause fewer behavioural side-effects such as lowered mood, caused by the withdrawal of the drug.

Stacking

The use of more than one anabolic steroid at a time. In its simplest form this regime involves the simultaneous use of both an orally administered steroid and an injectable one. More 'sophisticated' patterns involve intricate schedules of administration using many different steroids each with supposedly different pharmacological profiles. The aim of this technique is to avoid *plateauing*, that is, the development of tolerance to a particular drug. According to the amateur pharmacologists of locker rooms and gymnasia, these 'super stacking' programmes allow more receptor sites to be stimulated. This is very dubious pharmacology since the number of intracellular testosterone/DHT steroid receptors is stable and all are probably saturated under normal physiological conditions. Exact doses tried by abusers are almost impossible to establish. What is certain is that doses used by weight-lifters and body builders are at least 100 times those indicated for therapeutic use (Rogol and Yesalis, 1992) and also those used in most scientific studies (Elashoff *et al.*, 1991). The dose–response studies of Forbes (1985) also indicate that the doses used in 'ethical/clinical' studies of anabolic steroid effects on athletic performance are only sufficient to cause modest improvements in lean body mass (Figure 5.5). It is claimed that endurance and sprint athletes who abuse steroids may use doses closer to clinical recommendations (Rogol and Yesalis, 1992).

The abuse cycles documented above are often followed in males by a dose of human chorionic gonadotrophin (hGG), which is used to stimulate endogenous testosterone production that has been suppressed by the chronic administration of testosterone or anabolic steroids (Evans, 1997). Abuse of hCG is covered in Chapter 6.

Extent of usage

It is difficult to calculate which anabolic steroid is most often abused worldwide. Some anabolic steroids are not available in every country, some are stolen veterinary preparations and some have been illicitly manufactured. Many athletes will also be 'stacking' several preparations at once. The most popular abused drugs in the US college survey of Pope *et al.* (1988) are shown in Table 5.1, while in a survey of US power-lifters the most popular

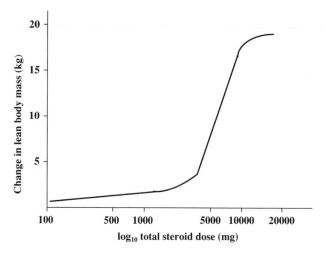

Figure 5.5 Semilog plot of relationship between steroid dose and change in lean body mass (from Forbes, 1985).

Table 5.1 The most popular anabolic steroids abused by a sample of 17 US college men (Pope *et al.*, 1988)

Drug	No. using drug*
Methandrostenolone	8
Testosterone esters	6
Nandrolone	5
Oxandrolone	4
Stanozolol	1
Methenolone	1

* More than one drug abused by some subjects.

drugs were methandrostenolone (93 per cent) and testosterone esters (80 per cent). The first British survey of anabolic steroid usage (Table 5.2) showed also that dianabol (methandrostenolone) at 69 per cent was the most frequently administered anabolic steroid (Perry *et al.*, 1992). In their study, published in 1994, Pope and Katz found that the majority of abusers reported taking testosterone, while 54 per cent admitted taking nandrolone. When the urine of the same athletes was tested, only 41 per cent were found to be abusing testosterone and 57 per cent nandrolone. This study illustrates the possible confusion of different drugs by abusers or the possibility of deception by drug suppliers. The study showed the tendency towards testosterone abuse. The supply, administration and abuse of the veterinary

Table 5.2 The most frequently abused anabolic steroids amongst 62 male gymnasia attenders in West Glamorgan, UK (Perry *et al.*, 1992)

Drug	No. abusing drug*
Dianabol	43
Deca Durabolin	37
Testosterone esters	32
Stanozolol	19
Equipoise	10

* More than one drug abused by some subjects.

steroid Equipoise (Table 5.2) has been identified by Perry *et al.* (1992). In 1994, Chinese athletes were alleged to be abusing dihydrotestosterone. Later surveys have shown minor changes in drug preferences and also for the first time the most popular anabolic steroids taken by females. The 1997 UK survey carried out by Korkia and Stimson at six separate sites in the UK, showed testosterone, nandrolone and dianobol were equally popular amongst male abusers while female abusers preferred oxandiolone, stanozolol and methandrostenlone. Though only 13 women (compared with 97 men) took part in the survey, it is interesting that women seemed to prefer orally active drugs. A local survey in the Clwyd area of North Wales also found differences in anabolic steroid preferences between males and females (Burton, 1996), though in this survey some women, of the eight surveyed, did use nandrolone, whereas the 62 males used three different injectable anabolic steroids and four different orally active drugs.

Data from the infamous GDR archives on the 'State' doping of athletes shows that both orally active and injectable anabolic steroids were used in their abuse programme. There is also the sinister documentation of coded, unnamed 'steroid substances' possibly indicating that some covert evaluations/clinical trials of drugs or new products were being undertaken (Franke and Berendonk, 1997).

Polypharmacy

The concurrent abuse of anabolic steroids with other drugs has also been a feature of surveys conducted twice since the 1980s. These additional abuses usually involve drugs taken to counteract the side-effects of anabolic steroids. In the 1992 survey of Perry *et al.*, 5 per cent of anabolic steroid abusers were additionally taking the anti-oestrogen tamoxifen. This was to counteract the feminizing effects produced by the conversion to oestradiol of the testosterone they were taking. Korkia and Stimson (1997) found 22.7 per cent of their abusers taking hCG, possibly for the reasons given earlier. A further 22.7 per cent were taking anti-oestrogens and 11.8 per cent were taking antibiotics, presumably to counteract acne. Several surveys (DuRant *et al.*, 1995; Burton, 1996; Evans, 1997; Korkia and Stimson, 1997; Meilman *et al.*, 1997) report alarming co-administration of anabolic steroids and stimulants. In their survey of US college students Meilman *et al.* (1997) found 44.7 per cent of steroid abusers also took amphetamine and 40.8 per cent cocaine. Both these drugs are stimulants, taken to aid weight loss or counteract negative psychological effects of steroid abuse. Diuretics are frequently co-abused with anabolic steroids and were noted in several surveys. Evans (1997) reported 22 per cent of anabolic steroid abusers in Glamorgan were taking diuretics, probably to counteract the water retention induced by anabolic steroids.

The epidemiology of anabolic steroid abuse

In response to the widespread view that anabolic steroid abuse was rife in the sporting population, several American investigators began surveys of athletes in order to establish the distribution and prevalence of anabolic steroid abuse. These useful investigations are continuing. In a summary of these early (1976–1984) findings, Pope *et al.* (1988) reported that as many as 20 per cent of intercollegiate athletes and fewer than 1 per cent of non-athlete students reported using anabolic steroids. This prevalence was much higher than the 2.5 per cent usage rate reported in a 1971 study. The review by Pope *et al.* (1988) also records a survey of students at a Florida High School where 18 per cent of male students but no females reported using anabolic steroids. This high prevalence of usage was suggested to be peculiar to Florida and could be related to so-called cosmetic factors discussed later.

From their own survey of 1010 college males, Pope *et al.* (1988) found that 2 per cent reported taking anabolic steroids, with university-standard athletes more likely to be taking steroids than non-athletes. Of this 2 per cent, 42 per cent reported that body building and appearance were their main reasons for anabolic steroid abuse; 58 per cent reported various reasons connected with sport for their abuse. High degrees of prevalence of abuse (6.6 per cent) were found by Buckley *et al.* (1988) in 1700 US high school students, while Windsor and Dumitru (1988) found a 3 per cent abuse level in 800 US college students. In this survey 5 per cent of males and 1.4 per cent of females admitted abusing steroids. Williamson (1993) has carried out the major British study of anabolic steroid abuse and found levels of 4.4 per cent in males, 1 per cent in females at a college of technology in Scotland.

When surveys of non-college athletes are conducted the percentage of abusers is much higher. Yesalis *et al.* (1988) found a current prevalence of 33 per cent amongst US powerlifters, which rose to 55 per cent when previous usage amongst non-users was included. In the UK, Perry *et al.* (1992)

reported a 38.8 per cent prevalence amongst weight-trainers in private gymnasia in their West Glamorgan survey area.

The figures for young abusers in GB and the USA – 3–6 per cent – may vary in different locations. In Britain, there is anecdotal evidence to suggest that anabolic steroid abuse is higher in areas with a macho culture, ample male leisure time (i.e. unemployment), low self-esteem and proximity to sandy beaches. Thus abuse may be said to be led by cultural pressure, feelings of social inadequacy and a suitable location to parade the results of your body-building. The high prevalence of steroid abuse in Florida (18 per cent according to Pope *et al.*, 1988) may well reflect this latter theory! In Australia, Handelsman and Gupta (1997) found that the 3.2 per cent of high school boys who abused anabolic steroids were frequently truants.

The prevalence of anabolic steroid abuse in international competition is difficult to judge. At the 1972 (pre-testing) Munich Olympics, 68 per cent of interviewed athletes in middle or short distance running or in field events admitted taking steroids. At the Mexico Olympics, all the US weightlifters admitted taking steroids (Wilson, 1988). Perhaps the introduction of mandatory testing for the 1976 Olympics in Montreal has led to a decline in steroid abuse rather than a switching to less detectable doping agents such as hGH. The official IOC figures in 2000 show that though anabolic steroid abuse at IOC accredited events as a percentage of total positive results was 38.1 per cent compared with 65.3 per cent in 1986, the actual numbers of positive anabolic steroid tests was up from 439 in 1986 to 946 in 2000. We may also have to regard the current generation of athletes as a lost cause and instead concentrate education and deterrent resources on the young. Up to 1992, progress in the USA (education programmes, legislation) had encouraged some experts to suggest that the availability and usage of steroids in the USA is decreasing (Catlin *et al.*, 1993). But analysis of the trends in the USA (1989–1997) by Yesalis and Bahrke (2000) shows that this optimism is unfounded as the abuse figures generally are static and in some surveys may be increasing. This was followed by the Mark McGuire 'androstenedione' baseball scandal; and in Europe the investigation of several Dutch footballers, including the ex-Manchester United footballer Jaap Stam, and the controversial 1998 Tour de France race.

Efficacy of anabolic steroids

Effects on muscle

Whether anabolic steroid treatment 'works' has been perhaps the most difficult question of all to answer satisfactorily since many of the early investigations that have been carried out were, in the main, poorly designed scientifically, clinically and statistically (see Ryan, 1981 for review). Increases in muscle strength are proportional to increases in the cross-sectional diameter of the muscles being trained but there is no way of showing conclusively, *in vivo*, that any increase in muscle diameter consists of increased muscle protein rather than increased content of water or fat. Advances in the use of ultrasound and NMR (nuclear magnetic resonance) techniques may make this possible early in the 2000s, and some progress has been made in the analysis of the effects of exercise and drugs on muscle structure (Blazevich and Giorgi, 2001). It is also apparent that different groups of athletes may wish to increase their muscle bulk for different purposes. For example, the American footballer or the wrestler may wish simply to increase his bulk and weight, whereas a weightlifter may want increased dynamic strength and the long distance runner may wish to accelerate muscle repair after an arduous and taxing run.

The first serious investigator of the question as to whether anabolic steroids work seems to be Ryan (1981) who reviewed a total of 37 studies between the years 1968 and 1977. He was confounded by the many different measurements being taken as indices of anabolic steroid activity. Some studies attempted to measure gains in strength of experimental subjects over controls, other studies measured the change in circumference of a limb. One study attempted to measure change in lean body mass. In 12 studies which claimed that athletes taking anabolic steroids gained in strength, the gains reported were often quite small. The majority of these 12 studies were not 'blind': that is either the investigator or the subject (or perhaps both!) knew when an active principle was being taken. In only five of the studies were protein supplements given and in none of the studies examined was there any dietary control or at least a listing of total protein and caloric intake for each subject. Other features of these studies were their poor design in matching control and experimental subjects and there were also errors in calculating the results. Ryan then examined 13 other studies in which valid matching of controls and experiments had occurred. Ten of these 13 studies were double blind (neither experimenter or subject knew when an active substance was being administered), the control and experimental groups contained at least six subjects in each and the average period of experimentation was some 50 per cent longer than in the early studies in which improvements were claimed. Also, in this second group of experiments, five different steroid groups were investigated compared with only two in the earlier group. Ryan's conclusion from examining these two groups of studies was that there was no substantial evidence for an increase in lean muscle bulk or muscle strength in healthy young adult males receiving anabolic steroids. Comparison of these studies is difficult because the various parameters used to assess improvement in strength were not the same. Though the majority of studies assessed by Ryan measured changes in gross body weight and 'improvement' in standard strength tests, the other tests employed included VO_{2max}, limb circumference, lean body mass and 'changes in blood chemistry'. One reason for the variety of measurements used and a possible explanation for the lack of agreement in assessing anabolic steroid efficacy is that different athletic groups each sought different parameters for improvement. As I have mentioned before, the American footballer or wrestler may be seeking increased bulk, the weightlifter or thrower an increase in strength or perhaps both.

Experiments with anabolic steroids, since 1975, have tended to be more carefully carried out, controlled and more sophisticated than those reviewed by Ryan. An example of an early, well-conducted trial is the frequently quoted study by Freed *et al.* (1975). In this experiment six standard strength exercises were used as a measure of increased strength. The study was carried out over a 6-week period in weightlifters who were given either 10 or 25 mg per day of methandienone. Drug treatment increased strength by 0.3–13 per cent during the 6-week study while those taking placebo showed strength gains of 0.3–2.3 per cent. Body weight increased only in the drug-treated athletes and those on the 25 mg dose showed no greater strength increase than those on 10 mg. A significant finding was that withdrawal of the anabolic steroid caused a loss of weight but no loss in strength gained, which suggested that anabolic steroid taking amongst athletes might be harder to detect since the drug could be withdrawn from an athlete well in advance of a meeting without significant loss of performance, thus allowing him to evade detection in any doping test. Further analysis of Freed's study shows that the doses of methandienone are some 75 per cent lower than those claimed to be used by some athletes. It might have been more useful to tailor the dose of the drug to the athlete's initial body weight, i.e. calculate the dose in terms of mg/kg body weight, and also to measure the actual free and bound plasma concentration of the drug. It is reasonable to conclude from Freed's work that only a proportion of people show a significant improvement in strength as a result of steroid treatment.

Studies should also determine who are the types of athlete or individual which 'benefit' from anabolic steroids. Another factor absent from the analyses of this and other earlier experiments is consideration of the subject's body build. The bodily changes induced by testosterone at puberty and indeed those that are produced *in utero* occur as a result of an interaction between testosterone and the individual genetic 'constitution' or genotype. Thus, the individual emerging from puberty with a lean, well-muscled body – the classic mesomorph somatotype – does so because of the expression of the genes controlling his muscularity rather than because he has higher testosterone levels than the more lightly muscled ectomorph. Thus, only certain somatotypes may benefit fully. An important early study on the influence of athletic experience and pre-training on the response of athletes to anabolic steroid treatment was researched by Wright (1980). He noted that inexperienced weightlifters showed no increase in strength or lean muscle mass while simultaneously taking anabolic steroids and protein supplements and undergoing short-term training. In contrast, weightlifters who trained regularly, i.e. to nearly their maximum capacity, did show increased strength compared with their pretreatment level. Though his results did not show consistent increases in strength amongst the steroid-treated trained athletes, Wright claimed to show that the trained athletes responded better to anabolic steroid treatment, a finding he could not explain adequately. However, the presence of a greater initial muscle mass in the trained athletes before anabolic steroid treatment might have been a factor. Another possibility is that trained muscles *are* different, i.e. they may produce some endogenous factor which enhances anabolic steroid action. It is already known that the muscles of trained athletes can increase their uptake of glucose by the production of an endogenous factor and that regular exercise regimes increase the responsiveness of skeletal muscle to insulin.

If the results of these studies, from 20 years ago, produce such inconsistent results, why do athletes continue to take anabolic steroids? One possible explanation was that the steroid trials discussed so far are based on dose levels which, while medically and ethically acceptable, are considerably less than those commonly taken by athletes. This factor coupled with the necessity of pre-drug intensive training and a high protein diet might explain the failure of anabolic steroids to produce a consistent increase in strength and performance.

The importance of training during and before a period of steroid treatment is apparently emphasized in a sophisticated series of experiments carried out by Hervey and colleagues between 1976 and 1981, and reviewed by Hervey (1982). The experimental design involved the administration of the anabolic steroid dianabol at 100 mg per day during one 6-week period and a placebo during the other 6 weeks. The two treatment periods (drug and placebo) were separated by a 6-week treatment-free period. The experiments were carried out double blind. All volunteers were athletes, one group being professional weightlifters. In each group, body weight, body fat, body density and the fat and lean tissue proportion were measured.

The non-weightlifting group of athletes showed the same improvement in weightlifting performance and leg muscle strength during both placebo and drug administration periods. In the group containing experienced weightlifters there was a significant improvement during drug administration when compared with the placebo period. Both weightlifters and other athletes exhibited weight gain and increases in limb circumference. Though the weightlifters were heavier than their non-weightlifting counterparts, the proportion of lean body mass was the same in both groups.

Hervey *et al.* (1981) concluded from these experiments that in athletes engaged in continuous hard-training regimes, anabolic steroids in the doses athletes claim to use cause an increase in muscle strength and athletic performance. The experimental design could be criticized in that it is possible that those subjects taking the drug in the first 6-week period were not completely drug free at the start of the placebo period 6 weeks later. Thus, the residual effect of the steroid could have affected measurements during the placebo period of evaluation and could have masked any apparent difference between the placebo and treatment periods.

These are two examples of well-conducted trials carried out in the early 1980s. Summarizing the evidence gained from these and earlier trials, Haupt and Rovere (1984) concluded that abuse of anabolic steroids will consistently result in a significant increase in strength if all of the following criteria are satisfied.

1. They are given to athletes who have been intensively trained in weight-lifting immediately before the start of the steroid regimen and who continue this intensive weightlift training during the steroid regimen.
2. The athletes maintain a high protein diet.
3. The changes in the athletes' strength are measured by the single repetition/maximal weight technique for those exercises with which the athlete trains.

Studies demonstrating significant increases in body size and body weight during the anabolic steroid regimen were consistently those studies that demonstrated statistically significant increases in strength.

Studies that did not demonstrate significant increases in body size and body weight during the anabolic steroid regimen were consistently those studies that did not demonstrate statistically significant increases in strength.

Janet Elashoff and her colleagues at Cedars Sinai Medical Centre, Los Angeles have provided an even more sophisticated analysis of 30 of these early studies in which athletes received two or more doses of anabolic steroid and in which changes in muscular strength were measured. They made use of the statistical technique known as meta-analysis and also analysed for the statistical power of the study. In addition to the study defects described previously, Elashoff et al. (1991) found marked evidence of poor statistical design and computation in many of the 30 studies examined; for example, the use of standard instead of paired t tests when comparing paired data. They queried whether any of the studies were truly blind and whether checks for compliance were carried out properly. Their conclusions were that, in many cases, it must be obvious to both experimenter and athlete who is on an active preparation since it should be possible to see who develops greater acne, beard growth and weight gain and the athletes will almost certainly experience the psychopharmacological effects of 'being on steroids'. As in previous reviews the authors question whether further analysis of these studies is worthwhile since the amounts administered are obviously below the amounts used by the abusing adult. Referring to the studies of Forbes (1985) quoted previously, it is obvious that the maximum dose of 7245 mg used in the experiments reviewed by Elashoff is at the start of the drug dose/lean body mass curve and thus only just at the threshold of producing an observable improvement in lean body mass (see Figure 5.5, page 154). The latest research seems to confirm that supraphysiological doses of anabolic steroids do have effects over and above low doses used in earlier studies.

In his 1997 computation of testosterone doses in relation to plasma level, Wu suggested that the responses to anabolic steroids obtained at the supraphysiological doses and plasma levels used by many abusers were part of a different/separate relationship than that obtained to physiological or clinical plasma levels. He doubted whether results obtained at ethical/clinical levels of dosage could be extrapolated to the high dosage levels used by many abusers. A year previously, Bhasin et al. (1996) designed a study incorporating many of the suggestions made by earlier reviewers. This well-controlled study recruited 43 volunteers and compared supraphysiological testosterone doses with placebo, with or without exercise, over a 10-week period. The dosing regime of the treated subjects was a 6000 mg injection of testosterone enanthrate per week. There was a strictly controlled exercise and dietary regime. Results showed an increase in muscle strength with exercise alone. Testosterone alone increased muscle size, strength and lean body mass, but each of these values could be increased further by simultaneous exercise. Supraphysiological doses of testosterone, and presumably also other androgens, according to this vital study do have an anabolic effect on muscle mass, strength and lean body mass in men and this can be enhanced by physical training regimes. In a later review of his own and other studies, Bhasin et al. (2001) concluded that testosterone supplementation increases maximal voluntary strength but that it does not improve specific tension. Thus testosterone would be expected to improve performance in weightlifting events as these activities are so dependent on maximal voluntary strength. No studies have yet demonstrated any effect of anabolic steroids on endurance exercise in man, but Tamaki et al. (2001) have shown a positive effect in rats.

What changes occur within the muscle itself? Blazevich and Giorgi (2001) have shown that certain changes in muscle architecture commonly associated with high-force production may be induced also by a combination of testosterone and heavy resistance training. Whilst that has little effect on muscle thickness, pennation (ability of muscle fibre to twist) and the length of muscle fibres were both increased by testosterone.

Following recent research we should then question whether (1) further analysis of studies carried out using low doses is worthwhile, and (2) more consideration should be given in studies to those anabolic steroid effects which are not directly concerned with increases in muscle strength, that is: lean body mass, psychological changes and even physical appearance. Again it must be emphasized that increases in lean body mass in runners and increased aggressiveness in American footballers and ice hockey players may be far more important to them, respectively, than improved muscle strength.

If anabolic steroid administration does produce increases in muscle strength, should this not be reflected in the progression of athletic records? Howard Payne analysed UK and world sporting records from 1950 to 1975.

The trend in all the events analysed, namely the 10 000 metres, pole vault, discus and shot shows a steady improvement year by year without a sudden upsurge in any event. Thus, anabolic steroids cannot be shown to have significantly improved performances in field events nor in the 10 000 metres, where competitors are, in some cases erroneously, assumed not to be steroid takers. A survey and review by Norton and Olds (2001) suggests that many other factors may be involved in these improvements in performance, such as improved training, selection and diet.

Effects on aerobic performance

Because anabolic steroids increase haemoglobin concentration, it has been suggested that they may be able to enhance aerobic performance by improving the capacity of the blood to deliver oxygen to the exercising muscle. However, only two out of ten recent studies support this hypothesis and one actually suggests that steroids may reduce aerobic power. Tamaki *et al.* (2001) showed that anabolic steroids could increase exercise tolerance in rats.

Effects on behaviour

If, even in the most careful experiments, the positive effects of anabolic steroids are seen only in maximally exercising individuals, why is it that so many claims are made for them? One reason is possibly that steroids make them 'feel better'. Some athletes claim they feel more competitive and aggressive, others may feel they *should* run faster as they are on anabolic steroids. The increase in body weight and in circumference of leg and arm muscles may improve the athlete's self-image. Whether anabolic steroids enhance aggression or competitiveness is hard to assess. It is difficult to demonstrate conclusively that steroids or indeed testosterone are responsible for aggressiveness since many behaviours are probably learnt. It is quite likely that behaviour if it is hormonally influenced is imprinted soon after birth. However, both male and female sexual behaviour are strongly influenced by androgens (see introductory section). Another possibility is that anabolic steroids may have a placebo effect – abusers may work or train harder because they expect anabolic steroids to work their magic! This has been investigated by Maganaris *et al.* (2000). They demonstrated moderate improvements in performance in athletes who believed they were taking anabolic steroids.

Effects on muscle repair

If it is agreed that anabolic steroids do increase athletic performance, albeit in strictly defined circumstances, what advantages do they confer on the taker? Obvious advantages are that the steroid taker may have stronger muscles with greater endurance, and a greater body mass with which to endure impact in sports like rugby, ice hockey or wrestling.

A further advantage conferred on the anabolic steroid taker is that their muscles and associated tissues *may* have greater reparative powers and so the athlete may be able to undertake more events in a short time. This observation has led to the increased use of steroids by both middle and long distance runners and marathon runners.

How does the anabolic steroid produce these effects? The original ideas that anabolic steroids simply stimulate muscle growth need to be revised following the results of the studies carried out in exercising individuals. From the results quoted previously it is possible to deduce that anabolic steroids may simply allow more intense exercise to take place thus stimulating muscle growth. Again, it could be that muscle produces an endogenous factor which stimulates further muscle growth *or* that exercise induces increased production of the hormones such as insulin, growth hormone and somatomedins, each of which is able to increase protein synthesis, particularly in muscle. It is interesting that most major studies involving anabolic steroids, with the exception of that by Hervey *et al.* (1981), have failed to measure other hormones simultaneously. This study by Hervey *et al.* measured testosterone and cortisol during the treatment of athletes with methandienone. They showed that as testosterone was suppressed by methandienone treatment by the end of the experiment so plasma cortisol concentration rose. It is not clear whether this is the free, or total cortisol in the plasma, but the deduction made was that anabolic steroid effects are possibly mediated via a rise in cortisol concentration. The authors claimed that the puffy facial and thoracic features produced by anabolic steroids are similar to those occurring in Cushing's Disease (CD) in which plasma cortisol is abnormally high as the result of either a pituitary or adrenocortical tumour causing adrenocortical overproduction of cortisol. There are many objections to this ingenious theory. The symptoms of CD and anabolic steroid administration are far from similar: CD patients have a characteristic moon face, abnormal fat distribution and distended abdomen. The limb muscles are *thin* and *wasted* – producing the characteristic 'lemon on sticks' appearance of CD. More importantly, the plasma cortisol levels in CD are much greater than those quoted by the authors at the end of the study. Following Hervey's original hypothesis, other theories have suggested that anabolic steroids may block the action of cortisol and corticosterone on muscle by competing with them for their intracellular receptors. Cortisol and corticosterone inhibit muscle protein synthesis and enhance muscle protein catabolism. If this action were inhibited then muscle protein anabolism would be enhanced. Evidence for anabolic steroid binding to glucocorticoid (GC) receptors has been summarized by Rockhold (1993). Such theories of anabolic effects produced by antagonism of GC receptors must account for the observation that androgen and GC receptor numbers increase during training regimes that increase muscle mass but not during those that increase endurance.

These theories have also been analysed by Wu (1997) who concluded that in cases where individuals are insensitive to androgens because of an androgen receptor defect, supraphysiological/clinical doses of testosterone were able to reverse the muscle wasting normally associated with the condition. Anabolic steroids clearly have pharmacological effects not associated with binding to androgen cytoplasmic receptors. Whether these effects, seen only at supraphysiological/clinical doses, are mediated via cell surface receptors, glucocorticoid receptors or from displacement of testosterone and other androgens from their plasma protein binding sites remains to be established.

5.6   Something special

The strange case of clenbuterol

Just before the start of the Barcelona Olympics in 1992, two British weightlifters, Andrew Saxton and Andrew Davis, tested positive for the drug clenbuterol. During the games the IOC acted swiftly to proscribe the drug.

Clenbuterol is classed as a β_2-agonist; it is structurally related to salbutamol and in some EC countries (but not the UK) is similarly licensed for the treatment of asthma. However, the reason for banning the drug was associated with claims that it increased muscle mass while simultaneously reducing body fat.

β_2-Agonists can promote normal skeletal muscle growth and experiments with clenbuterol show that it can increase muscle weight in rats by 10–12 per cent after 2 weeks treatment (Yang and McElliott, 1989) and can reduce amino acid loss from incubated muscle. It has been shown that clenbuterol can reverse experimentally induced muscle fibre atrophy by increasing muscle protein synthesis as well as inhibiting amino acid loss. In contrast, salbutamol has no significant effect on muscle protein, though this difference may be related to the short half-life of salbutamol, since continuous infusion of salbutamol causes similar anabolic effects to clenbuterol.

Clenbuterol does not produce its anabolic effects by interacting with testosterone, growth hormone or insulin (Choo et al., 1992), but via β_2-receptor stimulation. Similarly the fat mobilizing action of clenbuterol is also mediated via β_2-receptors. However, the dose of clenbuterol required in animal studies to bring about an 'anabolic' effect is approximately 100 times the maximum dose that humans can tolerate.

This clenbuterol mystery seems no nearer to being solved partly because of the dual difficulties of extrapolating animal studies to man and designing ethically suitable human studies. Spann and Winter reviewed the most recent clenbuterol experiments in 1995. They analysed data from the US Department of Agriculture which demonstrated increases in muscle mass and lean body mass in steers treated with clenbuterol; a result which has also been found in rats, poultry and sheep. Human studies are much more equivocal and show that clenbuterol produces no statistically significant increase in involuntary muscle strength but that certain type II or fast-twitch muscle fibres *may* benefit from the drug. There is also some weak evidence that clenbuterol may improve limb muscle strength rehabilitation after an ortho-paedic operation.

Therapeutic use of clenbuterol

Clenbuterol is not licensed in the UK, but in some EC countries it is licensed for the treatment of asthma. The fact that it increases lean body mass, decreases fat and may increase muscle protein synthesis suggests that the drug may be useful in weaning anabolic steroid abusers off their drugs.

Should clenbuterol be banned?

Most recent evidence suggests that clenbuterol does reduce body fat and increase muscle mass, though whether this leads to a consistent increase in strength does not seem to have been demonstrated yet. The important point to be considered here is whether clenbuterol confers any athletic advantage. It is assumed that reductions in body fat and increases in lean body mass will confer advantages to most athletes. The positive 'anabolic' effects, while not yet associated with increases in strength, may be advantageous in *maintaining* the anabolic effects of anabolic steroids when these are withdrawn before an athletic event so as to avoid detection by doping tests. The association between clenbuterol, other β_2-agonists and gains in muscle strength in athletes warrants further investigation.

5.7   Precursors, nandrolone and metabolites

Earlier in the chapter, I reviewed the biosynthesis and metabolism of testosterone, and it can be seen that testosterone is produced naturally in the testis and adrenal cortex by the conversion of dehydroepiandrosterone (DHEA) to androstenedione and then to testosterone. For some years, both these substances were suggested as possible anabolic agents in the knowledge that when administered, they could be converted to testosterone in the body (Johnson, 1999). Androstenedione was the major substance that Mark McGuire admitted to abusing in his quest for baseball fame in 1997–1998. Though several researchers, including the infamous East Germans, claimed that androstenedione and DHEA produced increases in serum testosterone concentration of up to 300 per cent in women and 200 per cent in men, this has not been correlated yet with any increases in muscle strength or athletic performance (Johnson, 1999). Despite this, DHEA and androstenedione were prohibited by the IOC in 1996. Brian Wallace and his colleagues showed in 1999 that compared with placebo, neither DHEA nor androstenedione was associated with a statistically significant increase in lean body mass, strength or testosterone levels. Since DHEA also disturbs the testosterone/epitestosterone ratio, the ability to cheat with the drug seems much reduced (Johnson, 1999). This lack of androstenedione efficacy may be associated with its rapid conversion to oestrogens in peripheral tissues (Wallace *et al.*, 1999).

DHT (5α-dihydrotestosterone)

This compound occurs naturally in males and females as a result of the action of the enzyme 5α-reductase on testosterone (Figure 5.2). DHT is reported to have 2–3 times the androgenic activity of testosterone (Ueki and Okana, 1999) and its production is necessary for normal male sexual development (see Section 5.2). As the 5α-reductase conversion is not readily reversible, the conversion of DHT to oestradiol via the 'aromatase' process is minimal, which therefore minimizes any possible feminizing effects in males, though it increases the likelihood of serious masculinizing side-effects in females (Ueki and Okana, 1999). It is for this reason that the 19-nor derivative of DHT (formed by the action of 5α-reductase on nandrolone) has been suggested as a possible drug of abuse in women, as it has much less androgenic activity than DHT (see below). Despite being promoted in the 1980s 'underground' literature as 'undetectable' doping, DHT abuse does not seem to have been identified until 1993. Following this single case, DHT abuse was detected in 11 Chinese swimmers at the 1994 Asian Games. According to Ueki and Okana (1999), detection is sometimes made more difficult by the simultaneous administration of 'traditional Chinese medicine', though it is unclear whether this is a deliberate attempt at masking drug abuse. DHT is still a licensed drug in some countries. It does not alter the testosterone/epitestosterone ratio but it can be detected by examining the ratio of the urinary concentration of DHT and its 5α-metabolites to non-5α-steroids.

Nandrolone

Nandrolone (Figure 5.2) was introduced as an anabolic steroid in the 1970s. It has structural modifications that allow it to be injected intramuscularly and which also reduce the likelihood of its conversion to oestrogen by aromatase enzymes (Mottram and George, 2000). In addition, nandrolone can be converted by the enzyme 5α-reductase to 'dihydro-19-nor-testosterone' (dihydro-nandrolone) which has even less androgenic activity and is therefore promoted as a potential 'drug of choice' for women athletes. Nandrolone is converted also to the metabolites norandrosterone and noretiocholanone by the same enzyme systems that metabolize testosterone (Figure 5.4) and these components, like their respective testosterone metabolites, may be detected in urine (Kinze *et al.*, 1999). The current controversy surrounding nandrolone does not only centre on the drug itself after being banned by the IOC in 1976, but on the possibility that it could be formed in the human body, by ingestion of one of its precursors, either deliberately or unintentionally (Mottram and George, 2000). In 1997, the US Drug Enforcement Agency noticed an increase in the importation of so-called nandrolone precursors norandrostenediol and norandrostenedione into the USA. Research showed that this seemed to be coupled to advertisements on the Internet claiming that these two compounds could be converted to nandrolone in humans (Ferstle, 1999a). In theory it should be possible to convert norandrostenedione to 19-nortestosterone (nandrolone) in humans (see Figure 5.2) and this has only recently been established (Wright *et al.*, 2000). As interest in nandrolone increased and even more sensitive analytical techniques appeared in the late 1990s, a new, short-acting, orally active form of nandrolone, nandrolone sulphate, was introduced. Suddenly, several high-profile nandrolone-positive test results appeared in the press involving the British Olympic Gold medallist Linford Christie, and the UK 400 m athlete Dougie Walker.

By the mid-1990s, it had been observed that the nandrolone metabolites norandosterone and noretiocholanone could be detected in the urine of previously drug-free monkeys (Ferstle, 1999b). Also the progestogen, norethisterone, an ingredient of some oral contraceptives, was shown to increase levels of nandrolone metabolites in urine and it has also been shown that the urinary concentration of norandrosterone and noretiocholanone increases in some pregnant women. Based on this and other analytical evidence the IOC set urinary concentration limits for nandrolone metabolites at 2 ng/ml for men and 5 ng/ml for women.

Several questions arise from this controversial era of abuse testing and regulation. Since testing for nandrolone abuse either from direct administration or from precursors depends on the detection of nandrolone metabolites, are the IOC threshold levels correct? The answer to this is not clear. Nandrolone metabolites are found in urine from previously drug-free human males at a concentration below the 2 ng/ml IOC threshold (Dehennin *et al.*, 1999). Evidence that this is a truly endogenous production comes from the demonstration that nandrolone metabolite levels in male urine can be increased following an injection of hCG which stimulates androgen release from the testis (Reznik *et al.*, 2001). However, in 1999 LeBizec *et al.* found that while nandrolone concentrations in half of the 40 samples they tested ranged from 0.05–0.6 ng/ml, these values could be increased by a factor of 2–4 after prolonged intense exercise. Recent research by Schmitt *et al.* (2002) has demonstrated that exhaustive exercise does not increase the excretion of nandrolone. Could nandrolone and its metabolites be formed in humans in other ways?

There was evidence in the 1980s that methosterone could be converted to a nandrolone metabolite (Ferstle, 1999a). Other studies have shown that pregnant women may produce increased amounts of the metabolites because of the action of hCG on the ovary. We know that hCG can stimulate production of nandrolone metabolites, but this may merely confirm that it is hCG that is being abused! (Reznik *et al.*, 2001). Other doubts concern the claim that some vitamin and food supplements may contain trace amounts of the nandrolone precursors norandrostenedione and norandronstenediol, which are metabolized to nandrolone and then to its metabolites, thus producing a positive, super-threshold test result. To test this explanation Catlin *et al.* (2000) administered trace amounts of androstenedione or 19-norandrostenedione to 41 healthy men. Twenty of the 24 men receiving androstenedione yielded urine samples containing norandrosterone at a concentration above the IOC limit. Some evidence of impurities and or norandrostenedione was found in the OTC samples.

In October 2000, the IOC commissioned the Institute of Biochemistry in Cologne to investigate nutritional supplementation in sport. A total of 634 non-hormonal nutritional supplements obtained from most EU countries and from the USA were examined and analysed. Twenty-three samples (24.5 per cent) contained precursors of nandrolone *and* testosterone, 64 samples (68.1 per cent) contained precursors of testosterone, while 7 samples contained nandrolone precursors only (Schänzer, 2002). Sample products that tested positive for anabolic steroid precursors originated from The Netherlands (25.8 per cent), Austria (22.7 per cent), the UK (18.9 per cent) and the USA (18.8 per cent). Analysis of the positive samples yielded anabolic steroid precursor concentrations of 0.01–190 µg/g (Schänzer, 2002). When positive-testing supplements were administered so that the total androgen intake exceeded 1 µg, the urine samples of the volunteers contained anabolic steroid levels in excess of IOC regulations. This has led to proposals for nutritional supplements to be controlled by the IOC.

We can summarize that

• nandrolone metabolites and possibly nandrolone are produced naturally in human males and females;
• norandrosterone and norandrostenedione can be converted in humans to nandrolone metabolites (via nandrolone); and
• the 2 ng cut off for nandrolone metabolites in the IOC test is fair but more studies need to be done on the effect of prolonged exercise on nandrolone secretion and the urinary concentration of nandrolone metabolites.

The questions still remain: why *should* exercise increase endogenous nandrolone (metabolite) production and why *are* there nandrolone precursors in some dietary supplements?

5.8   Anabolic steroid side-effects with particular reference to athletes

In the introductory section, the general side-effects of anabolic steroids were discussed. Of these side-effects some are of particular significance to athletes taking steroids, namely cardiovascular side-effects since exercise imposes a particular stress on the cardiovascular systems, and hepatic side-effects because anabolic steroids, particularly those with C-17 alkyl substituents are suspected hepatic carcinogens in the doses in which they are taken by athletes.

Cardiovascular

Blood volume

Rockhold (1993) has examined nine studies on the effect of anabolic steroids on blood volume. Eight of these studies were carried out on non-athletes and produced variable results. Some studies showed increases in blood volume while others demonstrated no change. In the single study carried out in athletes a 15 per cent increase in total blood volume in athletes taking methandienone was recorded. This study did not measure haematocrit and so any effect of the steroid on erythropoiesis could not be determined.

Salt and water retention

In the previous section, the effect of anabolic steroids on salt and water retention was discussed in relation to steroid-induced gains in body weight and muscle circumference. The increase in salt and water retention responsible for these changes has a deleterious effect on the cardiovascular system. Thus, the increased blood sodium concentration causes a rise in blood osmotic pressure. Since sodium ions cannot diffuse into cells, they remain in the extracellular fluid and blood unless excreted by the kidney, thus raising osmotic pressure and withdrawing water from the tissues. An expansion of the blood volume then occurs which imposes an increased workload on the heart. The heart increases its output and the blood pressure rises. The increased sodium concentration may also directly stimulate vasoconstriction, thus enhancing the hypertensive effect of the increased blood volume.

Hypertension

An increased incidence of potentially fatal hypertension in athletes on anabolic steroids is frequently mentioned in early reviews of anabolic steroid abuse in sport (Wright, 1980; Goldman, 1984). According to Rockhold (1993), the evidence for this is equivocal. He mentions three studies, two in athletes, one in healthy men, in which administration of either testosterone or oxandrolone for three months failed to cause an increase in blood pressure. An earlier study by Holma (1979) found a 15 per cent increase in blood volume in men taking methandienone but no increase in blood pressure. However, Kuipers *et al.* (1991) found mean increases in blood pressure of 12 mmHg in athletes self-administering various anabolic steroids. In a second double-blind study, using only nandrolone decanoate, no increase in blood pressure could be detected. The association between blood pressure and anabolic steroid abuse warrants further careful investigation, particularly in relation to the suggestion by Rockhold (1993) that an increased hypertensive effect might be associated with specific types of anabolic steroid molecule.

Ventricular function

Studies in animals on the effect of anabolic steroids on ventricular function and morphology have indicated an association between steroids and ventricular pathology which may have significance for humans (Lombardo *et al.*, 1991), particularly as the autopsy of an American footballer who was abusing anabolic steroids revealed significant cardiomyopathy. The technique of echocardiography has revolutionized non-invasive investigation of cardiac function and allows clinicians to measure accurately the dimensions of the ventricles during exercise and at rest at each stage of the cardiac cycle. A survey of six studies of ventricular function in athletes from different disciplines abusing anabolic steroids has been conducted by Rockhold (1993). The overall conclusion was that in intensely training athletes steroid administration induced left ventricular thickening, increases in end diastolic volume and relaxation index. Deligiannis and Mandroukas (1992) have shown that such changes occur in relation to increases in skeletal muscle mass. Nieminen *et al.* (1996) have reported similar cardiopathology in four young weightlifters with cardiac hypertrophy. Two patients additionally had symptoms of heart failure and one of these had a massive thrombosis in both ventricles. It should be noted that all the above studies were carried out in weightlifters and so may not be relevant to all athletes and it is interesting that while endurance athletes have a significantly greater life expectancy than non-athletes, this advantage is not shared by power athletes (Pärssinen and Seppälä, 2002). The fact that, so far, only isolated cases of cardiomyopathy have occurred in athletes abusing steroids should serve as a warning rather than a comfort.

Effects on blood lipids and lipoproteins

Anabolic steroids have important effects on the plasma levels of triglycerides, cholesterol and lipoproteins. Lipoproteins are large molecular conglomerates of lipids and specialized proteins called apolipoproteins. Their presence in the blood is to carry water-insoluble lipids from their site of production to tissues where they are utilized or stored. Anabolic steroids have been shown to increase blood triglyceride and cholesterol levels. They decrease the blood levels of high-density lipoprotein (HDL), especially the HDL_2 and HDL_3 fractions, while increasing the level of low-density lipoprotein (LDL). In addition, there is a significant rise in the ratio of free cholesterol to HDL-bound cholesterol following anabolic steroid administration, though the effect is less pronounced with testosterone (Alén and Rahkila, 1988). These changes appear to be induced by an action of anabolic steroids on key liver enzymes such as lipoprotein lipase and hepatic lipase associated with lipoprotein metabolism. Several studies, especially the widely quoted Framingham study in the USA, have shown that a reduction of just 10 per cent in the blood concentration of HDL could increase the chances of coronary disease by 25 per cent. A more recent study by Costill et al. (1984) has shown that in athletes taking anabolic steroids, HDL fell by 20 per cent after only 102 days of treatment, while cholesterol concentration was unchanged; while Rockhold (1993) reports even greater percentage reductions, i.e. HDL down 52 per cent, HDLb down 78 per cent. In normal males 22 per cent of cholesterol is in the form of HDL while in steroid takers only 7.8 per cent of cholesterol is found combined in this way.

There is wide agreement that anabolic steroids cause a reduction in the serum HDL cholesterol (Alén and Rahkila, 1988) and that this phenomenon is particularly associated with the abuse of orally administered steroids (Lombardo et al., 1991). At least two recent reviews of the literature concluded that this effect of HDL is reversible, i.e. HDL levels return to normal within 3–5 weeks of cessation of steroid administration (Lukas, 1993; Rockhold, 1993). A controlled study by Millar (1994) in which moderate doses of anabolic steroids were administered by physicians (140 mg per week of methenoline acetate) reported decreases in HDL and an increase in total cholesterol levels, which returned to normal 6–12 weeks after the end of dosage.

These reductions in HDL levels have been associated with increased incidence of cardiovascular disease (Alén and Rahkila, 1988; Wagner, 1991) in the general population. Low serum HDL is recognized as a risk factor for cardiac and cerebrovascular disease (Wagner, 1991). There are several well documented cases of coronary heart disease (CHD) in apparently fit, healthy athletes aged under 40, who have been taking anabolic steroids (Goldman, 1984). However, according to Lukas (1993), only one case of an athlete dying of coronary heart disease while abusing anabolic steroids had been reported up to 1992. It could be interpreted that low serum HDL is not a significant risk factor for steroid abusers, but it is also possible that such individuals may be fitter than the rest of the population so that any pathological changes are delayed. Street et al. (1996) in their review of anabolic steroid side-effects produced a table of individual cases of serious medical conditions associated with anabolic steroid abuse quoted in medical journals. Although, again, there was only one death due to myocardial infarction, there were several 'near misses' including five myocardial infarctions, one stroke, two cases of pulmonary embolism and one cerebral venous thrombosis. The statistics are also complicated by the different drug administration regimes used by abusers and complications arising from other risk factors such as smoking. This subject requires intensive long-term study.

Blood clotting

The increased risk of coronary and cerebrovascular disease in anabolic steroid abusers has prompted some physicians to consider whether there is increased risk of platelet aggregation leading to increased blood clot formation. Animal studies suggest that there is such a relationship, but so far there is only one report of an athlete taking steroids dying of a stroke (Lombardo *et al.*, 1991), though Street *et al.* (1996) quote three cases of near deaths from pulmonary embolism and one venous thrombosis. However, there is an association between increased platelet aggregation and age in weightlifters taking steroids (Lukas, 1993).

Carcinomas

The association between anabolic steroid administration and tumour formation, particularly of the liver and kidney, is now firmly established. Significant changes in liver biochemistry have been found in 80 per cent of otherwise healthy athletes taking anabolic steroids but without any signs of liver disease. In 1965, a detailed case study was published linking the death of an anabolic steroid-taking athlete with hepatocellular cancer (HC). Since then 13 other athletes taking anabolic steroids have been demonstrated to have HC and all were taking 17-alkylated androgens. A second more insidious liver pathology, petiocis hepatis was associated with anabolic steroids in 1977 (Goldman, 1984). In this disorder hepatic tissue degenerates and is replaced by blood-filled spaces.

Anabolic steroids have also been suspected of causing death from Wilm's Tumour of the kidney in at least two adult athletes (Pärssinen and Seppälä, 2002). The tumour is very rare in post-adolescent individuals. Surprisingly, in their survey of serious reported anabolic steroid side-effects, Street *et al.* (1996) could find only one case of prostate carcinoma. Three large case–controlled studies have found a much stronger though not unequivocal link between raised anabolic steroid levels and prostate cancer. In all three investigations, testosterone was associated significantly with an increased risk of prostate carcinoma (Pärssinen and Seppälä, 2002).

Sex-related side-effects

Fertility

In the introduction it was noted that spermatogenesis in human males is under the control of gonadotrophins and testosterone. Administration of anabolic steroids caused inhibition of gonadotrophin secretion followed by inhibition of testosterone. Holma (1979) administered 15 mg of methandienone to 15 well-trained athletes for 2 months. During the administration period sperm counts fell by 73 per cent and in three individuals azoospermia (complete absence of sperm) was present. In those individuals with sperm present in their sample there was a 10 per cent increase in the number of immotile sperm and 30 per cent decrease in the number of motile sperm. Thus fertility was severely reduced in males in this study, which provides confirmation of many clinical reports of the same phenomena. However, many of these effects were shown to be reversible. Though it is obviously unethical to test this, some clinical data suggest that long-term anabolic steroid-induced infertility might be permanent, though in their review of published work up to 1995, Street *et al.* (1996) found no evidence of long-term effects in fertility on young males given anabolic steroids to suppress excessive growth.

Effects on libido

The suppression of testosterone secretion in both males and females may well have effects on libido. As previously discussed, libido in males and females is thought to be influenced, at least in part, by testosterone. Thus, high levels of anabolic steroids in the blood suppress testosterone secretion and reduce libido. However, Yates *et al.* (1999) using doses of testosterone up to 500 mg per week could find no significant changes in male libido during a 14-week administration period.

Gynaecomastia

This is a paradoxical condition occurring in athletes attempting to increase their muscle mass, as it involves the development of mammary tissue. The most common cause of this condition in anabolic steroid abusers is that the agent they are administering is converted by liver aromatase enzymes (see Figure 5.2) to oestradiol, which then induces development of mammary tissue. Thus athletes who abuse anabolic steroids or testosterone (or hCG which releases testosterone) are at risk from developing gynaecomastia (Friedl and Yesalis, 1989). It is widely assumed by steroid abusers that use of an anabolic steroid which cannot be aromatized to oestradiol will reduce the incidence of gynaecomastia, but there is no evidence for this. Concurrent administration of the anti-oestrogen, tamoxifen, is thought by many abusers in both the US and Britain to be an effective antidote to gynaecomastia induced by steroids (Perry *et al.*, 1992). Though it is sometimes effective in reducing the pain associated with this condition, tamoxifen seems to have little effect on the size of breast tissue in steroid abusers (Friedl and Yesalis, 1989).

Specific actions in female athletes

Considering the side-effects mentioned in the introduction, people often wonder why female athletes should take anabolic steroids. The simple answer is that women's athletics is now as competitive as men's and that, according to some reports, the effects of anabolic steroids on muscle strength and bulk in a female athlete are considerably greater than in men. This has been explained by the lower normal circulating level of testosterone in females compared with men. Thus some female athletes take anabolic steroids in the knowledge that they may produce greater muscle strength and bulk at the expense of irreversible change, such as deepening of the voice and clitoral enlargement.

In 1996, Korkia interviewed 15 female body builders who admitted to anabolic steroid abuse, nine of whom reported deepening of the voice, eight to menstrual problems and seven to clitoral enlargement. Three complained of reduction in breast size, while the other side-effects mentioned were similar to males. Side-effects such as menstrual problems are not necessarily indicative of anabolic steroid abuse as regular intense endurance exercise is known to induce amenorrhoea as discussed by Warren and Shantha (2000).

Pricilla Choi (1998) described the case of a female bodybuilder who, as a result of chronic anabolic steroid abuse, became permanently masculinized and 8 years after cessation of anabolic steroid abuse, her enlarged clitoris and her deep voice remained and she appeared to be suffering psychologically from a gender identity crisis.

Tendon damage

Several researchers have noted the increased incidence of tendon damage in athletes taking anabolic steroids. A summary of the various tendon pathologies associated with anabolic steroid abuse has been provided by Laseter and Russell (1991). These include the quadriceps and rectus femoris tendons and the triceps; the four cases all involved powerlifters. This phenomenon has been explained in at least three different ways. First, that the increase in muscle strength acquired by a course of steroids, plus training, produces a greater increase in muscle power than in tendon strength since tendons respond slowly to strength regimes and anabolic steroids have little or no effect on tendon strength. Second, it is thought that anabolic steroids have, in common with corticosteroids (such as cortisol), the ability to inhibit the formation of collagen, an important constituent of tendons and ligaments. Third, anabolic steroids appear to induce changes in the arrangement and contractility of collagen fibrils in tendons, leading to critical alterations in physical properties known as the 'crimp angle'. The overall effect is to reduce the plasticity of the tendons. It should be pointed out that tendon ruptures also occur in athletes not abusing steroids. Weightlifters taking anabolic steroids appear to be particularly prone to muscle and tendon injuries. This has been explained by apologists for anabolic steroid abusers as evidence of greater weights being lifted. Sports doctors say it is the biochemical effects of anabolic steroids previously discussed, while other say that the increased aggressiveness and competitiveness induced by anabolic steroid administration causes athletes to attempt more and greater lifts with an increasingly reckless attitude to the actual mechanics of the lifting.

Glucose regulation

Anabolic steroid abuse has been shown to reduce glucose tolerance and increase insulin resistance. This could lead to the induction of type II diabetes (Cohen and Hickman, 1987). However, in this study, the glucose tolerance was still within normal limits.

Hobbs *et al.* (1996) found that testosterone at 300 mg per week had little effect on glucose uptake from the plasma, while the same dose of nandrolone enhanced glucose removal from the plasma. These differences were ascribed to the ability of testosterone to undergo aromatization to an oestrogen. This may be an important consideration in relation to other side-effects of anabolic steroids.

Immunological effects

Transient decreases in immunoglobulin IgA and IgG have been reported during steroid use.

Behavioural effects and addiction

Since the late 1940s it has been known that anabolic steroids have important influences on behaviour, but these have usually been acknowledged to be the stimulatory effects which anabolic steroids have on libido in both males and females (Greenblatt *et al.*, 1985). There is no evidence that troops of the Nazi Waffen-SS regiments were given anabolic steroids to increase aggressiveness before battle (Yesalis *et al.*, 2000). Studies in the 1980s have suggested that anabolic steroids have reduced the depression symptoms in a number of groups of depressed patients (Williamson and Young, 1992). Research by Alder *et al.* (1986) has shown that some women suffering from post-natal depression had abnormally low testosterone levels. It is surprising, given the frequency of anecdotal reports from athletes using steroids that they experienced euphoria, general feelings of well-being, increased confidence, self-esteem, libido and energy, that until the late 1980s little systematic research into the behavioural effects of anabolic steroids had been carried out. A review by Kashkin and Kleber (1989) cites many documented cases of increased aggression and violent behaviour, many of them reported by the abusers themselves. The same authors also report detailed cases of mild to severe psychiatric disturbances occurring in those abusing anabolic steroids ranging from impaired judgement, insomnia and agitation to panic attacks, grandiose ideas and paranoid delusions. Pope and Katz (1988) interviewed 41 body builders and football players who had used anabolic steroids. Nine of these fulfilled the DSMIIIR criteria for mood disorder and five displayed psychotic symptoms associated with steroid use. Williamson and Young (1992) describe several cases of manic episodes in athletes taking anabolic steroids. In a number of instances depressed steroid abusers attempting to withdraw from steroid administration became manic when treated with antidepressant drugs. Since the mid-1980s, there have been increasing reports of abusers maintaining steroid administration despite repeated attempts to stop them. There are similar reports in the literature of patients on high glucocorticoid doses being unable to stop their medication. Kashkin and Kleber (1989) also produce evidence of withdrawal symptoms in some individuals who stop taking steroids and cited several studies where steroid withdrawal had resulted in clinical depression. In a sample of men who stopped taking steroids, 12.2 per cent were diagnosed as depressed within 3 months of abstinence. Does anabolic steroid abuse lead to an increased risk of suicide? An examination of eight cases of suicide in anabolic steroid abusers by Thiblin *et al.* (2000) showed that depressive symptoms arising *after* anabolic steroid withdrawal were associated with suicide in five cases, while in the remainder depression during anabolic steroid abuse was implicated. Anabolic steroid abuse also appears to increase the risk of being murdered, as 9 of the 34 deaths among anabolic abusers quoted by Pärssinen and Seppälä (2002) had been the victims of homicide. In Britain the suicide of a Royal Marine guardsman taking anabolic steroids was reported (*Guardian*, 1994). These findings suggest that all anabolic steroid abusers who abstain should be carefully followed up.

There are a number of reports of steroid cravings associated with increased sympathetic nervous system activity in some abusers who attempt to refrain from anabolic steroids. There is also widespread fear, real and imaginary, of what I call 'muscle melt down', in those considering or attempting to withdraw from steroid abuse. This appears from the literature to involve feelings of loss of esteem, both social and sexual, if the well-developed torso is seen to 'melt away' after steroid withdrawal. Kashkin and Kleber consider that all the clinical evidence so far suggests the existence of a 'sex steroid hormone dependence disorder' which obeys the following established criteria for addiction:

1. The hormones are used over longer periods than desired.
2. Attempts are made to stop without success.
3. Substantial time is spent obtaining, using or recovering from the hormones.
4. Use continues despite acknowledgement of the significant psychological and toxicological problems caused by the hormones.
5. Characteristic withdrawal symptoms occur.
6. Hormones (or their supplements) are taken to relieve the withdrawal symptoms.

The evidence assembled by Kashkin and Kleber (1989) and Williamson and Young (1992) is substantial and convincing, but as Lukas (1993) has emphasized, the majority of athletes and body builders do not report major psychiatric symptoms, or perhaps refrain from doing so. It is interesting to note that, up to 2001, there is only one documented case of a female abuser of anabolic steroids suffering from dependency (Copeland *et al.*, 1998).

Why does dependency occur, and only in some abusers? To answer this question Kirk Brower (2000) has summarized the theoretical biochemical and physiological and psychological factors that he thinks may influence the development of dependency. He has divided these into:

1. Positive reinforcement mechanisms involving brain centres that mediate sexual function and pleasure including central opioid and dopaminergic systems, which are reinforced by
2. Muscular development giving rise to psychological, social and vocational benefits. There are then in parallel:
3. Negative reinforcement mechanisms – avoidance of depressive and other withdrawal symptoms which may be biologically mediated via testosterone deficiency or reduced activity of the opioid and/or dopaminergic sytems in the brain coupled with
4. Psychosocially mediated mechanisms – as a psychological response to loss of muscle and loss of social/vocational rewards.

One of the major reasons proposed by steroid abusers for the use of these drugs in their sport is that it increases their aggression. A number of studies have failed to find any relationship between endogenous testosterone levels and aggression (Archer, 1991) and a review of studies of aggression and hostility comparing anabolic steroid with placebo in several groups of athletes revealed both positive and equivocal results (Williamson and Young, 1992). It would be interesting to know whether increased aggression *is* required in the successful sportsperson and how far this differs from that found in the unsuccessful or non-athletic population. Behavioural factors in sport are discussed in a comprehensive review by Raglin (2001). When anger scores were compared between successful and non-successful qualifiers for the 1976 US Olympic wrestling team, the highest scores occurred in those selected, suggesting that anger may be a positive feature of wrestling but not necessarily in other sports.

Pope and Katz (1994) showed that anabolic steroid abuse was associated with increased incidence of recklessness and aggressiveness. Anecdotal reports from women published in magazines and also a number of criminal cases involving evidence of male anabolic steroid abusers towards female parties prompted Choi and Pope (1994) to examine whether anabolic steroids increased the likelihood of violent behaviour of abusers towards women. They found a significant increase in fighting behaviour, verbal aggression and violence inflicted on females by their steroid-abusing partners compared with either non-abusers or when the abusers were not taking anabolic steroids. However, Yates *et al.* (1999) could detect no increases in hostility (as measured by a rating scale) in male volunteers administered with testosterone in randomized doses of 100–500 mg for 14 weeks. The same study showed there were insignificant effects of anabolic steroids on mood, libido and sexual interest. The doses here were, however, well below those normally administered by many anabolic steroid abusers.

Perhaps the most disturbing reports of all are those linking anabolic steroids with serious crime, including murder. Lubell (1989) has documented three cases of murder where anabolic steroids were cited by the defence as the causes of their clients' behaviour, and one case in Florida where the defence (unsuccessfully) entered a plea of 'not guilty by reason of insanity' for a client who committed murder while abusing anabolic steroids. The effects of anabolic steroids on behaviour and their association with psychiatric illness and criminality appear strong, but most studies reviewed here have not demonstrated clear or quantitative relationships and none has been prospective. It is therefore impossible to know the personality or even the psychiatric profile of the person *before* they began abusing steroids. It is possible that body builders and even some athletes may have psychological problems, abnormal personalities or personality disorders before they begin steroid abuse. Thus body builders may suffer from body dysmorphic syndromes (feelings that their body size/shape is inadequate). Harrison Pope's research group (1997) think they can identify a 'muscle dysmorphic syndrome' in which affected individuals become 'pathologically pre-occupied with their degree of muscularity'. This new syndrome does not fit the accepted criteria in DSM IV (American Psychiatric Association, 1994) for body dysmorphic disorder as it involves dissatisfaction with the whole body rather than a particular structure or part. It is also unclear whether some of the symptoms described are delusional, but there does seem to be some commonality with eating disorders and some types of anxiety. Athletes may also form obsessional/perfectionist desires to be the best at all costs. John Porcerelli and Bruce Sandler (1995) have started to investigate this by attempting to construct a psychological profile of anabolic steroid users. They were particularly interested in narcissistic personality traits in anabolic steroid abusers and compared 26 steroid-abusing and 16 non-abusing weightlifters. They found significantly higher narcissism scores and lower empathy scores amongst anabolic steroid abusers, but could not detect whether these abnormalities of personality were present before abuse took place. It was unclear whether personality disorder which would meet DSM IV criteria was present among the abusers.

We also know very little about the cultural, social and psychological influences which affect both the developing and the adult athlete and also which of these influences may lead to psychiatric disturbance and/or drug abuse. In 1992, David Begel reviewed the most recent research in sport psychiatry and concluded that the close relationship between mental and physical phenomena in sport may account for the psychiatric problems associated with poor performance. John Raglin's recent (2001) review has suggested that the psychological profile of unsuccessful athletes is not significantly different from the normal population. Among American athletes a decrease in athletic performance is termed 'slump'. It would be interesting to know what the relationship was between 'slump' and anabolic steroid taking and whether abuse of the drugs was associated with attempts to pre-empt it.

A detailed and highly perceptive review of the social factors leading to anabolic steroid abuse and its increased prevalence has been carried out by Anna Wroblewska (1997). She noted the influence of cultural icons, i.e. the change in the appearance of Hollywood heroes from the simply tall and athletic to the lean, tall, wide-shouldered, muscular torso of the present day. The body dimensions of the 'Action Man' toy have changed also from tall and athletic to broad-shouldered, tall and lean – and steroidal! Her review concludes that the relationship between anabolic steroid abuse in athletes and non-athletes is complex and is driven by numerous factors relating to athletic success and social success to self-perception of body dimensions and potential attractiveness. She has hypothesized that the lure of 'winning (be it a race or an attractive partner) is very powerful at any age and especially so in adolescence and young men'. As an aside she notes that 'research into appearance anxiety is mainly focused on women' and presumably should include both sexes.

Michael Bahrke (2000) has summarized the current evidence for anabolic steroid-induced behavioural change and psychiatric disorder. He states that because a steroid user feels more aggressive and self-reports more aggression, it does not mean that he/she is going to behave violently or develop a mental disorder. His review also emphasizes that only a small percentage of anabolic steroid users appear to experience symptoms of mental illness. Of those that do, the majority recover without relapse when the anabolic steroids are withdrawn. It appears from this review that many methodological issues concerning this type of research need to be resolved, including sample size, dose and method of assessment.

The association between anabolic steroid abuse and all aspects of behaviour, personality and psychiatric disorder, in sport, should be the subject of continuing and further careful study.

Long-term risks of anabolic steroid abuse

Exactly how long the Anabolic Steroid Sorcerer has cast his spell (or curse) is unknown, but if 50 years is a reasonable estimate then we should now be investigating or realizing the long-term effects of their abuse. Mortality studies are notoriously difficult to control and in the case of anabolic steroid abuse the confirmation of abuse and its intensity is difficult to verify. A study of 62 elite powerlifters in Finland emphasizes the apparent long-term effects of anabolic steroid abuse. These athletes were the prizewinners in the Finnish championships (1977–1982) and were followed up for 12 years and compared with a control population. Premature death was 4.6 times higher in the powerlifters than in the control population (Pärssinen et al., 2000). As powerlifting does not itself cause an increase in mortality, the increase in mortality in this group was ascribed to anabolic steroid abuse (Pärssinen and Seppälä, 2002).

Indirect consequences of anabolic steroid abuse

Many of the surveys quoted (Pope et al., 1988; Lamb, 1991; Perry et al., 1992) suggest that abuse of orally active steroids is declining in favour of the injectable varieties. This may be due to better awareness of the toxicity of the oral compounds or to the supposedly lower risk of detection with injectable compounds once treatment is stopped. It is surely no coincidence that this switch appears to be associated with the appearance of HIV among steroid abusers, the first case of which was reported in the USA 18 years ago (Sklarek et al., 1984). There have been several further cases reported subsequently in body builders in the USA (Yesalis et al., 1988). The potential for the spread of HIV by this route in Great Britain has been highlighted by Perry et al. (1992) who reported high-risk behaviour, i.e. needle sharing and drug sample sharing, with all the attendant risks of cross-contamination of drug supplies and abusers' blood in their sample of body builders in Swansea.

Other related high-risk behaviour such as abuse of other more dangerous drugs, drink-driving, reckless driving behaviour and high-risk sexual activity have been catalogued in anabolic steroid abusers by Middleman and DuRant (1996).

Another unforeseen consequence of anabolic steroid abuse by injection is tissue and organ damage caused by inexperienced and untrained injectors. There are several anecdotal cases reported to me by local GPs of 'steroid limp'. This condition is characterized by the patient who can only raise his affected leg to walk by using his abdominal adductor muscles. It is caused by damage to the sciatic nerve by injection of anabolic steroids in the buttocks either into or close to the sciatic nerve resulting usually in permanent neuromuscular impairment.

5.9 Educational and social aspects

Though the number of positive steroid tests at Olympic events appear to be static, the high level of anabolic steroid usage by body builders and weightlifters and the disturbing level of abuse by the young in the USA and Britain shows that much remains to be done to counteract the anabolic steroid problem. The imposition of mandatory testing while possibly contributing to the decline in anabolic steroid usage in top class athletes will have little influence on the school or college abuser. In the USA mandatory testing measures have been introduced at school and college level resulting in a number of positive tests (Leach, 1993). How can the abuse be combated and how should the abuser be treated? It seems that we must first understand who is abusing and why. Though it cannot be condoned, it is easy to understand why athletes are tempted to cheat in order to run faster or throw further, particularly with the substantial financial rewards that go with winning. It is less easy to understand why athletes will risk disqualification and gamble on their own health to achieve this. European soccer appeared to be steroid free until the detection of anabolic steroid abuse by Dutch soccer players in 2001, including the ex-Manchester United player Jaap Stam. Perhaps it is the potential loss of all this, consequent on being tested positive, which is a disincentive. The abuse of anabolic steroids by body builders and others for cosmetic reasons is also difficult to understand, especially when they are well acquainted with the long- and short-term side-effects and have even expressed concern about them recently (Yesalis *et al.*, 1988).

In the USA the problem has been tackled by utilizing education programmes in colleges, schools and gymnasia and encouraging medical practitioners to adopt a sympathetic attitude to steroid abusers, particularly by advising on and treating side-effects of anabolic steroids (Frankle and Leffers, 1992). Central to this has been a planned intervention for abusers proposed by Frankle and Leffers (1992) including psychiatric intervention, group education at gyms, schools and colleges, drug testing for competitive athletes at all levels and a problem-related counselling approach emphasizing the relationship between steroid use and side-effects. They concluded that legal restraints on anabolic steroid supply are necessary, but more stringent legislation should be kept in the background. A similar approach has been adopted in the UK. Perry *et al.* (1992) have described a local project in West Glamorgan in which powerlifters in private gymnasia have been counselled, in order to prevent the spread of HIV by the sharing of contaminated drug samples and infected needles. They also advocate a sympathetic approach by GPs involving counselling, advice and support, the option of routine health checks and the admission of steroid abusers to needle-exchange schemes. An enlightened and thoughtful local scheme for education about, and the containment of, the anabolic steroid problem in the Durham area of North-East England has been described by Dawson (2001). This project's aim was risk awareness and harm minimization rather than stricture. It was found that 60 per cent of participants in the local needle-exchange scheme were anabolic steroid abusers rather than heroin addicts! It was discovered that people seeking help from the scheme were in four major categories:

1. Sport performance enhancers.
2. Those absorbed recently into 'gym' culture.
3. Occupational users, club door-men, police, prison warders.
4. Cosmetic users.

This service provides direct contact between doctors and patients/abusers allowing the communication of non-judgemental advice on harm reduction, e.g. moving towards less toxic/damaging drug forms and eventually away from anabolic steroids altogether. How successful this has been we do not know, but it may be a way forward, in particular if it invokes improved trust between physician and abuser and at last includes recognition by local and governmental authorities that there is a joint problem that we can solve together.

Have the education schemes worked? The answer appears to be a rather dejected 'no' from Yesalis and Bahrke (2000) in their review of adolescent anabolic steroid abuse. They conclude emphatically that 'scare tactics' have no role in persuading youth not to abuse steroids. When 3–12 per cent of adolescent US males continue to abuse steroids (Yesalis *et al.*, 2000) any complacency is misplaced. They feel targeting social influences may be more beneficial. Some support for this comes from the report by Goldberg *et al.* (2000) on the effectiveness of the 'Adolescents training and learning to avoid steroids programme' in the USA. Though at the end of the first year of the programme anabolic steroid abuse had not fallen significantly in the 3207 adolescent athletes surveyed, there were reductions in the abuse of alcohol, amphetamines and use of supplements, indicating that progress could be made here using sex-specific, team-centred education. The continuing mean prevalence of anabolic steroid abuse of 1.1 per cent in the US adolescent athletic population indicates that there is much still to be done. According to the survey by Faigenbaum *et al.* (1998) 54 per cent of US high school students who abused anabolic steroids knew they were harmful. With the age of first use being as low as 12–13 years in some studies (Yesalis and Bahrke, 2000) it is obvious that these educational programmes must start at a very early age. Many longitudinal studies are now active in the USA to study trends in drug abuse, including the MTF (monitoring the future) study, the Youth Risk and Behavior Surveillance System (YRBSS) and the National Household Survey on Drug Abuse (NHSDA), and their techniques and reports have been analysed by Yesalis *et al.* (2000). It is hoped that the information they gather may be used to plan future strategies.

Anabolic steroids were reclassified as controlled drugs in Great Britain in 1994, but this may not be the answer to the UK problem (Dawson, 2001). A sensible compromise might be the compulsory licensing of all local authority leisure centres and private gymnasia. The worrying trend of increasing anabolic steroid abuse in schools and colleges in the USA has been noted (Buckley *et al.*, 1988; Pope *et al.*, 1988; Yesalis and Bahrke, 2000), but until the 1990s has been unrecognized in Great Britain. The survey in Scotland by Williamson (1993) emphasized that such complacency was misplaced as 56 per cent of those admitting to steroid abuse began doing so when 17 or younger. It was also important that this survey identified a significant number (50 per cent) who were regular rugby union players, athletes who were previously 'not usually recognized' as steroid abusers. The 1998 survey of secondary age school children in Sefton, Merseyside, quoted by Dawson (2001), revealed 6.4 per cent of boys and 1.3 per cent of girls had been *offered* anabolic steroids. More studies in Great Britain need to be carried out and an immediate intensive education programme centred on schools and colleges should be instigated.

Perhaps also, exercise scientists should be prepared to take the lead and adopt a more high-profile role in the fight against drug abuse in sport as suggested by Kuipers (2001). Doctors and members of the paramedical professions are also sometimes placed in an invidious position: knowing that a patient is a sports cheat and yet bound to do their utmost to care for them and maintain confidentiality. This situation is discussed comprehensively in a recent review by the British Medical Association (Conway and Morgan, 2002) and concludes, perhaps understandably, that the doctor's first duty is to his/her patient, not to society or sport!

5.10   The future

Are we wasting our time? Athletes are getting bigger, taller, heavier and so is the general adult population world-wide according to Kevin Norton and Tim Olds (2001). Increasingly, athletes are being selected for size, bigness/tallness equals success and this is mirrored in society as a whole. They state that in some sports where *small* stature is important, this is reducing the pool of talent available. The next trend they suggest is genetic manipulation by direct or eugenic means. Is this the end of steroids? Will the Sorcerer return?

5.11 References

Alder, E.M., Cook, A., Davidson, D., West, C. and Bancroft, J. (1986) Hormones, mood and sexuality in lactating women. *Br. J. Psychiat.*, **148**, 74–79.

Alén, M. and Rahkila, P. (1988) Anabolic-androgenic steroid effects on endocrinology and lipid metabolism in athletes. *Sports Med.*, **6**, 327–332.

American Psychiatric Association (1994) *Diagnostic and Statistical Manual of Mental Disorders*, 4th Edn Revised (DSM IV).

Archer, J. (1991) The influence of testosterone on human aggression. *Br. J. Psychol.*, **82**, 1–28.

Bahrke, M.S. (2000) Psychological effects of endogenous testosterone and anabolic-androgenic steroids. In: Yesalis, C. (ed.), *Anabolic Steroids in Sport and Exercise*, pp. 94–106. Champaign, IL; Human Kinetics Publishers.

Begel, D. (1992) An overview of sport psychiatry. *Am. J. Psychiat.*, **149**, 606–614.

Bhasin, S., Storer, T.W., Berman, N. *et al.* (1996) The effects of supraphysiologic doses of testosterone on muscle size and strength in normal men. *N. Engl. J.Med.*, **335**, 1–7.

Bhasin, S., Woodhouse, L. and Storer, T.W. (2001) Proof of the effect of testosterone on skeletal muscle. *J. Endocrinol.*, **170**, 27–38.

Blazevich, A.J. and Giorgi, A. (2001) Effect of testosterone administration and weight-training on muscle architecture. *Med. Sci. Sport Exerc.*, **33**, 1688–1693.

Brower, K.J. (2000) Anabolic steroids: potential for physical and psychological dependence. In: Yesalis, C. (ed.), *Anabolic Steroids in Sport and Exercise*, pp. 279–304. Champaign, IL; Human Kinetics Publishers.

Buckley, W.E., Yesalis, C.E., Friedl, K.E., Anderson, W.A., Streit, A.L. and Wright, J.E. (1988) Estimated prevalence of anabolic steroid use among male high school seniors. *J. Am. Med. Assoc.*, **260**, 3441–3445.

Burton, C. (1996) Anabolic steroid use among the gym population in Clwyd. *Pharm. J.*, **256**, 557–559.

Catlin, D., Wright, J., Pope, H. and Kiggett, M. (1993) Assessing the threat of anabolic steroids. *Phys. Sports Med.*, **21**, 37–44.

Catlin, D.H., Leder, B.S., Ahrens, B. *et al.* (2000) Trace contamination of over-the-counter androstenedione and positive urine tests results for a nandrolone metabolite. *J. Am. Med. Assoc.*, **284**, 2618–2621.

Choi, P.Y.L. (1998) Illicit anabolic androgenic steroid use in women: a case of pseudohermaphroditism. *J. Perform. Enhanc. Drugs*, **2**, 24–26.

Choi, P.Y.L. and Pope, H.G. (1994) Violence towards women and illicit androgen-anabolic steroid use. *Ann. Clin. Psychiat.*, **6**, 21–25.

Choo, J-J., Horon, M.A., Little, R.A. and Rothwell, N.J. (1992) Clenbuterol and skeletal muscle are mediated by β_2 adrenoceptor activation. *Am. J. Physiol.*, **263**, 50–56.

Cohen, J.C. and Hickman, R. (1987) Insulin resistance and diminished glucose tolerance in powerlifters ingesting anabolic steroids. *J. Clin. Endocrinol. Metab.*, **64**, 960–963.

Conway, L. and Morgan, D. (2002) *Drugs in Sport: The pressure to perform*. London: BMJ Books.

Copeland, J., Peters, R., and Dillon, P. (1998) Anabolic-androgenic steroid dependence in a woman. *Austr. N.Z. J. Psychiat.*, **32**, 589–591.

Costill, D.L., Pearson, D.R. and Fink, W.J. (1984) Anabolic steroid use among athletes. Changes in HDC-C levels. *Phys. Sports Med.*, **12**, 113–117.

Daigle, R.D. (1990) Anabolic steroids. *J. Psychoact. Drugs*, **22**, 77–80.

Dawson, R.T. (2001) Drugs in sport – the role of the physician. *J. Endocrinol.*, **170**, 55–61.

Dehennin, L., Bonnaire, Y. and Plou, P. (1999) Urinary excretion of 19-norandrosterone of endogenous origin in man: quantitative analysis by gas chromatography mass spectrometry. *J. Chromatogr.*, **B721**, 301–307.

Deligiannis, A.P. and Mandroukas, K. (1992) Noninvasive cardiac evaluation of weight-lifters using anabolic steroids. *Scand. J. Med. Sci. Sports*, **3**, 37–40.

DuRant, R.H., Escobedo, L.G. and Heath, G.W. (1995) Anabolic steroid use, strength training and multiple drug use among adolescents in the United States. *Pediatrics*, **96**, 23–28.

Elashoff, J.D., Jacknow, A.D., Shain, S.G. and Braunstein, G.D. (1991) Effects of anabolic-androgenic steroids on muscular strength. *Ann. Int. Med.*, **115**, 387–393.

Elliot, D.I. and Goldberg, I. (2000) Women and anabolic steroids. In: Yesalis, C. (ed.), *Anabolic Steroids in Sport and Exercise*, pp. 225–240. Champaign, IL: Human Kinetics Publishers.

Evans, N.A. (1997) Gym and tonic: a profile of 100 male steroid users. *Br. J. Sports Med.*, **31**, 54–58.

Faigenbaum, A.D., Zaichkewsky, L.D., Gardner, D.E. and Micheli, L.J. (1998) Anabolic Steroid use by male and female middle school students. *Pediatrics*, **101**, 1–6.

Ferstle, J. (1999a) The nandrolone story. *Athletics Weekly*, 15th September, 16.

Ferstle, J. (1999b) Nandrolone Part 2. *Athletics Weekly*, 22nd September, 26–27.

Forbes, G.B. (1985) The effect of anabolic steroids on lean body mass. The dose response curve. *Metabolism*, **34**, 571–573.

Franke, W.N. and Berendonk, B. (1997) Hormonal doping and androgenisation of athletes: a secret program of the German Democratic Republic government. *Clin. Chem.*, **43**, 1262–1297.

Frankle, M. and Leffers, D. (1992) Athletes on anabolic androgenic steroids. *Phys. Sports Med.*, **20**, 75–87.

Freed, D.L.J., Banks, A.J., Longson, D. and Burley, D.M. (1975) Anabolic steroids in athletes: cross-over double blind trial in weightlifters. *Br. Med. J.*, **2**, 471–473.

Friedl, K.E. and Yesalis, C.E. (1989) Self-treatment of gynaecomastia in body builders who use anabolic steroids. *Phys. Sports Med.*, **17**, 67–79.

George, A.J. (1994) Drugs in sport – chemists v cheats – a score draw! *Chem. Rev.*, **4**, 10–14.

George, A.J. (1996) Anabolic steroids. In: Mottram, D.R., (ed.), *Drugs in Sport*, pp. 173–218. London: E. and F.N. Spon.

Goldberg, L., MaKinnon, D.P., Elliot D.L., Moe, E.L., Clarke, G. and Cheong J. (2000) The adolescents training and learning to avoid steroids program – Preventing drug use and promoting health behaviors. *Arch. Ped. Adol. Med.*, **154**, 332–338.

Goldman, B. (1984) *Death in the locker room: Steroids and sports.* London: Century Publishing.

Green, G.A., Uryasz, F.D., Petr, T.A., and Bray, C.D. (2001) NCAA Study of substance use and abuse habits of college student-athletes. *Clin. J. Sport. Med.*, **11**, 51–56.

Greenblatt, R.B., Chaddha, J.S., Teran, A.Z. and Nezhat, C.H. (1985) Aphrodi-
siacs. In: Iverson, S.D. (ed.), *Psychopharmacology: Recent Advances and Future
Prospects.* British Association for Psychopharmacology Monograph No. 6, pp. 290–
302. Oxford: Oxford University Press.

Handelsman, D.J. and Gupta, L. (1997) Prevalence and risk factors for anabolic-
androgenic steroid abuse in Australian high school students. *Int. J. Androl.*, **20**,
159–164.

Haupt, H.A. and Rovere, G.D. (1984) Anabolic steroids: A review of the literature.
Am. J. Sports Med., **12**, 469–484.

Hervey, G.R. (1982) What are the effects of anabolic steroids? In: Davies, B. and
Thomas, G. (eds) *Science and Sporting Performance: Management or Manipulation?* pp. 121–136. Oxford: Oxford University Press.

Hervey, G.R., Knibbs, A.V., Burkinshaw, L. *et al.* (1981) Effects of methandione on
the performance and body composition of man undergoing athletic training. *Clin.
Sci.* **60**, 457–461.

Hobbs, C.J., Jones, R.E. and Plymate, S.R. (1996) Nandrolone, a 19-nortestosterone,
enhances insulin dependent glucose uptake in normal men. *J. Endocrinol. Metab.*,
81, 1582–1585.

Holma, P.K. (1979) Effects of an anabolic steroid (methandienone) on spermatogenesis. *Contraception*, **15**, 151–162.

Johnson, R. (1999) Abnormal testosterone: epitestosterone ratio dehydroepian-
drostenedrine supplements. *Clin. Chem.*, **45**, 163–164.

Kashkin, K.B. and Kleber, H.D. (1989) Hooked on hormones? An anabolic steroid
addiction hypothesis. *J. Am. Med. Assoc.*, **262**, 3166–3170.

Kicman, A.J., Coutts, S.B., Cowan, D.A. *et al.* (1999) Adrenal and gonadal contributions to urinary excretion and plasma concentration of epitestosterone in men –
effect of adrenal stimulation and implications for detection of testosterone abuse.
Clin. Endocrinol., **50**, 661–668.

Kinze, P., Cirimele, V., and Ludes, B. (1999) Norandrosterone et noretiocholanolone:
les métabolites révélateurs. *Acta Clin. Belg.*, **S1999–1**, 68–73.

Korkia, P. (1996) Anabolic steroid use in adolescents. *Sports Exerc. Inj.*, **2**, 136–140.

Korkia, P. and Stimson, G.V. (1997) Indications of prevalence, practice and effects
of anabolic steroid use in Great Britain. *Int. J. Sports Med.*, **18**, 557–562.

Kuipers, H. (2001) Doping in Sport – Exercise scientists have to take responsibility.
Int J. Sports Med., **22**, 545.

Kuipers, H., Wijnen, J.A.G., Hartgens, F. and Willems, S.M.M. (1991) Influence of
anabolic steroids on body composition, blood pressure, lipid profile and liver
functions in bodybuilders. *Int. J. Sports Med.*, **12**, 413–418.

Lamb, D.R. (1991) Anabolic steroids and athletic performance. In: Laron, Z. and
Rogol, A.D. (eds), *Hormones and Sport*, pp. 259–273. New York: Raven Press.

Laseter, J.T. and Russell, J.A. (1991) Anabolic steroid-induced tendon pathology: a
review of the literature. *Med. Sci. Sports Exerc.*, **23**, 1–3.

Leach, R.E. (1993) Anabolic steroids – round 4. *Am. J. Sports Med.*, **21**, 337.

LeBizec, B., Monteau, F., Gaudin, I. and Andre, F. (1999) Evidence for the presence
of endogenous 19-norandrostenedione in human urine. *J. Chromatog. B*, **723**,
157–172.

Lombardo, J.A., Hickson, P.C. and Lamb, D.R. (1991) Anabolic/androgenic steroids
and growth hormone. In: Lamb, D.R. and Williams, M.H. (eds), *Perspectives in*

Exercise Science and Sports Medicine, Vol. 4: *Ergogenics – Enhancement of Performance in Exercise and Sport*, pp. 248–278. New York: Brown and Benchmark.

Lubell, A. (1989) Does steroid abuse cause – or excuse – violence? *Phys. Sport Med.*, **17**, 176–185.

Lukas, S.E. (1993) Current perspectives on anabolic-androgenic steroid abuse. *Trends Pharmacol. Sci.*, **14**, 61–68.

Maganaris, C.N., Collins, D., and Sharp, M. (2000) Expectancy effects and strength training: Do steroids make a difference? *Sports Psychol.*, **14**, 272–278.

Meilman, P.W., Crace, R.K., Presley, C.A. and Lyeria, R. (1997) Beyond performance enhancement: polypharmacy among collegiate users of steroids. *Int. J. Sports Med.*, **18**, 557–562.

Middleman, A.B. and DuRant, P.H. (1996) Anabolic steroid use and associated health risk behaviours. *Sports Med.*, **21**, 251–255.

Millar, A.P. (1994) Licit steroid use – hope for the future. *Br. J. Sports Med.*, **28**, 79–83.

Mottram, D.R. and George, A.J. (2000) Anabolic steroids. *Clin. Endocrinol. Metabol.*, **14**, 55–69.

Mulligan, K., Tai, V.W. and Schambelan, M. (1999) Use of growth hormone and other anabolic agents in AIDS wasting. *J. Parent. Ent. Nutr.*, **23**, 202–209.

Musshoff, F., Daldrup, T. and Ritsch, M. (1997) Black market in anabolic steroids – analysis of illegally distributed products. *J. Forensic Sci.*, **42**, 1119–1125.

Nieminen, M.S., Ramo, M.P., Viitasalo, M. *et al.* (1996) Serious cardiovascular side-effects of large doses of anabolic steroids in weight lifters. *Eur. Heart J.*, **17**, 1576–1583.

Norton, K. and Olds, T. (2001) Morphological evolution of athletes over the 20th century. *Sports Med.*, **31**, 763–783.

Pärsinnen, M., Kinjala, U., Vartiainen, E., Sarna, S., and Seppälä, T. (2000) Increased premature mortality of competitive powerlifters suspected to have used anabolic agents. *Int. J. Sports Med.*, **21**, 225–227.

Pärssinen, M. and Seppälä, T. (2002) Steroid use and long-term health risks in former athletes. *Sports Med.*, **32**, 83–94.

Payne, A.H. (1975) Anabolic steroids in athletics. *Br. J. Sports Med.*, **9**, 83–88.

Perry, H.M. and Hughes, G.W. (1992) A case of affective disorder with the misuse of anabolic steroids. *Br. J. Sports Med.*, **26**, 219–220.

Perry, H.M., Wright, D. and Littlepage, B.N.C. (1992) Dying to be big: a review of anabolic steroid use. *Br. J. Sports Med.*, **26**, 259–261.

Pope, H.G. and Katz, D.L. (1988) Affective and psychotic symptoms associated with anabolic steroid use. *Am. J. Psychiat.*, **145**, 487–490.

Pope, H.G. and Katz, D.L. (1994) Psychiatric and medical effects of anabolic-androgenic steroid use. *Arch. Gen. Psychiat.*, **51**, 375–382.

Pope, H.G., Katz, D.L. and Champoux, R. (1988) Anabolic-androgenic steroid use among 1010 college men. *Phys. Sports Med.*, **16**, 75–81.

Pope, H.G. Gruber, A.J., Choi, P., Olivardia, R. and Phillips, K.A. (1997) Muscle dysmorphia. *Psychosomatics*, **38**, 548–557.

Porcerelli, J.H. and Sandler, B.A. (1995) Narcissism and empathy in steroid users. *Am. J. Psychiat.*, **152**, 1672–1674.

Raglin, J.S. (2001) Psychological factors in sport performance. *Sports Med.*, **31**, 875–890.

Reznik, U., Dehennin, L., Coffin, C., Mahocideau, J. and Leymane, P. (2001) Urinary nandrolone metabolites of endogenous origin in man: A confirmation by output regulation under human chorionic gonadotropin stimulation. *J. Clin. Endocrinol. Metab.*, **86**, 145–150.

Rockhold, R.W. (1993) Cardiovascular toxicity of anabolic steroids. *Ann. Rev. Pharmacol. Toxicol.*, **33**, 497–520.

Rogol, A.D. and Yesalis, C.E. (1992) Anabolic-androgenic steroids and athletes: What are the issues? *J. Endocr. Metab.*, **74**, 465–469.

Ryan, A.J. (1981) Anabolic steroids are fool's gold. *Fed. Proc.*, **40**, 2682–2688.

Schänzer, W. (2002) Analysis of non-hormonal nutritional supplements for anabolic-androgenic steroids – An international study. www.olympic.org (accessed May 2002).

Schmitt, N., Flament, M.-M., Goubalt, C., Legros, P., Grenier-Loustalot, M.F. and Denjean, A. (2002) Nandrolone secretion is not increased by exhaustive exercise in trained athletes. *Med. Sci. Sports Exerc.*, **34**, 1436–1439.

Sklarek, H.M., Mantovani, R.P., Erens, E., Heisler, D., Niederman, N.S. and Fein, A.M. (1984) A.I.D.S. in a bodybuilder using anabolic steroids. *N. Engl. J. Med.*, **311**, 861–862.

Spann, C. and Winter, M.E. (1995) Effects of clenbuterol on athletic performance. *Ann. Pharmacother.*, **29**, 75–77.

Street, C., Antonio, J. and Cudlipp, D. (1996) Androgen use by athletes: A re-evaluation of the health risks. *Can. J. Appl. Physiol.*, **21**, 421–440.

Tamaki, T., Uchiyama, S., Uchiyama, Y., Akatsuka, A., Roy, R.R. and Edgerton, V.R. (2001) Anabolic steroids increase exercise tolerance. *Am. J. Physiol.*, **280**, E973–E981.

Tanner, J. (1962) *Growth at Adolescence*. Oxford: Blackwell.

Thiblin, I., Lindquist, O. and Rajs, J. (2000) Cause and manner of death among abusers of anabolic androgenic steroids. *J. Forensic Sci.*, **45**, 16–23.

Tucker, R. (1997) Abuse of anabolic-androgenic steroids by athletes and body builders: a review. *Pharm. J.*, **259**, 171–179.

Ueki, M., and Okana, M. (1999) Doping with naturally occurring steroids. *J. Toxicol. – Toxin Revs*, **18**, 177–195.

Wagner, J.C. (1991) Enhancement of athletic performance with drugs. *Sports Med.*, **12**, 250–265.

Wallace, M.B., Lim, J., Cutler, A. and Bucci, L. (1999) Effects of dehydro epiandrosterone vs androstenedione supplementation in men. *Med. Sci. Sports Exerc.*, **31**, 1788–1792.

Warren, M.P. and Shantha, S. (2000) The female athlete. *Clin. Endocrinol. Metab.*, **14**, 37–54.

Williamson, D.J. (1993) Anabolic steroid use among students at a British college of technology. *Br. J. Sports Med.*, **27**, 200–201.

Williamson, P.J. and Young, A.H. (1992) Psychiatric effects of androgenic and anabolic-androgenic steroid abuse in men: a brief review of the literature. *J. Psychopharmacol.*, **6**, 20–26.

Wilson, J.D. (1988) Androgen abuse by athletes. *Endocrinol. Rev.*, **9**, 181–199.

Windsor, R.E. and Dumitru, D. (1988) Anabolic steroid abuse by athletes. *Postgrad. Med.*, **84**, 37–49.

Wright, J.E. (1980) Anabolic steroids and athletics. *Exerc. Sport Sci. Rev.*, **8**, 149–202.

Wright, F., Bricout, V., Doukani, A. and Bongini, M. (2000) Nandrolone et norsteroids: substances endogenes ou xenobitiques? *Sci. Sports*, **15**, 111–124.

Wroblewska, A.-M. (1997) Androgenic-anabolic steroids and body dysmorphia in young men. *J. Psychosomat. Res.*, **42**, 225–234.

Wu, F.C.W. (1997) Endocrine agents of anabolic steroids. *Clin. Chem.*, **43**, 1289–1292.

Yang, Y.T. and McElliott, M.A. (1989) Multiple actions of β-adrenergic agonists on skeletal muscle and adipose tissue. *Biochem. J.*, **261**, 1–10.

Yates, W.R., Perry, P.J., MacIndoe, J., Holman, T. and Ellingrad, V. (1999) Psychosexual effects of 3 doses of testosterone cycling in normal men. *Biol. Psychiat.*, **45**, 254–260.

Yesalis, C.E. and Bahrke, M.S. (2000) Doping among adolescent athletes. *Clin. Endocrinol. Metab.*, **14**, 25–35.

Yesalis, C.E., Herrick, R.T., Buckley, W.E., Frieck, K.E., Brannon, D. and Wright, J.E. (1988) Self-reported use of anabolic androgenic steroids by elite power lifters. *Phys. Sports Med.*, **16**, 91–100.

Yesalis, C., Courson, S. and Wright, J. (2000) History of anabolic steroid use in sport and exercise. In: Yesalis C. (ed.), *Anabolic Steroids in Sport and Exercise*, pp. 54–56. Champaign, IL: Human Kinetics Publishers.

Chapter 6

Peptide and glycoprotein hormones and sport

Alan J. George

6.1 Human growth hormone (hGH)

Introduction

Human growth hormone (hGH) is one of the major hormones influencing growth and development in humans. Such is the complexity of human growth, a period extending from birth to the age of 20 years, that a very large number of hormones influence it, producing many complex interactions. Besides hGH, the hormones, testosterone, oestradiol, cortisol, thyroxine and insulin have important roles at different stages of growth and development. The exact role of hGH is difficult to evaluate exactly, because of the many different developmental and metabolic processes which hGH can influence.

Release of human growth hormone

hGH secretion is episodic, the highest levels (0.5–3.0 mg/l) occurring 60–90 minutes after the onset of sleep. hGH is metabolized in the liver; the plasma half-life is only 12–45 minutes. The physiological regulation of hGH release is complex. Systemic factors stimulating hGH secretion include hypo-glycaemia, a rise in blood amino acid concentration, stress and exercise, while conversely hGH secretion is inhibited by hyperglycaemia. Both endur-ance exercise and resistance training have been shown to cause an increase in hGH secretion in female athletes (Consitt *et al.*, 2002).

The anterior pituitary, a small endocrine gland at the base of, but not part of, the brain, contains somatotroph cells which secrete growth hormone. Release of hGH is under the control of two hypothalamic hormones: somatostatin, which inhibits secretion, and somatocrinin, which stimulates its secretion. Oestradiol also stimulates hGH secretion while testosterone has very little effect. Various brain neurotransmitter systems also influence hGH secretion. This is thought to occur via a controlling influence on the hypothalamic production of somatostatin and somatocrinin, but direct effects on the somatotroph cells cannot be ruled out. Drugs such as clonidine that stimulate α_2-adrenergic receptors cause increases in hGH secretion, while drugs that stimulate β_2-receptors such as salbutamol decrease hGH secretion. The factors influencing hGH secretion have been reviewed in detail by Macintyre (1987) and Muller (1987).

Human growth hormone action

The most obvious action of hGH is that it stimulates somatic growth in pre-adolescents, but it also has metabolic effects. The importance of these metabolic actions in homeostatic regulation of fuel usage and storage is unclear as is the overall role of hGH in the adult; this is discussed in detail by Macintyre (1987). Receptors for hGH are present on the surface of every cell in the body. Discussion of the actions of hGH is further complicated by the involvement of the plasma growth factors or somatomedins in the action of hGH. hGH stimulates the release mainly from the liver of two hormonal polypeptides, somatomedin C (or insulin-like growth factor I) and somatomedin A (insulin-like growth factor II), and a full account of this is provided by Macintyre (1987) and Kicman and Cowan (1992).

In this chapter somatomedin C (insulin-like growth factor I) will be known as IGF-I and somatomedin A (insulin-like growth factor II) as IGF-II. IGF-I is the most important of these IGFs but there is still doubt whether many, if any, of the important metabolic effects of hGH are mediated via IGFs (Sonksen, 2001).

In addition, the liver produces three binding proteins with affinity for insulin-like growth factors. These are called (IGFBP-1, 2, 3) of which IGFBP-3 seems to be the most important (Sonksen, 2001). IGFs are carried in the plasma in two different forms: as ternary complexes and simpler low-molecular-weight complexes (Boisclair et al., 2001). The ternary complexes which contain the IGF in combination with IGFB-3 and a protein called ALS (acid-labile subunit) render the IGF biologically inactive, unable to enter tissue spaces and resistant to metabolism. The simple complexes, however, allow the IGFs to enter tissue spaces from the blood capillaries (Boisclair et al., 2001). Very little IGF remains free in the blood.

Effects on muscle

hGH seems to have some effects on muscle growth but the effect of IGF-I is greater. This action *appears* similar to that of insulin in that it promotes amino acid uptake and stimulates protein synthesis resulting, in children, in an increase in the length and diameter of muscle fibres, while only the latter growth occurs in adults. This stimulation of muscle protein synthesis and growth is qualitatively different to that induced by work, since insulin is required for hGH-stimulated muscle growth but not for that induced by work (Macintyre, 1987). However, the action of insulin is more likely to be an anti-catabolic effect on muscle protein rather than a direct stimulatory effect on muscle protein synthesis (Sonksen, 2001).

Effects on bone

hGH stimulates directly and via the IGFs the elongation of bone in pre-adolescents. This is achieved by a stimulation of cartilage proliferation in the epiphyseal plates situated at each end of each long bone. Cartilage cells possess receptors for hGH and IGFs.

Effects on metabolism

The actions of hGH on metabolism are complex at both the cellular and organ level and appear to be biphasic. In the first or acute phase, which seems to involve the action of hGH alone, amino acid uptake into muscle (via mobilization of muscle membrane amino acid transporters) and liver is stimulated, and there is increased glucose uptake into muscle and adipose tissue together with reduced fat metabolism (Smith and Perry, 1992). During the second, chronic phase, mediated by the IGFs, there is increased lipolysis (triglyceride breakdown) in adipose tissue resulting in a rise in the plasma concentration of fatty acids and increased fatty acid utilization, thus sparing glucose.

Effects on adipose tissue

Treatment of GH-deficient adults has shown that GH can increase lean body mass by several kilograms and decrease fat mass, especially visceral fat, by an equivalent amount (Marcus and Hoffman, 1998). Whether the same effect would be achieved in someone with normal GH secretion is unknown.

Treatment with hGH causes a rise in blood free fatty acid levels or rise in the blood glucose level and a reduction in the triglyceride content of adipose tissue which contributes to a decrease in adipose tissue mass and an increase in fat-free weight (Kicman and Cowan, 1992).

Effects of exercise on hGH

It is worth considering the hGH response to exercise in more detail. Within 20 minutes of beginning exercise to 75–90 per cent VO_{2max}, hGH levels rise. The intensity of the response depends on age, level of fitness and body composition. The type of exercise undertaken also produces varying hGH responses. Intense exercise produces earlier hGH secretion, endurance exercise produces hGH peaks in mid-term, while intermittent intense exercise is claimed to result in the highest hGH levels (Macintyre, 1987).

Administration and supply of hGH

hGH is a peptide and must be injected. The same problems of possible contamination of samples and infection of needles apply as with injection of anabolic steroids (see Chapter 5). Human GH is now produced synthetically, as hGH from human sources has been withdrawn because of possible contamination with the prion agent that is thought to spread the degenerative brain disorder, Creutzfeld–Jacob disease (CJD). Initially, synthetic, injected hGH was associated with the stimulation in the recipient of hGH antibodies. This problem has been solved by increased purification procedures. Therapeutically, hGH administration is usually recommended as either three single injections, intramuscularly (i.m.) or subcutaneously (s.c.), or daily s.c. injections in the evening.

The supply of hGH is controlled by law in the UK under the Medicines Act 1968. In the USA, hGH is regulated by the Food Drug and Cosmetic Act but Congressional hearings have taken place with a view to making it a schedule II controlled substance (Smith and Perry, 1992). One of the major limitations on hGH supply is its price. It was claimed in the 1990s that abusers in the US had to spend $30 000 per year (£20 000) to obtain worthwhile effects (Smith and Perry, 1992). There is also some evidence that much of the hGH reaching the abuser is either counterfeit, adulterated, of animal origin or some other product (Cowart, 1988; Smith and Perry, 1992). Thus, abusers are being sold bovine hGH stolen from farms (useless in humans), other peptide hormones such as human chorionic gonadotrophin (hCG), which actually stimulates testosterone production, or even anabolic steroids themselves (Cowart, 1988; Taylor, 1988; Smith and Perry, 1992). Many hGH supplies are known to be illicitly obtained by theft from pharmaceutical company production lines and from retail pharmacies (Sonksen, 2001).

According to Macintyre (1987) a number of artificial stimuli have been used to increase hGH secretion. The ones used most frequently in clinical situations are clonidine, arginine and insulin-induced hypoglycaemia, but abusers are also known to administer gamma(γ)-hydoxybutyrate (GHB), a drug which is used as an anaesthetic in some parts of Europe but which is unlicensed in the UK (George, 1996b).

Attempts to counteract the embargo on hGH and the increasingly prohibitive price have included administering drugs which stimulate hGH release such as clonidine, propranolol and bromocriptine (Smith and Perry, 1992). More legitimate means include the ingestion of the amino acids arginine, ornithine, lysine and tryptophan. Arginine is the most potent of a number of amino acids which stimulate hGH secretion. As it is a normal constituent of protein and of a balanced diet its 'abuse' would be difficult if not impossible to detect. Some dietary products for athletes claim to be rich in arginine so as to promote hGH secretion. The long-term effectiveness of arginine and other amino acids in promoting or maintaining increases in hGH levels remains to be investigated, along with the claims made for γ-hydroxybutyrate (George, 1996b).

Growth hormone disorders

Inadequate secretion of hGH is one of the causes of the condition known as dwarfism. This disorder is usually recognized in childhood when the *rate* of growth is below the 90 per cent percentile for that child's age, race and sex. Further tests involve 'challenges' to the pituitary in the form of arginine, clonidine or insulin. If these fail to evoke adequate hGH secretion then a diagnosis of dwarfism, due to inadequate hGH, can be made. The treatment is regular administration of synthetic hGH until the end of puberty. Treatment after adolescence is ineffective in stimulating growth in stature because by this time the epiphyseal plates in the long bones have fused, terminating any further bone growth. Overproduction of hGH as a result of a tumour may occur in puberty and adolescence when it gives rise to gigantism; the individual is well above average adult height for their age, sex and race, and the limbs and internal organs are also enlarged.

In late adulthood, a tumour of the anterior pituitary causing increased hGH secretion causes the condition known as acromegaly. The affected individual does not grow any taller because the epiphyses have fused, but their internal organs enlarge (especially the heart), the fingers grow and the skin thickens. Metabolic disorders occur which often precipitate type II diabetes mellitus.

In the past 10 years, a deficiency in hGH secretion in adulthood has been recognized in elderly people, some of whom have responded favourably to hGH therapy (Marcus and Hoffman, 1998). The investigations of this syndrome while providing interesting data on the effects of hGH have not indicated a universal benefit for the elderly of hGH treatment.

Therapeutic use of hGH

hGH is used to treat pituitary dwarfism when it must be administered to the affected individual before the end of puberty. The administration must be carefully monitored to prevent diabetes and/or hyperplasia (overgrowth) of the skin. Synthetic growth hormone is now used instead of hGH obtained from human autopsies.

It has also been suggested by a number of geriatricians that hGH might be used to reverse some of the bodily changes occurring in old age. Normal ageing is associated with a reduction in lean body mass, an increase in fat mass and a reduction in skin thickness. Trials of hGH treatment in the elderly have shown that the hormone is able to reverse these changes (Jorgensen and Christiansen, 1993), but a recent review of world-wide clinical trials of hGH in the elderly was not favourable (Marcus and Hoffman,

1998). A possible role for the hormone in patients with severe burns and even AIDS is also under investigation.

6.2   The abuse of hGH in sport

There appear to be four major abuses of hGH in sport: (1) to increase muscle mass and strength, (2) to increase lean body mass, (3) to improve the 'appearance of musculature', and (4) to increase final adult height. Scientific evidence from controlled trials that hGH increases muscle strength is controversial. There is some evidence to support the claim that hGH administration may increase lean body mass. Lombardo *et al.* (1991) describe experiments where hGH administration has caused significant reductions in 'fat weight', and increases in fat-free weight compared with placebo.

As early as 1988, Cowart reviewed anecdotal reports by body builders of increases in strength following hGH administration. There are also several positive findings of increased muscle growth, strength and protein synthesis in hGH *deficient* adults treated with human growth hormone (Marcus and Hoffman, 1998). When Taaffe *et al.* (1996) examined the effects of growth hormone treatment on muscle strength and lean body mass in elderly men they found no increases in strength but an increase in lean body mass and a decrease in fat mass. Similarly when Yarasheski *et al.* (1993) examined resistance training schedules before and during hGH administration in elderly men they found hGH did not further enhance muscle strength improvements induced by exercise regimes. In younger adult men there is a similar picture. Sixteen healthy men, 21–34 years, who had not previously trained were given hGH (0.56 IU/kg per week) or placebo during 12 weeks of heavy resistance training. At the end of the study, lean body mass and total body water increased in the hGH group compared with placebo, but there was no difference in muscle strength or limb circumference (Yarasheski *et al.*, 1992). Negative results have also been obtained with seven weightlifters who were given hGH at 0.56 IU/kg per week during a 14-day heavy session. Muscle protein synthesis did not increase and there was no change in whole body protein breakdown. When slightly higher doses (0.63 IU/kg per week) were administered to 22 male power athletes aged 20–28 for 6 weeks no increases in biceps or quadriceps maximal strength occurred in the hGH group compared with placebo (Deyssig *et al.*, 1993).

What conclusions can we draw from the above evidence, which conflicts with positive anecdotal reports (Cowart, 1988) and the continuing popularity of hGH abuse suggested by surveys and from the infamous confiscation of hGH in the 1998 Tour de France (Bidlingmaier *et al.*, 2000)?

By 1992, Kicman and Cowan had stated that several 'underground' advocates of hGH were commenting adversely on its usefulness and yet the abuse continues. Ehrnborg *et al.* (2000) reviewed the experiments previously described and concluded that possibly the studies are 'too short and included too few subjects'. As with early studies on anabolic steroids (Chapter 5) the doses used may have been too low and some of the hGH abusers may also have been concurrently abusing anabolic steroids. Another conclusion advanced by Wirth and Gieck (1996) is that the experiments did use suitable subjects but that hGH is simply not a suitable ergogenic aid for weightlifters and similar athletes. It may therefore be beneficial to other athletes via mechanisms or processes not yet investigated. Yarasheski *et al.* (1993) also concluded that increases in lean body mass can occur without increases in strength if it is non-contractile protein that is produced. A further complication has been advanced by William Kraemer. He is quoted by Schnirring (2000) as stating that athletes may well be combining low doses of hGH with low doses of anabolic steroids and gaining an additive effect.

It is claimed that hGH administration because of the above effects improves the appearance of the bodybuilder making his/her muscles more salient or 'sculpted' and improving their photogenicity. There is no way this effect can be measured directly or objectively but it appears to be a logical development associated with loss of fat tissue. This may be the most important effect that some abusers are seeking. Its basis needs further research, particularly in relation to psychiatric and personality factors described for anabolic steroids in Chapter 5.

The desire to produce tall offspring for cosmetic reasons, 'so that their athletic potential is increased' where height is an advantage or so that they can qualify for a vocation where there is a minimum height limit has prompted hGH abuse amongst children in the USA. Despite the ethical problems that it presents in relation to sport, children may later resent their tallness, particularly if later they fail to qualify as professional sportspersons for other reasons. Also, it is difficult to gauge exactly how much hGH should be given so as not to produce an overly tall individual. Other potential problems of child treatment relate to side-effects discussed in the next section. An apparent relentless drive for 'bigness' and 'tallness' in sport and society by selective and drug-induced means is discussed in a recent review by Norton and Olds (2001).

Side-effects associated with hGH abuse in sport

The potential risks of hGH therapy in children have been mentioned together with the close monitoring required in paediatric patients. In the UK, the recommended standard *replacement* dose of hGH is about 0.6 IU/kg body weight per week. It is widely assumed that athletes who abuse the drug are taking 10 times this dose (Smith and Perry, 1992). Major side-effects include skeletal changes, enlargement of the fingers and toes, growth of the orbit and lengthening of the jaw. The internal organs enlarge and the cardiomegaly which is produced is often one of the causes of death associated with hGH abuse. Although the skeletal muscles increase in size, there are often complaints of muscle weakness. Biochemical changes include impaired glucose regulation (usually hyperglycaemia), hyperlipidaemia and insulin resistance. At least one report, however, has found that clinical doses of hGH did not produce diabetic symptoms in children with short stature (Walker *et al.*, 1989). These changes described above contribute to the prevalence of diabetes in hGH abusers. Arthritis and impotence often occur after chronic hGH abuse (Kicman and Cowan, 1992).

A weird consequence of the increased protein synthesis during hGH abuse is changes to the skin. This includes thickening and coarsening – the so-called 'elephant epidermis' which has been known to make the skin almost impenetrable by standard gauge syringe needles (Taylor, 1988). Other skin effects include activation of naevocytes and an increase in dermal viscosity (Ehrnborg *et al.*, 2000). This combination of side-effects, particularly the cardiomegaly, hyperlipidaemia and hyperglycaemia, almost certainly contributes to the shortened life span seen in those suffering from overproduction of hGH (Smith and Perry, 1992). The effect of hGH on blood lipids seems equivocal: whereas long periods of abuse may cause elevation of blood lipids, abuse for up to 6 weeks may decrease plasma cholesterol and apolipoproteins (Zuliani *et al.*, 1989).

Who abuses hGH and why?

There are few scientific studies available on the prevalence of hGH abuse in sport. Macintyre (1987) has identified American football players and body-builders as the most likely abusers based on laboratory reports from accredited testing agencies. Significantly, the UK investigation into drug abuse by athletes in South Wales by Perry *et al.* (1992) revealed no hGH abuse.

By 1997, Korkia and Stimson reported that 2.7 per cent of the anabolic steroid abusers in their UK survey were also abusing hGH, while Evans (1997) also found concordant abuse of anabolic steroids and hGH in 12.7 per cent of abusers in his gymnasia survey. Presumably the co-abuse here was for the reasons cited previously; that is, possibly to reduce hyperlipidaemia side effects of anabolic steroids and for a co-operative effect on muscle strength whilst preventing the 'expected' loss of muscle strength when anabolic steroids are withdrawn.

The reasons for hGH abuse appear to be based on some false premises that it is as effective as anabolic steroids, with fewer side-effects and is less easily detected. Abusers believe hGH may protect the athlete who has abused anabolic steroids and who wishes to stop 'muscle meltdown', when anabolic steroids are withdrawn.

If abuse is difficult to identify in adults, this is not the case in adolescents. Five per cent in a recent survey (Rickert *et al.*, 1992) admitted using hGH and 24.5 per cent claimed to know of someone who was abusing it. Fifty per cent of the abusers could not name one side-effect of hGH. Those who abused hGH were most likely to be involved in wrestling or American football and to have obtained their information about hGH from another person such as a coach. There was also some evidence of co-abuse of anabolic steroids and hGH in the same adolescent sample.

Detection of hGH abuse

It is beyond the scope of this chapter to discuss detection of hGH abuse in detail but some consideration of it is important because of the widespread belief that it remains undetectable. Ben Johnson, for example, only confessed to abusing hGH *after* he had been banned for doping with anabolic steroids! Cheating with hGH is based on the observations that administered hGH is indistinguishable from endogenous hGH and that the plasma half-life of hGH is only 15–28 minutes and less than 0.01 per cent of hGH is excreted in urine (Kicman and Cowan, 1992). Despite this there is a good correlation between plasma and urinary hGH concentrations which *might* enable recent hGH abuse to be detected during random urine sampling.

Lack of a suitable test almost certainly led to the 1996 Atlanta Olympics being labelled the 'Growth Hormone Games' by Charles Yesalis, quoted in an article by Schnirring (2000). Advances in the detection of illicit hGH administration have been made since the last edition of this book and are reviewed in detail by Bidlingmaier *et al.* (2000) and Sonksen (2001). One method relies on immunological differences between endogenous and recombinant (biosynthetic) hGH and their detection by radioimmunoassay (RIA). However, the test will not distinguish hGH which has been injected after extraction from human cadavers or hGH released by the action of drugs that stimulate hGH release. A separate assay detects increases in plasma factors or constituents known to be influenced by hGH secretion or injection. Both these tests, unfortunately, require blood samples, which has legal and religious implications in many countries.

The two plasma factors deemed most suitable are IGF-I and IGCBP-3 (Wallace *et al.*, 1999) and possibly also the so-called acid labile subunit (ALS) described recently by Boisclair *et al.* (2001). It should be obvious that extreme care must be taken before a cheat-proof hGH/IGF test is inaugurated. Recent research shows that hGH and IGF-1 plasma levels can be elevated following a resistance training programme (Consitt *et al.*, 2002). After the Sydney Olympics, the Italian evening newspaper *Corriere della Sera* claimed that five of their country's Gold medallists had abnormally high hGH levels before the Olympic competition. Later, when one of the female Olympic cycling champions was tested under normal and stressed conditions, it was found that stress caused a significant increase in her hGH to 1.5 times the normal level, while IGF-1 remained normal (Armanini *et al.*, 2002). In 1993, the possible development of orally active hGH-releasing peptides with similar actions to somatocrinin was described (Jorgensen and Christiansen, 1993). If these compounds are developed, manufactured, and marketed, they will further complicate the picture. Future alternatives to hGH may well be IGFs themselves. These are not yet available commercially, but being much smaller and simpler molecules than hGH, their synthesis by 'designer' chemists is possibly more feasible. They could be used to circumvent hGH/IGF-I/IGFBP-3 tests, or by themselves. Much will depend on how accurately clinical biochemists can distinguish the many metabolic effects of hGH from those of IGF-I alone.

Social factors associated with hGH

The hGH 'problem' *appeared* to be mainly confined to the USA in the early 1990s, but this may be because this is the major source of information on hGH abuse in athletes. The prevalence of hGH abuse in the young (5 per cent in the survey of Rickert et al., 1992) suggests that hGH abuse is taking a hold in a small group of obsessed athletes. It is also prevalent in the UK, mainly amongst co-abusers of anabolic steroids (Evans, 1997; Korkia and Stimson, 1997). Educational programmes similar to those advocated for steroids in Chapter 5 are obviously required. However, according to Cowart (1988) much pressure on physicians to prescribe hGH comes from parents, who will also need educating. In the USA there have already been Congressional inquiries into the law relating to hGH and a number of state legislatures such as Texas have enacted laws classifying hGH as a controlled drug (Taylor, 1988).

6.3   Adrenocorticotrophic hormone (ACTH)

The use and abuse of corticosteroids in sport is discussed in Chapter 8. It is relevant here to discuss the abuse of the peptide hormone ACTH. ACTH is produced and secreted by the corticotroph cells of the anterior pituitary. It is a polypeptide consisting of 39 amino acids, of which only the 24 N-terminal amino acids are necessary for its biological activity. ACTH stimulates the reticularis and fasciculata cells of the adrenal cortex to synthesize and secrete corticosteroids such as cortisol and corticosterone.

Administration of ACTH

ACTH itself is never used for treatment or abuse; instead a synthetic derivative, the peptide tetracosactrin consisting of the first 24 N-terminal amino acids of ACTH, is administered by injection. Tetracosactrin administration stimulates a rise in blood cortisol and corticosterone concentration within 2 hours.

Abuse of ACTH

ACTH abuse is limited to short-term boosting of plasma cortisol and corticosterone in an attempt to reduce lethargy and produce 'positive' effects on mood during training and competition. It is for this reason that it is banned by the World Anti-Doping Agency (WADA) along with corticosteroids. ACTH and corticosteroids are unsuitable for chronic use because they decrease muscle protein synthesis, leading to skeletal muscle wasting.

Detection of ACTH

Tetracosactrin abuse and endogenous ACTH are difficult to detect in urine samples. In the blood a rise in ACTH levels and therefore of corticosteroids occurs naturally during exercise. Kicman and Cowan (1992) investigated blood analysis for tetracosactrin, which should enable abuse to be detected.

6.4 Insulin and its use in sport

An innocent enquiry by a Russian medical official at the Nagano Winter Olympics in 1998 led to the investigation of insulin by sports authorities and its subsequent prohibition in non-diabetic athletes by the IOC. There are no published, scientific/clinical studies on the effects of insulin on athletic performance and so much of the rationale to explain the 'street' knowledge that insulin *is* ergogenic in athletics is theoretical.

Insulin has powerful effects on carbohydrate, fat and protein biochemistry and simultaneously has a co-operative effect on these processes with other hormones particularly hGH and IGF-I.

Insulin enhances glucose uptake into muscle and aids the formation and storage of muscle glycogen. It inhibits glucose output from the liver; so encouraging liver glycogen storage. In adipose tissue, insulin encourages triglyceride formation and thus the formation of fat. The action of insulin on muscle and muscle protein is more complex. There has always been weak evidence that insulin increases muscle protein synthesis, but it now seems that in normal physiology, hGH and IGF-I are more important than insulin in stimulating this process. Insulin's role now seems to be inhibition of protein catabolism, an action it may share with supraphysiological doses of anabolic steroids! (see Chapter 5). So what is the basis for the 'underground' enthusiasm for insulin? This can be summarized briefly as follows:

1. Increasing muscle glycogen stores.
2. Enhancing muscle glycogen storage during training schedules to increase stamina.
3. As a co-operative muscle-building stimulant with hGH.

In example 3, insulin would enhance the effects of hGH while the latter would oppose the insulin-stimulated deposition of triglycerides in adipose tissue. A full account of the physiology of this new phase of doping is provided by Sonksen (2001).

6.5   Human chorionic gonadotrophin (hCG)

Human chorionic gonadotrophin (hCG) is produced by placental trophoblast cells during pregnancy and also by a number of different types of tumour cell. Its major physiological role is stimulation of the corpus luteum in pregnant females to maintain synthesis and secretion of the hormone progesterone during pregnancy. However, when injected into males, hCG also stimulates the Leydig cells of the testis to produce testosterone and epitestosterone, and so it can mimic the natural stimulation of testicular hormone produced by luteinizing hormone (LH). Administration of hCG stimulates secretion of testosterone and epitestosterone in a 'natural' ratio, allowing the testosterone/epitestosterone test to be circumvented (see below).

The Leydig cells of the testis possess receptors which when stimulated by LH or hCG bring about activation of testosterone synthesis. This increase in synthesis is rapid, a 50 per cent increase in plasma testosterone concentration has been measured 2 hours after i.m. injection of 6000 IU of hCG (Kicman *et al.*, 1991). Injection of hCG also stimulates production of nandrolone (19-nortestosterone) metabolites (see Chapter 5) and this may indicate that it can stimulate production of endogenous nandrolone itself (Reznik *et al.*, 2001).

Therapeutic use

hCG is used to stimulate ovulation in conjunction with follicle stimulating hormone (FSH) in infertile women. Occasionally, hCG is used to stimulate testicular hormone production when puberty is delayed.

hCG abuse in sport

The increasingly successful identification of anabolic steroid abusers by various IOC approved tests has led abusers to switch to testosterone abuse, which itself may be detected by measurement of the testosterone:epitestosterone ratio. hCG abuse has become popular because it stimulates the secretion from the testes of both testosterone and epitestosterone, resulting in a urinary excretion ratio of less than 4:1, below the limit set by WADA for further investigation.

A standard doping regime for hCG has been described (Brooks *et al.* 1989) in which the abuser first injects testosterone. Apart from any gains in strength or competitiveness the testosterone causes inhibition of LH secretion from the pituitary. When testosterone is withdrawn before competition (to avoid detection) the athlete would be at a disadvantage with lower than normal plasma testosterone levels. However, administration of hCG stimulates testicular testosterone secretion and also that of epitestosterone, so that apparent compliance with WADA regulations occurs. In a small, elegant experiment, Kicman *et al.* (1991) reproduced this situation in three normal men and showed that hCG can stimulate the testosterone substitution claimed by abusers and retain the testosterone/epitestosterone ratio within WADA limits. In all three cases, the hCG could be detected in the urine by radioimmunoassay as long as plasma testosterone levels were raised. Brower (2000) has described three separate regimes to restore endogenous testosterone secretion to normal following its suppression by administration of testosterone or anabolic steroids. He has recorded descriptions of hCG at 50 IU/kg producing a doubling of endogenous testosterone secretion within 3–4 days of administration. Despite the availability of a highly specific radioimmuno-assay for hCG, it does not reproduce the discriminating power of GC-MS and so it is as yet unacceptable to WADA.

Side-effects of hCG in sport

The side-effects of hCG will be similar to those described for anabolic steroids in Chapter 5. However, the incidence of gynaecomastia may be greater as hCG also stimulates oestradiol production by the Leydig cells. The increase of oestradiol may be linked to nandrolone metabolite production in the process of aromatization (Reznik *et al.*, 2001).

Prevalence of hCG abuse

Though hCG abuse is mentioned in the survey by Yesalis and Bahrke (2000), it is not quantified. In two UK surveys the prevalence of hCG abuse was 22.7 per cent (Korkia and Stimson, 1997) and 49 per cent (Evans, 1997). In an earlier UK survey in the same area as Evans (1997), Perry *et al.* (1992) did not record any hCG abuse, suggesting that in the UK its abuse has occurred or been detected only in recent years. WADA statistics for 2003 showed 14 cases of hCG misuse, worldwide.

6.6   Luteinizing hormone (LH) and its use in sport

Luteinizing hormone (LH) is produced by the gonadotroph cells of the anterior pituitary in both males and females. In males LH stimulates testicular sperm production and the synthesis and secretion of testosterone, while in females it stimulates ovulation and the production of progesterone. There are structural similarities between LH and hCG and a detailed comparison is made by Kicman and Cowan (1992). LH secretion is subject to negative feedback control by testosterone, i.e. as plasma testosterone levels rise, so LH secretion is reduced.

   In the previous edition of this book, LH was cited as a *potential* drug of abuse because its stimulation of testosterone production by the testis also produces epitestosterone such that the normal testosterone to epitestosterone ratio is maintained in plasma and urine. Its abuse is limited by its scarcity and its high cost and because its plasma half-life is 50 per cent less than hCG (Kicman and Cowan, 1992). 'Designer' synthesis of LH, a dual chain peptide, is probably impossible owing to the complexity of its structure.

It is much more likely that LH-releasing hormone, the substance regulating LH release, will become a drug of abuse. It could be used to stimulate endogenous LH release, which will in turn stimulate the testes to secrete testosterone in males withdrawing from anabolic steroid abuse. Brower (2000) has described several LH treatment regimes, which could be used to restore testosterone secretion in males suffering anabolic steroid withdrawal syndromes or in those who need to restore normal testosterone before an event or test! WADA statistics for 2003 indicated just 7 cases of LH misuse from its 31 accredited laboratories.

6.7   References

Armanini, D., Faggian, D., Scaroni, C. and Plebani, M. (2002) Growth hormone and insulin-like growth factor I in a Sydney Olympic gold medallist. *Br. J. Sports Med.*, **36**, 148–149.

Bidlingmaier, M., Wu, Z. and Strasburger, C.J. (2000) Test method: GH. *Best Clin. Endocrinol. Metab.*, **14**, 99–109.

Boisclair, Y.R., Rhoads, R.P., Ueki, I., Wang, J. and Ooi, G.T. (2001) The acid labile subunit (ALS) of the 150 kDa IGF-binding protein complex: an important but forgotten component of the circulating IGF system. *J. Endocrinol.*, **170**, 63–70.

Brooks, R.V., Collyer, S.P., Kicman, A.T., Southan, G.J. and Wheeler, M.A. (1989) hCG doping in sport and methods for its detection. In: Bellot, P., Benzi, G. and Ljungavist, A. (eds), pp. 37–45. *Official Proceedings of Second IAF World Symposium on Doping in Sport*, London.

Brower, K.J. (2000) Assessment and treatment of anabolic steroid abuse, dependence and withdrawal. In: Yesalis, C. (ed.), *Anabolic Steroids in Sport and Exercise*, 2nd edn, pp. 305–332. Champaign, Illinois: Human Kinetics.

Consitt, L.A., Copeland, J.L. and Tremblay, M.S. (2002) Hormonal responses to exercise in women. *Sports Med.*, **32**, 1–22.

Cowart, V. (1988). Human grown hormone: the latest ergogenic aid? *Phys. Sports Med.*, **16**, 175.

Deyssig, R., Firsch, H., Blum, W.F. and Waldher, T. (1993) Effect of growth hormone treatment and hormonal parameters, body composition and strength in athletes. *Acta Endocrin.* (Copenhagen), **128**, 313–318.

Ehrnborg, C., Bengtsson, B.A. and Rosen, T. (2000) Growth hormone abuse. *Best Clin. Endocrinol. Metab.*, **14**, 71–77.

Evans, N.A. (1997) Gym and tonic: a profile of 100 anabolic steroid users. *Br. J. Sports Med.*, **31**, 54–58.

George, A.J. (1996a) Anabolic steroids and peptide hormones. In: Mottram, D.R. (ed.), *Drugs in Sport*, pp. 173–218. London: E. and F.N. Spon.

George, A.J. (1996b) Gamma-hydroxybutyrate – its social and sporting abuse. *Pharm. J.*, **256**, 503–504.

Jorgensen, J.O.L. and Christiansen, J.S. (1993) Brave new senescence, hGH in adults. *Lancet*, **341**, 1247–1248.

Kicman, A.T., Brooks, R.V. and Cowan, D.A. (1991) Human chorionic gonadotrophin and sport. *Br. J. Sports Med.*, **25**, 73–80.

Kicman, A.T. and Cowan, D.A. (1992) Peptide hormones and sport: Misuse and detection. *Br. Med. Bull.*, **48**, 496–517.

Korkia, P. and Stimson, G.V. (1997) Indications and prevalence, practice and effects of anabolic steroid use in Great Britain. *Int. J. Sports Med.*, **18**, 557–562.

Lombardo, J.A., Hickson, P.C. and Lamb, D.R. (1991) Anabolic/androgenic steroids and growth hormone. In: Lamb, D.R. and Williams, M.H. (eds), *Perspectives in Exercise Science and Sports Medicine*, Vol. 4, *Ergogenics – Enhancement of Performance in Exercise and Sport*, pp. 249–278. New York: Brown and Benchmark.

Macintyre, J.G. (1987) Growth hormone and athletes. *Sports Med.*, **4**, 129–142.

Marcus, R. and Hoffman, A.R. (1998) Growth hormone as therapy for older men and women. *Ann. Rev. Pharmacol. Toxcol.*, **38**, 45–61.

Muller, E.E. (1987) Neural control of somatotropic function. *Physiol. Rev.*, **3**, 962–1053.

Norton, K. and Olds, T. (2001) Morphological evolution of athletes over the 20th century. *Sports Med.*, **31**, 763–783.

Perry, M.H., Wright, D. and Littlepage, B.N.C. (1992) Dying to be big: A review of anabolic steroid use. *Br. J. Sports Med.*, **26**, 259–261.

Reznik, Y., Dehennin, L., Coffin, C., Mahoudeau, J. and Leymine, P. (2001) Urinary nandrolone metabolites of endogenous origin in man: A confirmation by output regulation under human chronic gonadotrophin stimulation. *J. Clin. Endocrinol. Metab.*, **86**, 146–150.

Rickert, V.I., Pawlak-Morello, C., Sheppard, V. and Jay, M.S. (1992) Human growth hormone: A new substance of abuse among adolescents? *Clin. Paediat.*, **31**, 723–726.

Schnirring, L. (2000) Growth hormone doping: the search for a test. *Phys. Sports Med.*, **28**, 1–6.

Smith, D.A. and Perry, P.J. (1992) The efficacy of ergogenic agents in athletic competition. Part II. Other performance enhancing agents. *Ann. Pharmacother.*, **26**, 653–659.

Sonksen, P. (2001) Insulin growth hormone and sport. *J. Endocrinol.*, **170**, 13–15.

Taaffe, D.R., Jin, I.H., Vu, T.H. *et al.* (1996) Lack of effect of recombinant human growth hormone (GH) on muscle morphology and GH-insulin-like growth factor expression in resistance trained elderly men. *J. Clin. Endocrinol. Metab.*, **81**, 421–425.

Taylor, W.N. (1988) Synthetic human growth hormone. A call for federal control. *Phys. Sports Med.*, **16**, 189–192.

Walker, J., Chaussain, J.L. and Bougneres, P.F. (1989) GH treatment of children with short stature increases insulin secretion but does not impair glucose disposal. *J. Clin. Endocrinol. Metab.*, **69**, 253–258.

Wallace, J.D., Cuneo, R.C., Baxter, R. *et al.* (1999) Responses of the growth hormone (GH) and insulin-like growth factors axis to exercise, GH administration, and GH withdrawal in trained adult males: A potential test for GH abuse in sport. *J. Clin. Endocrinol. Metab.*, **84**, 3591–3601.

Wirth, V.J. and Gieck, J. (1996) Growth hormone: myths and misconceptions. *J. Sport Rehab.*, **5**, 244–250.

Yarasheski, K.E., Campbell, J.A., Smith, K., Rennie, M.J., Hallozy, J.O. and Bier, D.M. (1992) Effect of growth hormone and resistance exercise on muscle growth in young men. *Am. J. Physiol.*, **262**, 261–267.

Yarasheski, K.E., Zachweija, J.J., Angelopoulis, T.J. *et al.* (1993) Short-term growth hormone treatment does not increase muscle protein synthesis in experienced weight-lifters. *J. Appl. Physiol.*, **74**, 3073–3076.

Yesalis, C.E. and Bahrke, M.S. (2000) Doping among adolescent athletes. *Best Clin. Endocrinol. Metab.*, **14**, 25–35.

Zuliani, U., Bernardini, B., Catapano, A. *et al.* (1989) Effects of anabolic steroids, testosterone and HGH on blood lipids and echocardiographic parameters in body builders. *Int. J. Sports Med.*, **10**, 62–66.

Chapter 7

Blood boosting and sport

David J. Armstrong and Thomas Reilly

7.1 Introduction

In sports events or strenuous exercise lasting more than 1 minute, the predominant mode of energy production is aerobic. This means that performance is limited by the oxygen that is delivered to and utilized by the active muscles. The level of performance is determined by the nature of training, which can affect both central and peripheral physiological factors. When the muscles are well trained, as in the case of elite endurance athletes, the limiting factors in determining the maximal oxygen uptake are the cardiac output and the oxygen-carrying capacity of the blood. The maximal cardiac output is also highly important when exercise is conducted in the heat since it then subserves two functions – the distribution of blood to the skin for thermoregulatory purposes and the supply of oxygen to the active muscles for energy metabolism.

The oxygen-carrying capacity of the blood is determined by the haemoglobin content, which helps bind oxygen within the red blood cells. It is the total body haemoglobin rather than its relative concentration which is correlated with the maximal oxygen uptake. When the total haemoglobin level falls, exercise performance is impaired. Athletes and their mentors are cognizant of this relationship and many performers regularly take iron supplements to prevent anaemia. Often this practice of supplementation is unnecessary as haemoglobin levels are normal and iron stores are adequate. It is also well recognized by sports practitioners that 'blood boosting' can enhance endurance performance. Consequently, various ways have been devised of augmenting the oxygen-carrying capacity of the blood of athletes. These methods include the so-called procedures of 'blood doping' as well as altitude training.

The mechanisms by which blood doping and altitude might work are analogous. They operate by elevating the number of red blood cells, either by infusion or increased production via the process of erythropoiesis. The haematological background to erythropoiesis is first presented before the various practices of blood boosting are described in an exercise context.

7.2   Erythropoiesis

Erythropoiesis, the production of the red blood cells, takes place in haemo-poietically active bone marrow. Nearly all bones contain haemopoietically active 'red' marrow for the first 2–3 years of life. In a normal adult the only sites of haemopoietically active marrow are to be found in the skull, bony thorax, vertebrae, iliac crests and the upper ends of the femur and humerus. The majority of bone marrow consists of fatty or 'yellow' marrow, which is haemopoietically inactive. It can become active again in times of pathologic-ally elevated demand for production of red blood cells.

Although erythropoiesis takes place within the bone marrow (i.e. medull-ary) it is extravascular, that is it occurs outside the blood vessels that supply and drain the bone marrow. The most primitive stem cells, which are found in the endothelial lining of the medullary sinusoids, are totipotential haematopoietic stem cells (HSC) which are self-regenerating and can de-velop into any type of blood cell, either lymphoid or non-lymphoid. The HSCs give rise to pluripotential myeloid stem cells or colony-forming units-spleen (CFU-S). These in turn are stimulated to mature into unipotential, committed precursor cells (e.g. burst-forming units erythroid; BFU-E) by a number of cytokines including interleukin-1 (IL-1), interleukin-6 (IL-6) and granulocyte colony-stimulating factor (G-CSF). Under the influence of interleukin-3 (IL-3), granulocyte–macrophage colony-stimulating factor (GM-CSF) and erythroid-promoting factor (distinct from erythropoietin), which are produced in the bone marrow and act locally, BFU-E cells become committed to the formation of erythrocytes. They then give rise to discrete colony-forming unit-erythrocyte (CFU-E) cells which, in turn, generate dis-crete colonies of developing erythrocytes. The CFU-E is the first red cell precursor to possess receptors for erythropoietin (Bick et al., 1993).

The BFU-E compartment contains thousands of erythroblasts. The cells reach a maximum size by 14 days and produce 3–6 CFU-E. Each CFU-E forms clusters of erythrocytes (approximately 20–25) within 7 days. The BFU-E cells develop as islands of erythroblasts centred about a single histiocyte or macrophage. This cell, which has processes extending between the developing erythroblasts, is responsible for engulfing the extruded nuclei of the late normoblasts as they mature into reticulocytes (Bick et al., 1993).

The first recognizable precursor of an erythrocyte is a pronormoblast. This cell is 15–20 µm in diameter, with a nucleus containing one or two nucleoli, mitochondria but no haemoglobin. It divides mitotically three times, giving three generations of normoblasts: early or basophilic, intermediate or neutrophilic, and late or eosinophilic. The terms baso-, neutro- and eosinophilic refer to the affinity for histological stains. As the normoblasts develop they synthesize haemoglobin, which stains with eosin and confers a pink tinge upon the cytoplasm. The development of normoblasts is also characterized by a decrease in cell diameter and condensation of nuclear material, such that the cytoplasm:nucleus ratio increases from early to inter-mediate to late normoblast. The late normoblast is approximately 10–12 μm in diameter, has a dense pyknotic nucleus and is almost fully haemoglo-binized. It is incapable of mitotic division and further development occurs by maturation. Intramedullary development from pronormoblast to late normoblast takes approximately 3 days.

Development to this stage has been intramedullary but extravascular. The developing erythrocyte must now enter the circulation. The late normoblast loses its nucleus by extrusion. The residue of the cell passes between the junctions of the medullary capillaries by diapedesis (amoeboid-like move-ment) and enters the circulation as a reticulocyte. This cell is slightly smaller than a late normoblast (8–10 μm diameter) and lacks a nucleus. It contains residual ribosomal material and mitochondria which have an affinity for haematoxylin and which confer a blue reticular appearance upon the cyto-plasm, hence the name of the cell. Final maturation to the mature erythro-cyte involves completion of haemoglobinization and loss of reticular material. This occurs either during sequestration in the spleen or in the circulation and takes 24–48 hours.

The mature red blood cell is a biconcave disc, diameter 6.7–7.7 μm, volume 85 ± 8 fl containing an average of 29.5 ± 2.5 pg of haemoglobin. Mature erythrocytes have neither a nucleus, RNA nor mitochondria. They are unable to synthesize enzymes or to produce adenosine triphosphate (ATP) aerobically. They metabolize glucose by glycolysis, to produce ATP for maintenance of cationic pumps, and by the hexose monophosphate pathway for generation of reduced NAD^+P for maintenance of haemoglobin in the reduced state (Bick et al., 1993). They have a finite lifespan of 120 days. After that time, they are removed by the reticulo-endothelial system, principally the spleen. If anaemia is not to develop, the rate of production of new erythrocytes must equal the rate of destruction. Consequently, 0.83 per cent of the circulat-ing red cell mass must be replaced each day. Since the total red cell mass, the erythron, is approximately 3×10^{13} cells, that means that some 2.5×10^{11} eryth-rocytes must be produced and released each day, i.e. some 3×10^6/s. The total body haemoglobin contained in 3×10^{13} cells is approximately 900 g.

The normal red cell indices by which anaemia is diagnosed and classified are shown in Table 7.1.

Regulation of erythropoiesis

Erythropoietin in health

The rate of production of red blood cells must be closely regulated because of the huge number of cells involved (3×10^6/s). Erythropoiesis is controlled by the circulating level of **erythropoietin**, a glycoprotein hormone which con-sists of 165 amino acids with a molecular mass of 18 kDa and a carbohydrate

Table 7.1 Normal red cell indices (x ± 2 s.d.)

		Male	Female	Units
Red cell count	(RBC)	5.5 ± 1.0	4.8 ± 1.0	$10^{12}/l$
Haemoglobin concentration	(Hb%)	15.1 ± 2.5	14.0 ± 2.5	g/dl
Mean corpuscular volume	(MCV)	85 ± 8	85 ± 8	fl
Mean corpuscular haemoglobin	(MCH)	29.5 ± 2.5	29.5 ± 2.5	pg
Mean corpuscular haemoglobin concentration	(MCHC)	33 ± 2	33 ± 2	g/dl
Packed cell volume or haematocrit	(PCV or HCT)	0.47 ± 0.07	0.42 ± 0.05	l/l

entity with a mass of 30 kDa. In adults, it is produced primarily in the kidney (90 per cent) with a minor contribution from the liver (10 per cent). It has a half-life of 6–9 hours and is inactivated in the liver. Normal serum concentration is approximately 20 mU or 10 pmol, although this value can vary considerably for different subjects with the same number of red blood cells. There is often diurnal variation in serum levels with the highest levels recorded around midnight (Rivier and Saugy, 1999).

The stimulus for the production of erythropoietin is reduced oxygen delivery to the kidney. This may happen as a result of either altitude-induced hypoxia (including training-induced, see Section 7.3), haemorrhage, cardiovascular disease, respiratory disease or anaemia. A reduction in tissue oxygen pressure can increase red cell production by as much as 6–9 times by stimulation of erythropoietin secretion. Secretion is facilitated by the action of catecholamines upon ß-adrenergic receptors. Androgens increase erythropoiesis and have been used with some success to treat aplastic anaemia. Cobalt, thyroid hormone (by an indirect effect upon metabolic rate and oxygen requirement), adrenal corticosteroids (directly), growth hormone and stimulation of peripheral chemoreceptors all increase erythropoietin production (Hoffbrand and Lewis, 1989; Ganong, 2001).

The site of production of erythropoietin is in the endothelial cells of the peritubular capillaries within the renal cortex. The hypoxaemia-sensitive receptor contains a haem moiety. The deoxy form of the haem moiety stimulates, and the oxy form inhibits, the transcription of the erythropoietin gene to form erythropoietin mRNA (Ganong, 2001). The system is extremely sensitive. A decrease in haematocrit below 20 per cent results in a hundred-fold increase in erythropoietin.

Mode of action of erythropoietin

Erythropoietin stimulates proliferation of late BFU-E cells and controls the rate at which the erythropoietin-sensitive cells (CFU-E) give rise to pronormoblasts. The effect is receptor mediated. Within minutes there is a burst of RNA synthesis. This is followed after several hours by an increase in DNA synthesis. Stimulation of nucleic acid synthesis increases the number of committed stem cells, the rate of cell division and the rate of synthesis of haemoglobin, whilst also decreasing the maturation time of more mature cells. The net effect is an increase in the number of erythrocytes that are produced and the rate at which they are released into the circulation.

Erythropoietin in disease

Increased secretion of erythropoietin causes a rise in the number of circulating erythrocytes, secondary polycythaemia, characterized by elevated haemoglobin and haematocrit. The increases can be of both renal and extra-renal origin. Renal causes include renal cell carcinoma, renal cysts, hydronephrosis and renal graft rejection. Extra-renal causes include hepatoma, phaeochromocytoma and cerebellar haemangioblastoma. Secondary polycythaemia can also be caused by increased erythropoietin secondary to decreased tissue oxygenation, caused by low arterial oxygen saturation consequent upon chronic lung disease, right–left shunts and altitude exposure or, alternatively, normal oxygen saturation consequent upon sleep apnoea, high affinity haemoglobins and abnormal 2,3-bisphosphoglycerate (2,3-BPG) metabolism.

Recombinant erythropoietin

The gene responsible for the synthesis of erythropoietin has been located and characterized on chromosome 7. Recombinant erythropoietin (r-HuEPO) is licensed in the UK for the treatment of anaemia associated with chronic renal failure. Before erythropoietin is prescribed, other possible causes of anaemia or chronic renal failure should be excluded, e.g. iron and folate deficiency should be corrected. Erythropoietin can be administered either subcutaneously or intravenously. The dose is adjusted according to the patient's response. The aim is to increase haemoglobin concentration at a rate not exceeding 2 g/100 ml per month to a stable level of 10–12 g/100 ml (British National Formulary, 2004). A typical regimen for Epoetin Alfa (human r-HuEPO) would be 50 units/kg three times weekly, increased according to response in steps of 25 units/kg three times weekly at intervals of 4 weeks. The maximum dose is 600 units/kg weekly in three divided doses. The maintenance dose is usually 33–100 units/kg weekly in 2–3 divided doses.

Treatment requires careful supervision because of the risk of a dose-dependent increase in blood pressure. This may evoke an acute hypertensive crisis which necessitates urgent medical attention (British National Formulary, 2004).

7.3 Exercise at altitude

As altitude increases, the barometric pressure falls. At sea level the normal pressure is 760 mmHg, at 1000 m it is 680 mmHg, at 3000 m it is about 540 mmHg and at the top of Mt Everest (height 8848 m) it is 250 mmHg. So high-altitude conditions are referred to as low-pressure or hypobaric conditions.

The main problem associated with hypobaric environments is hypoxia. Although the proportion of oxygen in the air at any altitude is constant at 20.93 per cent, as ambient pressure decreases (with increase in altitude) the air is less dense. As a result there are fewer oxygen molecules in a given volume of air, and, if we were to inspire the same volume of air as at sea level, less oxygen would be inspired. Thus the uptake of oxygen into the body by the lungs is decreased and there is a decreased rate of oxygen delivery to the tissues where it is needed. However, the body is able to show some adaptive responses which compensate for the relative lack of oxygen in the air. Although these responses begin immediately on exposure to hypobaric conditions, for some people the full response is not manifested until weeks or months at altitude. It is to be noted, however, that even with complete acclimatization, the sea-level visitor to altitude is never as completely adapted as the individual born and bred at altitude. This becomes apparent with endurance sports events in particular.

The hypoxia of altitude is probably more widely recognized in mountaineering than in any other sporting activity. Mountaineers need to have very good aerobic fitness levels to climb the high peaks. The conventional practice has been to use oxygen to compensate for the reduced alveolar oxygen tension. In 1978, it was shown that Mt Everest could be climbed without supplementary oxygen. This was possible with mountaineers who had a high VO_{2max}, were acclimatized and were favoured by the day-to-day variations in atmospheric pressure on the peak. At this level of altitude, prior acclimatization at medium altitude is essential. Nevertheless the ascents need to be planned so that the time above 6000 m is restricted to avoid inevitable high-altitude deterioration. Above an altitude of 5200 m (the highest permanent settlement in the Andes) acclimatization is replaced by a steady deterioration. Appetite is suppressed, leading to a negative energy balance. Furthermore, there is an increased risk of 'mountain sickness' and medical emergencies at these higher altitudes.

7.4 Adaptations to altitude

Physiological adaptations

An immediate physiological response to exercise in hypobaric conditions or lack of oxygen is respiratory compensation. This is achieved by an increased tidal volume (depth of breathing) and/or an increased respiratory frequency. An increase in depth of respiration is the main response, especially relevant during sports such as swimming and running where the breathing rate is synchronized with stroke or stride patterns.

The hyperventilation (increase in breathing) that occurs on exposure to altitude causes a problem in that more carbon dioxide is 'blown off' from blood passing through the lungs. Elimination of carbon dioxide, which is a weak acid in solution in the blood, leaves the blood more alkaline than normal because of an excess of bicarbonate ions. The kidneys compensate by excreting bicarbonate over several days, which helps return the acidity of the blood towards normal. The outcome is that the alkaline reserve is decreased, and so the blood has a poorer buffering capacity for tolerating entry of additional acids into it. Consequently lactic acid diffusing from muscle into blood during exercise at altitude will be more difficult to neutralize. High-intensity performance will decline earlier than at sea level because of this, and the intensity of training will need to be reduced for exercise to be sustained.

The low oxygen tension (partial pressure) does not significantly affect the uptake of oxygen by the red blood cells until the oxygen pressure declines to a certain point. However, with adaptation to altitude the critical oxygen pressure falls. This results from increased production of 2,3-BPG by the red blood cells, and is beneficial in that it aids the unloading of oxygen from the red cells at the tissues. The oxygen-carrying capacity of the blood is enhanced by an increase in the number of red blood cells. This process begins within a few days of altitude, and is stimulated by erythropoietin secreted by the kidneys which later causes increased red blood cell production by the bone marrow. As a result, the bone marrow increases its iron uptake to form haemoglobin after about 48 hours at altitude. If the individual remains at high altitude, it takes 2–3 weeks to secure a true increase in total body haemoglobin and the red cell count continues to increase for a year or more but does not attain the values observed in high-altitude natives. The haemoglobin concentration also increases, and there is a rise in haematocrit, the percentage of blood volume occupied by red blood cells.

On first exposure to altitude there is an increase in heart rate. Later, successful adaptation to altitude results in a reduction in the heart rate to a near normal level.

Within a few days of reaching an altitude location a rise in haemoglobin concentration is apparent, but this initial increase in haemoglobin is a result of haemoconcentration due to the drop in plasma volume. Nevertheless there is a gradual true increase in haemoglobin which is mediated by stimulation of the bone marrow to overproduce red blood cells in the course of erythropoiesis, as explained earlier. This requires that the body's iron stores are adequate and may, indeed, mean supplementation of iron intake prior to and during the stay at altitude.

Upon return to sea level it will take a few days for the acid–base status to be re-established. Hypoxia no longer stimulates erythropoiesis and the elevated red cell count will slowly come down. The decreased affinity of red blood cells for oxygen, which facilitated unloading to the active tissues by means of the activity of 2,3-BPG, is soon lost on return to sea level. Any exploitation of the haematological adaptation must be carefully timed to occur before the red blood cell count returns to normality: this may take up to 6 weeks. Otherwise, repeated sojourns to altitude are needed.

The use of altitude training camps for enhancement of sea-level performance received renewed interest in the 1990s amongst British coaches. A symposium convened by the British Olympic Association (1993) represented an attempt to co-ordinate the experiences of the various sports and provided an opportunity to consider the relevance of altitude training for its athletes.

The British middle and distance runners used a range of altitude locations from Albuquerque (1500 m) to Mexico City (2300 m). The difference in these two exposures was reflected in a significant increase in haemoglobin concentration at Mexico and no change after Albuquerque. It does seem that an altitude in excess of 2000 m, when the reduction in ambient pressure takes the oxygen-saturation curve of haemoglobin into a steep decline, is needed to induce an appreciable effect on red cell mass.

The most comprehensive monitoring of athletes was of the rowers. Particular attention was given to reducing the training load on early exposure to avoid acute mountain sickness. Later, individuals were carefully programmed with increased training loads and metabolic responses were recorded (Grobler and Faulmann, 1993). The programme took into account the competitive schedule following return to sea level. It has proved to be effective in the gold medal winning men's teams at the 1996 and 2000 Olympic Games.

There is not complete consensus on the timing of this return to sea level before participation in major competition. A study of Swedish skiers was carried out for a 3-week period at 1900 m with a subsequent long-term follow-up. Ingjer and Myhre (1992) reported that a strict liquid intake regimen was effective in reducing the fall in plasma volume associated with dehydration at altitude. The blood lactate response to a sub-maximal exercise test was lowered on immediate return to sea level. This decrease was correlated with the improvement in haemoglobin and haematocrit that occurred at altitude. It seems that those that benefit most from altitude training are those with the greatest room for elevating oxygen-carrying capacity.

The level of altitude seemingly influences the stimulatory effect of erythropoietin. At about 1900 m the rise in serum erythropoietin is about 30 per cent higher than at sea level after 2–3 days, but at 4500 m this increase is about 300 per cent. Serum erythropoietin concentrations decrease after approximately 1 week at altitude, and this may be associated with increased oxygenation of the tissues due to an increase in red cell 2,3-BPG. The average true rise in haemoglobin approximates to 1 per cent each week, at least at altitudes between 1.8 and 3 km (Berglund, 1992).

Best estimates are that optimal haematological adaptations to altitude take around 80 days. This may be accelerated by periodic visits to higher altitude (up to about 3 km) but not training there. The inability to tolerate high training loads at altitude may lead to a drop in aerobic fitness which offsets the positive effects of the altitude sojourn. The answer may be a combination of living at altitude for a sustained period but frequently returning to near-sea level (locally if possible) for strenuous exercise training. This strategy has been referred to as 'live high, train low' (Levine, 1995).

Altitude simulation

Altitude training to enhance subsequent performance capability at sea level is widely used by sea-level natives in a range of sports. Such a manoeuvre is legal and has spawned the development of training camps based at altitude resorts. It has even encouraged many professional endurance athletes to reside at altitude. The so-called 'training camp' atmosphere cannot be replicated in environmental simulators. Nevertheless the benefits of the haematological adaptation to altitude will depend on a host of factors. These include the nature of the sport, the training and nutritional state of the athlete, the duration of the sojourn, the frequency of visits to altitude (or its simulation) and the timing of the return to sea level. The opportunity to take advantage of altitude training depends either on an accident of birth or the financial support available to the sea-level dweller. Even then, exposure to altitude demands careful attention to physiological detail so that adverse effects (such as acute mountain sickness) are avoided and the training stimulus carefully matched to the prevailing capability of the individual.

A recent development has been the simulation of altitude at sea level by means of 'hypoxic huts', so-called normobaric hypoxia. Hypoxia is achieved by reducing the partial oxygen content in the inspired air and increasing the nitrogen content of the room air, the ambient pressure remaining normal. Athletes may sleep in this environment but train normally, thereby living 'high' and training 'low' (Ekblom, 1997).

Hypobaric environmental chambers provide opportunities also for athletes to spend time training in hypoxic conditions in attempts to promote the physiological adjustments associated with altitude exposure. The hypoxic stimulus is accentuated by sleeping in such an environment, whether hypobaric or normobaric but hypoxic, as the alveolar pO_2 drops during sleep. This is also the basis for the 'hypoxic tents' used by some cyclists designed for their homes. These devices have replaced the portable altitude simulators of the 1980s in which the inspired pO_2 was reduced by recirculating part of the athlete's own expired air. These designs were effective in altering the ventilatory response to exercise but any further adaptive benefits were questionable (Clucas *et al.*, 1985). Ashenden *et al.* (2001) compared the physiological response to simulated altitude exposure with r-HuEPO administration. The group mean increase in serum erythropoietin (422 per cent for r-HuEpo v. 59 per cent for simulated altitude), per cent reticulocytes (89 per cent v. 30 per cent) and VO_{2max} (6.6 per cent v. −2.0 per cent) indicated the changes induced by simulated altitude were relatively modest compared with those obtained with r-HuEPO. Based on the different magnitude of these responses, the authors concluded that simulated altitude facilities should not be considered unethical based on the tenet that they provide an alternative means of obtaining the benefits sought by illegal r-HuEPO doping.

7.5   Blood doping

Blood doping is defined by the IOC (2001) as the administration of blood, red cells and/or related blood products to an athlete, which may be preceded by withdrawal of blood from the athlete, who continues to train in such a blood-depleted state. It is referred to colloquially as 'blood boosting' and is known physiologically as induced-polycythaemia. It can be achieved in an ever increasing number of ways. The first methods to be adopted involved blood transfusions. These were either by transfusion of matched blood from a donor, in much the same way as compatible blood for therapeutic transfusions is drawn from a blood bank (non-autologous blood); or by drawing an amount of blood from an athlete, storing the frozen red cells for 4 to 5 weeks or longer and later reinfusing them to augment the extra cells produced naturally in the meantime to compensate for those withdrawn earlier (autologous blood).

Transfusional polycythaemia was used in the 1970s to correct for anaemia in a Finnish 3000 m steeplechaser who broke the world record soon after receiving a transfusion but otherwise made little impact on the track. Since that time a number of notable Finnish and Italian distance runners have admitted to using blood doping, whilst the ploy was also linked with US cyclists at the 1984 Olympics and with Italian runners and cyclists. The improved performance capability is achieved virtually overnight. Once the excess fluid is excreted, the blood is left with a supranormally high red cell count. This elevates the oxygen-carrying capability of the blood, which delivers more oxygen to the active muscles. The same end result is achieved from reinfusing one's own blood after a few weeks' storage, a ploy which avoids risks associated with any error in matching blood donations.

The early experiments on blood reinfusion did not all agree that this manoeuvre was effective as an ergogenic measure. The main reason for inconclusive findings was that the refrigerated blood cells aged in storage. Glycerol freezing is used to preserve the oxygen-carrying capacity of the erythrocytes, if the storage time exceeds 3 weeks (Birkeland and Hemmersbach, 1999). Storage of packed cells from 900 to 1000 ml of blood with special freezing techniques can provoke a 10 per cent increase in hae-moglobin when the cells are reinfused. Some experimenters have reinfused up to 1.5 litres of freeze-preserved blood, but it is usual to infuse only the packed cells. Mostly, volumes of 800 to 900 ml have been withdrawn (usu-ally two separate phlebotomies), but reinfused volumes of 400 to 500 ml have proved effective in enhancing performance; improvements have been shown in maximal oxygen uptake and in endurance performance of runners and skiers. After thawing and reconstituting with physiological saline, the red blood cells are reinfused 1 to 7 days prior to competition.

Runners over 10 km have displayed improvements of over 1 minute in their times (Figure 7.1), whilst experiments have also indicated improvements in 1500 m running. The runners also showed a decrease in sub-maximal heart rate in response to a set treadmill run (Brien and Simon, 1987). The charac-teristic change in performance is that the runners do not slow down during the later parts of their races but can maintain a steady pace to the end without relenting. The improvement in performance was retained over at least a 2-week period.

7.6   The use of erythropoietin in blood boosting

The natural improvement in oxygen transport with acclimatization to altitude is due to increased synthesis of erythropoietin. The result on return to sea level is an increased oxygen-carrying capacity of the blood and an improved potential for endurance performance in trained individuals. It is possible to simulate the benefits of altitude training upon secretion of erythropoietin by administration of synthetic or human r-HuEPO. Amgen received a licence for r-HuEPO in 1984. The first clinical reports of EPO were published in 1987. There were several newspaper articles about this time which linked the deaths of 18 European cyclists with rumours of EPO abuse in the peleton (Leith, 1992). In 1990, EPO was implicated in the death of one such cyclist, Johannes Draaijer, by his widow. At that time, it was unlikely that the magnitude of the increase in red blood cell production was accurately controlled and the haematocrit (Hct) may have been raised to dangerously high levels. Values of 60 per cent were rumoured. This concen-tration would cause significant increases in both systolic blood pressure and blood viscosity. In the short term there would be an increased risk of throm-bosis and stroke. In the long term, chronically elevated Hct and blood viscosity could lead to left ventricular hypertrophy and, ultimately, to left ventricular failure.

The ergogenic effects of recombinant human EPO (r-HuEPO) were com-pared with those of transfusional polycythaemia by Ekblom and Berglund (1991). These authors reported that r-HuEPO increased Hb concentration from 152 g/l to 169 g/l and VO_{2max} from 4.52 to 4.88 litre/min. These effects did not differ significantly from those evoked by reinfusion of 1350 ml of

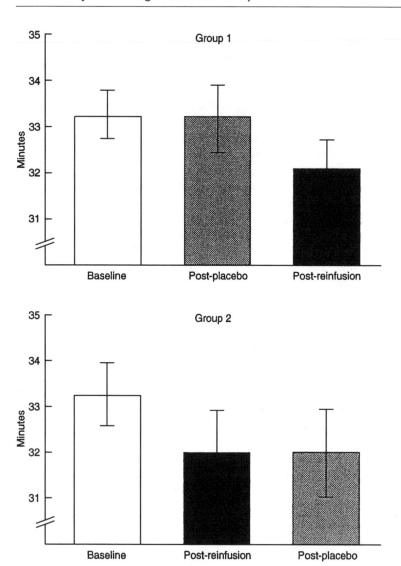

Figure 7.1 The relation between 10 km times and reinfusion or placebo. In Group 1, running time fell after infusion but not after placebo. In Group 2, time fell after reinfusion and the improvement was maintained 13 days afterwards at the time of a placebo infusion (Brien and Simon, 1987).

autologous blood. Significantly, systolic blood pressure was increased whilst cycling at 200 W from before to after r-HuEPO. In a later study, time to exhaustion was also increased from 493 ± 74 to 567 ± 82 s following identical doses of r-HuEPO (Ekblom, 1997). These improvements occurred without any change in biochemical characteristics of the leg muscles. In 1990, the IOC added EPO to the list of banned substances (IOC, 1990). There was much conjecture about abuse of EPO at this time. The former professional cyclist, Paul Kimmage, referred in his book *Rough Ride* (Kimmage, 1998) to such suspicions within the peleton. He also referred to the Donati dossier (1994) which was an account of EPO abuse involving elite Italian cyclists. The curriculum vitae of Sandro Donati is a fascinating insight into the politics of anti-doping in top level sport (Donati, 2001). Proof of the widespread abuse of EPO did not exist until the 1998 Tour de France and what became known as the 'Festina Affair'. Subsequent detention of the Festina *soigneur*, Willy Voet, prompted him to publish a personal account of drug abuse within the peleton (Voet, 2001). He stated that provision and administration of EPO were formalized within the team. Riders had deductions made from salary according to the cost of drugs administered. It is difficult to imagine that other teams could compete with Festina without recourse to EPO, not least because there is undisputed evidence in sport-specific investigation of the ergogenic benefit derived from EPO (e.g. Ekblom and Berglund, 1991; Birkeland *et al.*, 2000).

The abuse of EPO must not be seen as the prerogative of cycling. It is possible that the first cases of EPO abuse occurred in the 1988 Calgary Winter Olympics, among cross-country skiers. Indeed, the International Skiing Federation (FIS) was the first to establish health checks in the form of Hb concentrations. This was followed in 1997 by the International Cycling Union (UCI) setting haematocrit limits above which cyclists were barred from competition for 15 days for the sake of their health. More recently, seven Chinese rowers were withdrawn from the team for the Sydney Olympics after testing positive for EPO before the Games. The first tests for EPO at the Olympic Games were introduced in Sydney in 2000. To be deemed culpable, the athlete had to test positive in both blood (Parisotto *et al.*, 2001) and urine tests (Lasne and de Ceaurriz, 2000). Since then, there have been two high profile cases. The Russian middle distance runner, Olga Yegorova tested positive for EPO after winning the 3000 m at the Golden League meeting in Paris, April 2001, but was not banned as only one of the laboratory tests was conducted. In August 2002, Brahim Boulami tested positive for EPO after breaking his own world record in the 3000 m steeple-chase. The preceding cases are in no way exhaustive but merely illustrative of the spectrum of sports which have been shown to be abusing EPO. It is not known the extent to which they represent the tip of the iceberg.

In September 2001, the US Food and Drug Administration granted a licence to Amgen for the use of darbepoetin alfa (Aranesp™) in the treat-ment of anaemia of chronic renal failure. Darbepoetin is a modified form of EPO. It has a longer half-life than EPO, which is an advantage for legit-imate users because it need only be injected once a week. It is also 10 times more potent which means that less drug is needed for the same therapeutic response (Amgen, 2001). There were three positive tests for Aranesp at the 2002 Winter Olympics in Salt Lake City. Johann Muelegg (representing Spain) had to return his gold medal after testing positive before the 50 km cross-country race. He retained two gold medals that he had won in earlier events. Two Russian skiers, Larissa Lazutina and Olga Danilova, were sent home from the Olympics after testing positive. The former returned a gold medal but retained two silvers whilst the latter retained one gold and one silver. The first two positive tests for abuse of Aranesp in cycling occurred in the 2002 Giro d'Italia. Italian Roberto Sgambelluri (team: Mercatone Uno) and Russian Faat Zakirov (team: Panaria) subsequently withdrew from the race.

In addition to the risk to health posed by the more obvious increase in blood viscosity and the risk of thromboembolism, there is perhaps a more sinister and long-term potential side-effect of blood doping. The risks of thromboembolism will decrease with time as the Hct falls. However, EPO-stimulated erythropoiesis vastly augments the demands of the sportsperson for ferrous iron for the synthesis of haemoglobin. Excess iron within the body is toxic. The body can protect itself to a certain extent from increased oral intake of iron by decreasing absorption from the gastrointestinal tract. Such are the requirements engendered by EPO administration that iron must be injected, thus by-passing the gastrointestinal regulation and leading to iron overload. There is evidence from both France and Italy that elite cyclists have ferritin levels indicative of severe iron overload. Thus recent investigations in Italy revealed that a large proportion of professional cyclists had elevated ferritin levels, often in excess of 1000 ng/ml (Cazzola, 2001). A study of elite riders in France revealed a mean ferritin level of 806 ng/ml with a range of 534–1997 ng/ml (Dine, 2001). These values are equivalent to those seen in congenital haemochromatosis. This condition is characterized by iron deposition in various tissues and organs leading to multiple organ failure, including cirrhosis. It also increases the risk of hepatic carcinoma. Thus not only is EPO banned by the World Anti-Doping Agency (WADA), but also it poses significant short- and long-term health problems to the abuser, inadvertent or not (WADA, 2005).

7.7   Blood substitutes

As WADA is seeking to eliminate EPO abuse and to protect the athletes, the latter are thought to be looking to advances in medicine and pharmacology to maintain their competitive advantage. Because of problems with the availability of blood for transfusions and the associated risk of infections (e.g. hepatitis C and variant Creutzfeldt–Jakob disease, vCJD) from transfusions, there has been much research into blood substitutes and into drugs which can increase tissue oxygenation. The market in blood substitutes is potentially enormous. It is estimated that approximately 4 million patients in the USA and 8 million patients world-wide will receive 2 or more units of blood each year during surgery (Alliance Pharm. Corp., 2001). The value of that market is estimated to be $2b (Wadler, 1999).

There are two major types of blood substitutes, perfluorocarbons (PFCs) and haemoglobin oxygen carriers (HBOCs). The PFCs are synthetic, highly fluorinated, inert organic compounds that can dissolve large volumes of oxygen and other respiratory gases (Lowe, 2001). They are immiscible with aqueous solutions and must be injected into the bloodstream as an emulsion. The PFCs are unreactive in the body and are excreted as a vapour by exhalation (Lowe, 2001). The first-generation compounds were withdrawn because of problems including activation of complement, short half-life and the necessity for concurrent administration of high inspired oxygen concentration (American Society of Anaesthesiologists, 1999). A second generation of PFCs (e.g. Oxygent™) is currently undergoing clinical trails. The HBOCs are either cross-linked or microencapsulated haemoglobin molecules. Cross-linking is required to decrease the oxygen affinity and to stabilize the molecule and hence reduce potential renal toxicity. The haemoglobin is derived from a variety of sources including aged human red cells, bovine cells and recombinant human haemoglobin, r-HuHb (Hill, 2001). One HBOC, Hb raffimer, is currently undergoing phase II and phase III clinical trials (Cheng, 2001).

Abuse of blood substitutes has been rumoured for some time (Schamasch, 1998). In 1998, a Swiss cyclist was withdrawn from a stage in the Tour of Romandie, Switzerland and treated for a mysterious and near fatal illness which was initially diagnosed as an infection. The symptoms were difficulty in breathing, muscle pain, gastroenteritis and 'intravascular coagulation'. Doctors from Lausanne hospital suspected that he had been given PFCs without his knowledge (Gains, 1998). The 2001 Giro d'Italia was subjected to a raid upon team hotels in San Remo, by 200 drug squad officers. An Italian cyclist, who was lying second overall at the time of the raid, withdrew from the race after it was revealed that banned substances (including Hemassist™) had been found in his hotel room (Anon, 2001). Hemassist™ is a synthetic haemoglobin, an HBOC, which was developed by Baxter Pharmaceutical Healthcare. However, a clinical trial was stopped after adverse results (Baxter Pharmaceuticals, 1998).

Haemoglobin modifiers

Another approach to increasing oxygen delivery to the tissues is to decrease the oxygen affinity of Hb, i.e. shifting the oxyhaemoglobin dissociation curve to the right. This is achieved physiologically by increases in $[H^+]$, pCO_2, temperature and 2,3-BPG. RSR13 is a new drug that mimics the effects of 2,3-BPG and decreases the oxygen affinity of Hb by binding allosterically to the Hb tetramer. It augments the effects of other naturally occurring allosteric inhibitors, e.g. 2,3-BPG. The drug, which must be given by slow intravenous infusion, is in clinical trials in Canada and the USA. The peak pharmacological effect occurs immediately at the end of the infusion and lasts for 3–6 hours. The drug has obvious potential for abuse in sport. However, the manufacturer, Allos Therapeutics, Denver, Colorado, has reported that sensitive and validated methods of detection exist for both human blood and urine (Paranka, 2001).

Plasma expanders

Finally, plasma expanders, which can be used to mask the raised Hct caused by EPO, are banned as a Prohibited Method, M1 Enhancement of Oxygen Transfer). Hydroxyethyl starch (HES, Hespan™) is a synthetic polymer derived from starch amylopectin. It has a high molecular weight and causes plasma volume expansion for 24 hours. It can be detected in plasma for up to 17–24 weeks. It has numerous side-effects including increased coagulation (American Society of Anaesthesiologists, 1999). Nevertheless, it is a drug of abuse in sport. Jari Isometsä (Finland) was disqualified from the Men's Classic Cross-Country skiing race on 15th February 2001 and lost the silver medal that he had won in the men's pursuit event held on 17th February 2001 after testing positive for HES (WADA, 2001).

7.8   Actovegin

Actovegin is a deproteinized haemodialysate of calf blood and contains peptides, oligosaccharides and nucleic acid derivatives (Schaffler et al., 1991). It has been the subject of clinical investigation for at least 20 years. Actovegin has been shown to improve glucose tolerance in diabetics but not in patients with normal carbohydrate metabolism (Heidrich et al., 1979). More specifically, Actovegin increased insulin-stimulated glucose disposal in type II diabetes (non-insulin dependent diabetes, IDDM) (Jacob et al., 1996). These authors speculated that this could have been caused by supplementation of inositol-phosphate-oligosaccharides. Actovegin improved pain-free and pain-limited walking times in patients with Fontaine stage IIb peripheral arterial occlusive disease (Streminski et al., 1992). Perhaps of more immediate relevance to sport, intramuscular injection of Actovegin reduced the time of recovery to full sports activity after acute muscle injury (Pfister and Koller, 1990). In a later placebo-controlled, double-blind study of patients with Achilles paratendinitis, Actovegin was shown to evoke a significant reduction in severe pain on full athletic activity after 3 weeks of treatment (Pforringer et al., 1994).

It is the drug at the centre of allegations against the US Postal Service cycle team. Allegedly, it was recovered from items discarded by the team during the 2000 Tour de France. Numerous national teams brought Actovegin into Australia for the 2000 Sydney Olympics. It was added to the list of banned substances by the IOC in December 2000 under the category of blood doping agents. It was suspected of being an oxygen-carrying agent. Two months later, the IOC announced that it was unclear about the mode of action of the drug and uncertain as to whether Actovegin enhanced performance. Actovegin is prohibited under WADA rules (WADA, 2005).

7.9   Testing for blood doping

The history of testing for blood doping reflects concerns both for the ethics of sport and the health of participants. The International Olympic Committee (IOC) added 'blood doping' to its banned procedures in 1985. Berglund and co-workers (1987) reported the detection of autologous blood doping by combining measurements of EPO, Hb, bilirubin and iron. The principle was that the transfusion of one's own blood increased Hb but suppressed endogenous production of EPO, and the retransfused red blood cells were more fragile with the result that an increase in haemolysis post-exercise was detected by elevated serum levels of iron and bilirubin. Birkeland and Hemmersbach (1999) outlined the limitations of this approach, including its detection of only 50 per cent of positive cases.

In 1988 the Federation Internationale de Ski (FIS) classified EPO as a doping substance. The FIS was the first federation to introduce blood sampling for detection of heterologous erythrocyte infusions in 1989. Samples were analysed for blood groups, EPO and haemoglobin concentration. Erythropoietin was banned by the IOC in 1990. In 1997, the UCI and the FIS accepted random blood testing before competition and fixed maximum haematocrit and haemoglobin levels. These tests were instigated in part for the benefit of the riders and skiers. Indeed, they were called health checks. However, the scandal of the 'Festina Affair' of 1998 happened not because of positive drug tests or health checks but because of the actions of French custom officials. It is difficult to believe that this check occurred by chance rather than by design and suggests that concerns about EPO abuse had spread beyond the realm of the sporting world. Development of a direct test for EPO was not successful for a further two years. On 28th August 2000, the IOC voted to use a combination of blood and urine tests for the detection of EPO at the Sydney Olympics. Three hundred and seven tests for EPO were performed out-of-competition and began when the Olympic village opened and continued until the end of the Games. The only positives that were reported were for samples provided for internal quality control (IOC, 2000). These results might be interpreted as evidence that the threat of testing had been sufficient deterrent to eradicate the abuse of EPO.

Whilst it could be argued that that was the case at the XXVII Olympiad in Sydney, it is certainly not the case outside the Olympics. The

Danish cyclist, Bo Hamburger (silver medallist in the 1997 World Road Race Championship) became the first sportsman to test positive for EPO at the end of the Belgian one-day classic, the 2001 Fleche-Wallonne. That was just 10 days after cycling became the first sport to adopt blood and urine tests for EPO abuse. He was subsequently suspended by his team (Denmark's CSC-World Online) after the 'A' urine sample was declared positive on May 10th. However, the Danish federation's anti-doping committee reversed the decision on August 9th. Apparently, two samples of the 'B' urine sample were tested at the approved laboratory in Lausanne on June 11th and gave different results, one positive and one negative. Allegedly, this cast doubt upon the reproducibility of the testing technique (Fotheringham, 2001). Implementation of the anti-doping regulations is plagued not only by uncertainties concerning the analytical techniques but also by simple human error. Olga Yegorova was faced with a 2-year suspension after testing positive for EPO following the Golden League meeting in Paris in July 2001. The IAAF was later forced to reinstate her before the World Championships in Edmonton 2001 because of human or administrative error in the sampling process. It was found that the Parisian officials had only taken a urine sample from Yegerova and not a blood sample. The IAAF protocol requires both positive urine and blood tests before the athlete can be considered positive and subject to suspension (Fendrich, 2001). A month later, Yegorova went on to become the World Champion at 5000 m in Edmonton.

7.10 Conclusions

The maximal oxygen uptake of aerobically trained sportspersons is limited largely by their cardiac output and the oxygen-carrying capacity of their blood. The latter is determined by the total body haemoglobin. Since it is not possible to increase, artificially, the haemoglobin content of individual red cells, the strategy of practitioners has been to increase the total number of red cells and hence the overall quantity of haemoglobin that the 'erythron' contains. This led to the introduction of altitude training into the programmes of elite aerobic sportsmen and women. The cost in terms of time, inconvenience and money led to the search for alternative methods for augmenting the total red cell count. The first approach was to reinfuse the subjects' own packed red cells. However, the lifespan of reinfused cells was relatively brief, a couple of weeks at the most. The advent of r-HuEPO provided a means of directly stimulating erythropoiesis without the need for withdrawal and subsequent reinfusion of red blood cells. The administration of r-HuEPO would appear to confer an unfair advantage upon the recipient. It is contrary to the ethos of sport, is banned by WADA and has been linked to the death of elite professional cyclists. Unfortunately blood doping cannot as yet be detected with total confidence, hence it is likely to continue until such time as detection does become foolproof.

7.11   References

Alliance Pharmeutical Corporation (2001) Oxygent™: Product fact sheet. http://www.allp.com/Oxygent/ox_fact.htm (accessed 27/03/2001).

American Society of Anaesthesiologists (1999) Blood substitutes and pharmacological alternatives. http://www.asahq.org/ (accessed 29/03/01).

Amgen Inc. (2001) New Aranesp (darbepoetin alfa). Prescribing information. http://www.aranesp.com/prescribing_info.html (accessed 29/01/2002).

Anon (2001) Editorial: Frigo comes clean. *Cycling Weekly*, 7th July, 5.

Ashenden, M.J., Hahn, A.G., Martin, D.T., Logan, P., Parisotto, R. and Gore, C.J. (2001) A comparison of the physiological response to simulated altitude exposure and r-HuEpo administration. *J. Sports Sci.*, **19**, 831–837.

Baxter Pharmaceuticals (1998) Baxter ends U.S. trauma study of Hemassist® (DCLHb) http://www.baxter.com/utilities/news/releases/1998/03-31hemassist.html (accessed 29/09/01).

Berglund, B. (1992) High altitude training: aspects of haematological adaptations. *Sports Med.*, **14**, 289–303.

Berglund, B., Hemmingson, P. and Biegegard, G. (1987) Detection of autologous blood transfusions in cross-country skiers. *Int. J. Sports Med.*, **8**, 66–70.

Bick, R.L., Bennett, J.M., Brynes, R.K. *et al.* (1993) *Haematology: Clinical and Laboratory Practice*. Mosby, St Louis, Missouri.

Birkeland, K.I. and Hemmersbach, P. (1999) The future of blood doping in athletes: issues related to blood sampling. *Sports Med.*, **28**, 25–33.

Birkeland, K.I., Stray-Gundersen, J., Hemmersbach, P., Hallen, J., Haug, E. and Bahr, R. (2000) Effect of r-HuEPO administration on serum levels of sTfR and cycling performance. *Med. Sci. Sports Exerc.*, **32**, 1238–1243.

BNF (2004) *British National Formulary*, Number 47, March 2004. British Medical Association and the Royal Pharmaceutical Society of Great Britain.

Brien, T. and Simon, T.L. (1987) The effects of red blood cell infusion on 10 km race time. *JAMA*, **257**, 2761–2765.

British Olympic Association (1993) The altitude factor in athletic performance. *Proceedings of International Symposium (Lilleshall), 13–15 December*, BOA, London.

Cazzola, M. (2001) Erythropoietin pathophysiology, clinical uses of recombinant human erythropoietin, and medical risks of its abuse in sport. *The International Society for Laboratory Hematology (ISLH) XIVth International Symposium*, p. 21.

Cheng, D.C.H. (2001) Safety and efficacy of o-raffinose cross-linked human haemoglobin (Hemolink™) in cardiac surgery. *Can. J. Anaesthesia*, **48(4)**, S41–S48.

Clucas, N., Reilly, T. and McLean, I.A. (1985) A portable simulator of altitude stress. In: I.D. Brown, R. Goldsmith, K. Coombes and M.A. Sinclair (eds) *International Ergonomics*, **85**. Taylor & Francis, London, pp. 535–537.

Dine, G. (2001) Biochemical and haematological parameters in athletes. *The International Society for Laboratory Hematology (ISLH) XIVth International Symposium*, p. 24.

Donati, S. (2001) Curriculum vitae. http://www.play-the-game.org/speeches/doping/antidoping.html (accessed 16/08/01).

Ekblom, B. (1997) Blood doping, erythropoetin and altitude. In: *The Clinical Pharmacology of Sport and Exercise* (eds T. Reilly and M. Orme). Elsevier, Amsterdam, pp. 199–212.

Ekblom, B. and Berglund, B. (1991) Effect of erythropoietin administration on maximal aerobic power. *Scand. J. Med. Sci. Sports*, **1**, 88–93.

Fendrich, H. (2001) Associated Press. http://www.sportserver.com/track_field/story/55898p-818396c.html (accessed 20/09/01).

Fotheringham, W. (2001) Danish cyclist's positive overturned. *The Guardian*, 11th August.

Gains, P. (1998) A new threat in blood doping. *New York Times*, 18th October.

Ganong, W.F. (2001) *Review of Medical Physiology*, 20th edn. Appleton and Lange, Connecticut, USA.

Grobler, J. and Faulmann, L. (1993) The British experience. *BOA Tech. News*, **1(5)**, 3–5.

Heidrich, H., Quednau, J. and Schirop, T. (1979) Reaction of blood sugar and serum insulin to intravenous long-term treatment with Actovegin. Clinical double-blind study (author's transl.). *Med. Klin.*, **74(7)**, 242–245.

Hill, S.E. (2001) Oxygen therapeutics – current concepts. *Can. J. Anaesthesia*, **48(4)**, S32–S40.

Hoffbrand, A.V. and Lewis, S.M. (eds) (1989) *Postgraduate Haematology*, 3rd edn. Heineman Medical Books, Oxford.

Ingjer, F. and Myhre, K. (1992) Physiological effects of altitude training on young elite male cross-country skiers. *J. Sports Sci.*, **10**, 49–63.

International Meeting of IOC, April 1990, Lausanne, Switzerland.

International Olympic Committee Medical Commission (2000) Post-Olympic public report on doping controls at the Games of the XXVII Olympiad in Sydney (Australia). Lausanne, 14th December 2000.

International Olympic Committee Medical Commission (2001) Prohibited classes of substances and prohibited methods, 1st September 2001.

Jacob, S., Dietze, G.J., Machicao, F., Kuntz, G. and Augustin, H.J. (1996) Improvement of glucose metabolism in patients with type II diabetes after treatment with hemodialysate. *Arzneimittelforschung*, **46(3)**, 269–272.

Kimmage, P. (1998) *Rough Ride*. Yellow Jersey Press, London.

Lasne, F. and de Ceaurriz, J. (2000) Recombinant erythropoietin in urine. *Nature*, **405**, 635.

Leith, W. (1992) EPO and cycling. *Athletics*, July, 24–26.

Levine, B.D. (1995) Training and exercise at high altitudes. In: *Sport, Leisure and Ergonomics* (eds G. Atkinson and T. Reilly), E. and F.N. Spon, London, pp. 74–92.

Lowe, K.C. (2001) Fluorinated blood substitutes and oxygen carriers. *J. Fluor. Chem.*, **109(1)**, 59–65.

Paranka, N. (2001) Haemoglobin modifiers: is RSR 13 the next aerobic enhancer? *The International Society for Laboratory Hematology (ISLH) XIVth International Symposium*, p. 23.

Parisotto, R., Wu, M., Ashenden, M.J. *et al.* (2001) Detection of recombinant human erythropoietin abuse in athletes utilizing markers of altered erythropoiesis. *Haematologica*, **86**, 128–137.

Pfister, A. and Koller, W. (1990) Treatment of fresh muscle injury. *Sportverletz Sportschaden*, **4(1)**, 41–44.

Pforringer, W., Pfister, A. and Kuntz, G. (1994) The treatment of Achilles paratendinitis: Results of a double-blind, placebo-controlled study with a deproteinized hemodialysate. *Clin. J. Sport. Med.*, **4(2)**, 92–99.

Rivier, L. and Saugy, M. (1999) Peptide hormones abuse in sport: State of the art in detection of growth hormone and erythropoietin. *J. Toxicol. Toxin Rev.*, **18(2)**, 145–176.

Schaffler, K., Wauschkuhn, C.H. and Hauser, B. (1991) Study to evaluate the encephalotropic potency of a hemodialysate. Controlled study using electro-retinography and visual evoked potentials under hypoxic conditions in human volunteers (preliminary communication). *Arzneimittelforschung*, **41(7)**, 699–704.

Schamasch, P. (1998) EPO and PFCs: Personal View. *Olympic Review, Lausanne*, **26(22)**, 8.

Streminski, J.A., de la Haye, R., Rettig, K. and Kuntz, G. (1992) Comparison of the effectiveness of physical training with parenteral drug therapy in Fontaine stage IIb peripheral arterial occlusive disease. *Vasa*, **21(4)**, 392–402.

Voet, W. (2001) *Breaking the Chain*. Yellow Jersey Press, London.

WADA (2001) Skier uses prohibited substance in world championships. WADA, 19.02.2001. http://www.wada-ama.org/ (accessed 28/03/01).

WADA (2005) World Anti-Doping Code 2005 Prohibited List. Available at http://www.wada-ama.org/ (accessed 02/02/05).

Wadler, G.I. (1999) The use of performance enhancing drugs in Olympic competition. Committee on Commerce, Science and Transportation. US Senate, 20th October.

Chapter 8

Drug treatment of inflammation in sports injuries

Peter Elliott

8.1 Introduction

All sports have developed from the natural capabilities of the human mind and body and so, when partaken at modest level, few sports involve great risk of physical injury. This situation changes dramatically when sporting pursuits are undertaken at higher competitive levels. As it becomes necessary to push the body further, in an effort to achieve greater performance, a point may well be reached where the stresses and strains exerted on the structural framework of the body may exceed that which the body is capable of withstanding, resulting in connective tissues being torn or joints being dislocated. Many sports carry their own peculiar additional risks of injury to the body; the boxer may suffer repeated blows to the face causing extensive bruising and laceration and the footballer may receive kicks to the legs resulting in bruising or even bone fracture.

Any traumatic injury to a competitor will result in a reduced level of performance capability and may require the abstention from sport for a period of recuperation. As well as the pain and personal discomfort associated with injury the individual's performance is likely to deteriorate during a period of inactivity. Muscle bulk may be lost and an extended training period will inevitably be required to regain peak fitness.

In a sport where a career may be of limited duration and where there is a short season of competition the result of even minor trauma may be devastating. To the keen amateur, years of training may be wasted by an inability to participate competitively in a once in a lifetime event. To the top international professional a day on the bench may represent the loss of vast sums of money to the individual or club.

Whatever the cause or nature of the injury one of its inevitable features will be the occurrence of an inflammatory reaction at the damaged site. If we are to appreciate the potential to treat sports injuries we must have some understanding of the inflammatory response.

8.2   The inflammatory response

The term inflammation is derived from the Latin *inflammare* which means to set on fire. It is a term widely employed to describe the pathological process that occurs at the site of tissue damage. A precise definition of the condition is difficult as its nature can vary quite significantly. If we accept that it is a process which is aimed at maintaining the integrity of the tissues and that the bloodstream carries a huge range of cells and chemicals which have a role in the protection of the body, then it is feasible to construct a useful, descriptive definition.

Inflammation is a process that enables the body's defensive and regenerative resources to be channelled into tissues which have suffered damage or are contaminated with abnormal material (such as invading micro-organisms). It is a process which aims to limit the damaging effects of any contaminating material, to cleanse and remove any foreign particles and damaged tissue debris, and allow healing processes to restore the tissues to some kind of normality. Inflammation is a process which is fundamentally important for survival.

Inflammation is a phenomenon that was well known to ancient civilizations. Examples of inflammatory conditions can be identified in early writings of Chinese, Egyptian, Greek and Roman origin. Hieroglyphs that can be translated as inflammation can be identified in an Egyptian manuscript, which is about 4000 years old. The classical description of inflammation was undoubtedly given by Celsus in the first century AD. In his *De re medicinia* he states that 'the signs of inflammation are four, redness and swelling with heat and pain'. To these four signs was added a fifth, loss of function, by Virchow (1858), the founder of modern cellular pathology. Loss of function is a consequence of the swelling and pain associated with inflammation and is clearly an indication that affected tissues require rest for rapid rehabilitation.

Prior to the 20th century the principal tool employed to study the processes of inflammation was the microscope. Defence mechanisms typical of those seen in mammals were found in many simple organisms and it was maintained that the primary movement of the inflammatory reaction was the direction of protoplasm to digest any noxious agent. This activity can be seen in many different phyla of the animal kingdom. In protozoans, phagocytic (engulfing) activity is exerted by the organisms as a whole, but in more complex animals this function is attributed to specialized cells. The phagocytic cells of multicellular organisms are able to move to the site of the noxious agent by amoeboid movement (a directional, flowing movement of the cytoplasm). This movement is greatly enhanced in, but not restricted to, those organisms having a vascular system for transport of these cells to the affected area. The ability to ingest and destroy foreign, non-self material such as bacteria and to remove damaged tissue debris is vitally important.

Nineteenth century physiologists recognized the importance of the circulation and proposed that it was the vascular system itself which was responsible for inflammation. Undoubtedly the vascular system is of fundamental importance in the inflammatory process of mammals, but it is well to remember that defensive reactions can occur in simple organisms which do not possess a vascular system. The reaction of such organisms to noxious stimuli will not, however, be accompanied by all the classic signs of inflammation. Without a vascular system there can be no redness or heat, and indeed with the exception of mammals and birds, which are warm blooded, inflammation of the tissues in animal species will not be accompanied by heat at the affected site.

Inflammation is a dynamic process, and this process may, on occasions, be capable of causing more harm to the organism than the initiating noxious stimulus itself. The necrotic lesions produced on dogs at the feeding site of a tick, for example, are brought about by the dog's defence system. The damage is not caused directly by the tick. The necrosis can be virtually eliminated by the prior destruction of polymorphonuclear leucocytes. (Polymorphonuclear leucocytes or polymorphs are blood cells which have a phagocytic role in the defence system.) Some allergic reactions to seemingly harmless agents result in tissue damage which is out of all proportion to the threat posed by the allergen. Hayfever can be very incapacitating and is the consequence of a reaction by our defence system to harmless, airborne pollen.

Clearly not all inflammatory reactions are useful. There is, for example, no obvious reason why the inflammatory reactions which occur in diseases such as rheumatic fever or rheumatoid arthritis benefit individuals. What is abundantly clear is that the combined effect of the components of the body's defensive mechanism may often be excessive. A study of inflammation tends to leave one with the distinct impression that the body generally overreacts to stimuli. If this is the case then we may be drawn to the view that inhibiting inflammatory reactions may in some circumstances be beneficial. Could it be that suppressing the inflammatory reactions associated with traumatic sports injuries falls into such a category?

Whilst there are many and varied kinds of inflammation, it is possible to consider that the basic components of the inflammatory reaction result from the combined effects of: changes in the microcirculation, alteration of permeability of the blood vessel walls to protein, and immigration of leucocytes and leucocyte-derived cells which exhibit activities such as phagocytosis.

Changes in the microcirculation during the inflammatory response

The immediate reaction of skin to a burn or irritant is to become reddened. This reddening will persist for a variable time depending on the severity of the stimulus. The redness is due to an increased volume of blood flowing through the inflamed area. Consequently the temperature of the inflamed skin rises and approaches that of the deep body temperature. This effect on the microcirculation is seen clearly if a firm line is drawn with a blunt point over a surface of the forearm. As Lewis demonstrated in 1927 a red line appears in the exact location of the stimulus. This dull red area is then surrounded by a bright red halo and a weal begins to form, first at the red line and then spreading outwards. Lewis confirmed earlier suggestions that many different types of injury could induce inflammation, including heat, cold, electric shock, radiation and chemical irritants, besides mechanical injury.

Detailed studies of vascular changes occurring during inflammation have been made by many physiologists who have observed vascular changes in sheets of living connective tissue arranged on microscope stages. Using this technique it is possible to observe mild inflammatory reactions over long periods of time. In this way it has been demonstrated that the whole capillary bed at the damaged site becomes suffused with blood at an increased pressure. Capillaries dilate and many closed ones open up. The venules dilate and there is an increased flow of blood in the draining veins. This rapid flow gradually slows in the central capillaries and venules even though the vessels are still dilated. This slowing may gradually spread to the peripheral areas of the lesion and the flow may even stop completely. Despite this stasis the capillary pressure remains high, probably due to a resistance to outflow. Two of the cardinal signs of inflammation (heat and redness) are caused by this increase in blood flow to the affected area.

Another of the cardinal signs, swelling, is also the consequence of a change in the vascular system. In this case it is a change in the permeability of the blood vessel wall to protein. Normally the fluid found outside the blood system, in the tissues, is composed of water with some low-molecular-weight solutes such as sodium chloride. The protein content of this fluid is very low whilst the protein content of blood is relatively high. This state of affairs is maintained by virtue of the fact that the blood vessel wall is permeable only to water and salts. Proteins can not normally move from the blood vessel through the vessel wall into the surrounding tissues.

Water is forced out of small blood vessels at the arteriolar end of capillary beds due to the internal pressure that is generated by the pumping action of the heart on the blood, which is enclosed in the vascular system. The colloid osmotic pressure exerted by the protein present in the blood counterbalances this force causing water to be drawn back into the blood system. Without the presence of the plasma protein, blood volume would very rapidly diminish due to the net movement of water from the blood to the tissues.

During an inflammatory reaction the fluid equilibrium is altered. The permeability of small blood vessels changes to allow plasma protein to leak out of the vessel into the surrounding tissue. This change in distribution of protein is followed by a net passage of water from the blood into the tissues giving rise to the oedema, which may ultimately be seen as a swelling. Electron microscopic examination of blood vessels to which vasoactive substances were applied revealed the production of gaps 0.1–0.4 μm in diameter between adjacent endothelial cells. These gaps are temporary and there is no apparent damage caused to the endothelium of the leaking vessel.

Another consequence of oedema formation is the development of pain. Pain is, at least in part, due to the increased pressure on sensory nerves caused by the accumulation of the oedematous fluid. The common experience of relief that occurs instantly following the rupture of a painful boil lends itself to support this idea; there is, however, some evidence to support the idea that pain may also be due to the release of pain-inducing chemicals at the site of the reaction. The cardinal signs of inflammation can thus be accounted for by the various changes that occur to the vasculature of the affected area. Vasodilatation results in the increased redness and temperature of the affected area whilst the change to the protein permeability of blood vessels results in the development of swelling and pain.

Even though each inflammatory reaction is unique, very similar reactions can be induced by widely differing stimuli. This has led to the idea that some intermediary control system exists to link the stimulus and the effect. The most popular idea is that the inflammatory insult activates or releases chemicals within the body, which then trigger the inflammatory reactions. This mediator concept was exemplified by Lewis (1927), who proposed that the local vasodilatation and increased vascular permeability observed in the triple response could be mediated by a substance, liberated by the tissue, which he termed H-substance. The search for chemical mediators of inflammation has been particularly directed towards finding substances capable of increasing vascular permeability, largely because this parameter may be quantified quite easily. It should be remembered, however, that mediators of increased vascular permeability might not necessarily be responsible for mediation of other aspects of the inflammatory reaction. The time course of vasodilatation and increased vascular permeability differ from each other markedly in many types of inflammatory reactions induced by chemical irritants. In general, investigations of permeability change mediation centre on endogenous substances which exhibit high permeability increasing potency and can be demonstrated in normal or inflamed tissues. Many such substances, including histamine and various metabolites of arachidonic acid, have been investigated to determine their possible role in the inflammatory responses.

Histamine

One of the first substances to be examined as a potential mediator of inflammation was histamine. Histamine is formed by the decarboxylation of the amino acid histidine and is a normal constituent of most tissues. The most abundant source of histamine in the body is to be found in the mast cells where it is stored in granules in association with the anti-coagulant substance heparin. Mast cells are found in high levels in the lungs, gastrointestinal system and skin. When released from the mast cell, or when injected, histamine produces vasodilatation and an increase in blood vessel permeability to protein. At high concentration histamine can also induce pain and so this particular locally acting hormone has the properties that could contribute to all four cardinal signs of inflammation.

Histamine has been found to be released following chemical, thermal, ionizing irradiation and immunological challenge. The contribution of histamine to most inflammatory reactions is limited, however, to the very early phase and in most cases, after the first few hours, anti-histamine drugs have no anti-inflammatory activity. The most notable exception is in the case of immunological reactions where histamine activity may persist throughout the reaction. In type I hypersensitivity reactions such as hayfever or urticaria, anti-histamine drugs represent an effective therapeutic approach throughout their duration.

Arachidonic acid metabolites

Perhaps the most studied potential chemical mediators of inflammatory reactions are the various products of arachidonic acid metabolism. Every cell in the body has the capacity to generate some products from arachidonic acid, which is a 20-carbon, straight-chain, polyunsaturated fatty acid. This substance is usually found only at very low levels in the free form, but an abundant supply is normally available in a bound form, principally as cell membrane phospholipid. Following hormone activity or perturbation of the cell, the phospholipids are split by the action of enzymes such as phospholipase A_2 causing the release of arachidonic acid and other, similar substrates. Once made available, arachidonic acid is metabolized in a way that is characteristic for the particular cell. This metabolism is generally rapid since it is the availability of arachidonic acid that is the rate-limiting factor. Two enzyme systems are available for this metabolism, a cyclo-oxygenase and a lipoxygenase. None of the biologically active products of these enzymes has a long half-life in the body and the products are not generally stored. They tend to exert their activities locally and it has become apparent that many of them exhibit opposing properties giving rise to the idea that they are involved in the local modulation of physiological processes.

The first class of these products to be discovered was the prostaglandins, so named because it was thought that they were secreted by the prostate gland, although it was subsequently found that the principal source of these substances (which are found in seminal fluid) was the seminal vesicles. Prostaglandins (PG) are formed by the action of the cyclo-oxygenase on arachidonic acid. This enzyme causes the oxygenation and internal cyclization of the fatty acid to give an unstable cyclic endoperoxide PGG_2. This unstable 15-hydroperoxy compound rapidly reduces to the 15-hydroxy derivative PGH_2, this change being accompanied by the release of a free radical. It is worthy of mention here that free radicals are extremely damaging to biological tissues and may be responsible for some of the tissue destruction that occurs in the course of inflammatory reactions (free radicals are also generated by cells during phagocytosis). The second stage of synthesis involves another enzyme, which is tissue specific and results in the conversion of the cyclic endoperoxide to either PGE_2, $PGF_{2\alpha}$, PGI or to a thromboxane depending on the tissue.

There appear to be two distinct cyclo-oxygenase enzymes, cyclo-oxygenase 1 and cyclo-oxygenase 2. The cyclo-oxygenase 1 is normally present in cells whilst the cyclo-oxygenase 2 appears to be an inducible enzyme which may have a very distinct role in the course of an inflammatory reaction.

Tremendous interest has been shown in these highly biologically active substances since the discovery of their presence in inflammatory exudates. Several properties exhibited by prostaglandins are compatible with the idea that these locally acting hormones are mediators of the inflammatory response. First, they can cause profound vasodilatation at very low concentrations and the erythema that they induce is very long lasting, persisting even after the prostaglandins have been broken down. Prostaglandins by themselves do not greatly affect vascular permeability nor do they evoke a pain response at physiological concentrations. Prostaglandins do, however, radically enhance the vascular permeability increasing and pain-provoking activity of other substances such as histamine and bradykinin. These properties, coupled with the fact that raised prostaglandin levels are readily detectable in a number of inflammatory conditions, make them ideal candidates for the role of mediators of inflammation.

Leucocytes in inflammation

Some types of inflammatory reaction such as acute allergic responses are restricted to changes in the microcirculation alone. More persistent inflammatory reactions of the type common to sports injuries, however, involve another major physiological change, that is the influx of leucocytes. The most significant leucocyte in the normal reaction to traumatic injury is the polymorph. There are several different kinds of polymorphs but the most abundant can be identified in a blood smear by virtue of their affinity to take up a neutral pH stain. These cells are sometimes referred to as neutrophils.

Normal tissues contain few extravascular polymorphs, but in an inflammatory reaction these cells may pass from the microcirculation into the damaged tissue site. Following an injury, blood polymorphs stick momentarily to the endothelium; they roll along the inside surface of the vessel wall, adhering briefly until they re-enter the circulation. After a few minutes, more and more cells adhere, and eventually these are not dislodged by the blood flow. In this way the endothelium comes to be lined with leucocytes, a process known as margination. Other leucocytes, platelets and red cells may also stick. Margination is promoted by the rapid deployment of selectins on the surface of the endothelial cells. Polymorphs have attachment sites on their cell surfaces for these selectins.

The marginated polymorphs leave the intravascular site by a process, which starts with a pseudopodium insinuating itself between two adjacent endothelial cells that form the blood vessel wall. The bulk of the polymorph, including the nucleus, then passes between the endothelial cells and comes to lie outside the endothelial cell but within the basement membrane. The cell then passes through the basement membrane.

These cells make an important contribution to the inflammatory process. The inflammatory response that occurs in experimental animals when their polymorphonuclear leucocytes have been depleted can be significantly reduced. To achieve this reduction the number of both circulating polymorphs and polymorphs that enter the circulation (presumably from the bone marrow) following an inflammatory stimulus must be reduced to very low levels.

Polymorphonuclear leucocytes are the first inflammatory cells to accumulate in large numbers in an injured area. These cells are phagocytic and play a protective role by ingesting and subsequently digesting invading microorganisms or tissue debris in the affected area. Polymorphs do not survive for more than a few hours outside blood vessels and when they die they release their contents, which include lysosomal granules that contain a wide range of catabolic enzymes, into the surrounding area. These highly destructive enzymes may be responsible for additional damage occurring to the tissues.

As well as the influx of polymorphonuclear cells from the blood there is also a movement of mononuclear cells. Monocytes begin to move into the affected site at the same time as the polymorphs but they are slower and are therefore generally outnumbered by polymorphonuclear cells at the start of a reaction. Mononuclear cells are, however, much more enduring than the polymorphs and in many reactions begin to predominate after a day or so. Outside of the circulation monocytes go through a maturation phase becoming macrophages which, as the name implies, are large phagocytic cells. These cells can undergo cell division, which also contributes to the large numbers of mononuclear cells that accumulate at the inflamed site. Mononuclear cells such as macrophages do have a number of other, significant roles. They are capable of secreting many different chemicals that affect defensive activities and they have a key role in determining whether the body mounts an antibody-generating response to a challenge.

In the same way that changes in the microcirculation are brought about by chemical mediation the influx of leucocytes is also subject to chemical control. The simplest explanation of the phenomena of cell migration is that a chemical stimulus originating from the damaged site is recognized by leucocytes that respond by moving along a concentration gradient of the chemical towards the highest concentration. This process is called chemotaxis. There are a number of chemotactic substances known to be released from inflammatory sites and whilst cells may respond in a minor way to the mediators which affect changes in the vasculature the most potent agents have little effect on the microcirculation.

Arachidonic acid can be metabolized by a lipoxygenase enzyme system to generate a range of hydroxyeicosatetraenoic acids, one of which is 5,12-dihydroxyeicosatetraenoic acid or leukotriene B_4 (LTB_4). LTB_4 is a potent chemotactic agent for polymorphonuclear leucocytes and mononuclear cells. LTB_4 also stimulates the general activity of leucocytes as well as inducing more rapid movement and the release of destructive enzymes into the area. Thus when arachidonic acid is released from cell membranes the resultant prostaglandins and leukotrienes produced may, between them, mediate the development of all the major processes involved in an inflammatory response.

Another important source of chemotactic agents is the complement system. This is a complex system of plasma proteins that can be activated by a variety of stimuli including antigen–antibody interaction and endotoxin release to produce a powerful cytolytic, membrane-attack unit. Complement activation is an example of a biological cascade in which a small stimulus results in a large response. (The complement system has much in common with the blood-clotting cascade.) In the course of activation a number of small fragments, split off from complement components, are released into the area and some of these are powerfully chemotactic. Examples include components $C3_a$ and $C5_a$, which are also potent histamine releasers and the aggregate C567 fraction. The complement system represents about 10 per cent of plasma protein and has been implicated in a variety of inflammatory reactions. Other chemotactic material can be released from the breakdown of the structural protein collagen and from the breakdown of the blood-clotting protein fibrin.

The contributions of the leucocytes to the inflammatory reactions are various. The presence of cells capable of phagocytosis at an injured site is an advantage. The removal of damaged tissues and any foreign material such as micro-organisms is of obvious importance. The local increase in leucocyte numbers at the site of inflammation results in a general increase in the concentration of proteolytic enzymes, because the lysosomes of the leucocytes contain cathepsins, hydrolases and other catabolic enzymes. Release of these enzymes may be an important factor in the maintenance of inflammation by the production of altered tissue proteins and by the non-specific activation of thrombin, kinin and plasmin systems. Polymorphs also provide a source of enzymes with more specific activities for maintaining the inflammatory reaction. The release of kininogenases from polymorphs has been reported, and the presence of a specific collagenase in human polymorphs has been noted. Polymorphs may also contribute to the generation of prostaglandins in the inflammatory site.

8.3   Acute and chronic inflammation

The initial reaction to most types of injury is an acute inflammatory response exhibiting the prominent feature of increased vascular permeability. This reaction will normally resolve in time and, if actual tissue necrosis is slight, no identifiable trace of the reaction will be left. In a more severe situation repair is effected by the synthesis of connective tissue to form a scar.

In some circumstances, however, inflammation may persist. This chronic reaction may be caused by the presence of some foreign material that is not easily removed from the inflammatory site. It has been found that the resolution of an inflammatory lesion is invariably associated with the disappearance of the inflammatory-inducing irritant, but persistent inflammation may not necessarily be caused by any detectable irritant. The aetiology of rheumatoid arthritis, for example, is uncertain. The characteristic feature of chronic inflammation is the presence of leucocytes at the site of reaction. Some acute inflammatory reactions may proceed without migration of phagocytic cells into the tissues, but chronic inflammation is invariably associated with large numbers of extravascular white cells. Chronic inflammation is also characterized by concurrent tissue destruction and resultant inflammation. The death of invading polymorphs at an inflamed site with the resultant release of all the cellular enzymes can give rise to a suppurative lesion. A suppurative lesion may continue at the site of some foreign material, but the necrotic area may become surrounded by a deposition of fibrous material and white cells to give rise to an abscess. A separation of degenerative and synthetic processes as in the case of an abscess is not always seen, the two processes often occurring simultaneously at the same site. Such a chronic inflammatory mass is called a granuloma.

Chronic inflammation can occur, however, without passing through an acute or suppurative phase by the gradual development of the chronic state. Histological examination of chronic inflammatory lesions reveals the presence of a variety of different types of white cell. In rheumatoid synovial fluids large numbers of white cells, principally polymorphs, can be found. These have extremely short half-lives of the order of only 3–4 hours and the variety of damaging agents which can be released from these cells has already been outlined. Polymorphs are also actively phagocytic, but this function may not be important in chronic inflammatory situations since their short life-span will frequently result in the release of any ingested material on the death of the cell. The predominant variety of polymorph is the neutrophil, but eosinophilic polymorphs, which share many of the properties of the neutrophil, also occur in inflammatory foci, possibly as a marker of general polymorph involvement, and in certain reactions the eosinophilic polymorph may predominate.

Most chronic inflammatory reactions are characterized by the presence of large numbers of mononuclear cells. Those mononuclear cells in a chronic inflammatory state may be derived either by emigration or division and the persistence of these cells may be due to their great longevity. Macrophages, like polymorphs, are phagocytic and this would seem to be an important function, the removal of foreign material and tissue debris being a pre-requisite for the resolution of a reaction.

Within an area of chronic inflammation macrophages may be transformed into two other cell types: epithelioid cells and foreign body giant cells. Epithelioid cells are a common feature of granulomatous inflammation and can be transformed into epithelial cells by natural maturation if they live long enough, and do not have undigested phagocytosed material within the cell. Giant cells are multinucleate and have been shown to be produced by cell fusion, although this fusion may be followed by nuclear division without cytoplasmic fission. These cells are found in large numbers around foreign bodies that are too large for macrophages to engulf. Other cells present in chronic inflammatory reactions are fibroblasts, which are probably derived from local connective tissue fibroblasts and are responsible for collagen deposition, and lymphocytes and plasma cells, which are responsible for the production of antibodies that facilitate the elimination of micro-organisms.

Our knowledge of inflammatory processes has largely been derived from observations made in humans with chronic inflammatory disease and in laboratory experiments in animals. The contribution that any of the factors described above may make in the inflammatory sequel to a sporting injury cannot be specified but undoubtedly there will be several predictable phenomena.

1. An influx of blood giving rise to the characteristic heat and redness.
2. A movement of plasma protein and associated water into the tissue, causing swelling.
3. An influx of phagocytic cells that have the potential to cause tissue destruction.
4. Pain, due perhaps to pressure on the nerve endings caused by the swelling or to the effect of chemical mediators of pain being released.
5. Finally, and perhaps most importantly to the sportsman, there will be a loss of function – Virchow's fifth cardinal sign.

The persistence of the problem depends on many factors, but certainly the influx of leucocytes and the release of their enzyme-rich content may compound the damage already caused and tend to prolong the duration of the reaction. Given that no further aggravation occurs and that there are no complications, resolution should occur within days or weeks and at worst months.

A pertinent question to ask at this point is whether the inflammation that follows a traumatic injury is necessary. Clearly the body automatically takes what it deems to be the safest course of action when injured. It directs its defensive systems to the area to make sure that no microbial invasion occurs and that all the necessary resources are made available to repair the damage. It is evident, however, that the body has a tendency to overreact. The response in many cases may be more serious than the stimulus.

8.4   The treatment of sporting injuries

The acronym 'RICE' will be familiar to those with experience of treating sports injuries. Rest, ice, compression and elevation are all of value. Rest enables healing and limits adding to the damage already sustained. Applying pressure to an affected area and the elevation of a limb above the level of the heart can influence the intravascular–extravascular fluid balance equilibrium with a resultant inhibition of oedema development.

Cooling a traumatized part of the body is also effective. A common sight these days is the arrival on the field of play of the trainer who reaches into his bag for the aerosol can with which he sprays some area of the prostrated participant being attended. The injured player stands gingerly and then cautiously runs on. The trainer collects up the bag with its 'magic' spray and walks off. These aerosol sprays contain volatile compounds that evaporate on the skin surface causing rapid chilling of the area. The practice of cooling an injured area whether by volatile spray, cold compress or ice-packs, if applied rapidly, may well reduce the immediate response to minor trauma by inhibiting the active processes which are involved in the initiation of an inflammatory reaction. Problems have arisen because of the abuse of these solvent-based products for 'sniffing'. Nevertheless cooling will undoubtedly reduce the immediate reaction to a traumatic stimulus. Given that the body does seem to have a natural inclination to overreact, inducing a delay in the response produced by cooling may well prevent, or at least limit, any subsequent inflammation.

Other non-specific topical applications that can be used successfully for the treatment of injured tissues include liniments. These preparations are rubefacients and are thought to act by counter-irritation. This is a phenomenon where mild or moderate pain can be relieved by irritating the skin. Counter-irritation is effective in providing relief from painful lesions of muscles, tendons and joints. There is, however, little evidence that the topical application of preparations containing adrenaline or aspirin is of value in the relief of pain.

A number of more specific, anti-inflammatory treatments are available to deal with sporting injuries. The reduction of pain and inflammation represents an obvious therapeutic target. It is clear, however, that great care must be taken in judging the severity of an injury. Pain is the cue that intimates the severity of a problem. There are many drugs which can reduce our appreciation of pain, but a reduction of pain sensation may lead to the induction of further damage to an injury by the failure to respond to the natural inclination to rest. Clear evidence of the dangers of masking pain sensation can be seen amongst those who suffer the peripheral mutilation common amongst people with impaired sensory nerve activity such as that which occurs in untreated leprosy victims. Anti-inflammatory drugs may nevertheless be of value.

The use of anti-inflammatory drugs to treat inflammatory conditions

Although the treatment of inflammation with anti-inflammatory agents was practised by Hippocrates, who recommended the chewing of willow bark for a variety of ailments, such sensible practices were largely forgotten during subsequent centuries. It was not until 1876 that a physician named MacLagan revolutionized the treatment of rheumatic fever (and, indeed, other inflammatory conditions) by the reintroduction of an extract of willow bark called salicin. MacLagan had been unimpressed with the treatments that were routinely used to treat rheumatic fever (a condition characterized by extensive inflammatory lesions) which even included such measures as blood letting. A synthetic analogue of this glycoside was soon produced and in 1899 a German pharmaceutical company, Bayer, introduced a more palatable derivative, acetylsalicylic acid under the trade name Aspirine. Over 100 years later we still have aspirin readily available as a simple, cheap and effective remedy for a wide variety of ailments. It has been the subject of innumerable clinical trials in many diverse areas of medicine ranging from the treatment of food intolerance to the prevention of heart attacks. Without doubt though, the bulk of the tens of thousands of tons of aspirin consumed each year is taken for the alleviation of pain, inflammation and fever.

Since the introduction of aspirin many other drugs with similar therapeutic profiles have been developed and there are now about 20 aspirin-like drugs available for clinical use in the UK, although only aspirin and ibuprofen are available for general purchase. These aspirin-like drugs, generally referred to collectively as non-steroidal anti-inflammatory drugs or NSAIDs, all have proven anti-inflammatory activity in the treatment of chronic inflammatory conditions such as rheumatoid arthritis. Countless clinical trials have demonstrated the efficacy of these agents in alleviating both objective and subjective symptoms of inflammatory disease. Whilst some of these agents are more popular than others, there is no clear indication that any particular example is more effective than the others. Indeed it is difficult to find convincing proof that any of the newer drugs in this class is more effective than aspirin. The assessment of activity of this type of drug is, however, fraught with difficulties. It is not easy to find large numbers of patients with similar disease states who are prepared to be subjected to the withdrawal of their effective therapy so that they may be used as controls in such trials. It is also very difficult to quantify a reduction in inflammation.

Given that these difficulties exist when testing drugs on common chronic conditions, it is not hard to appreciate that the difficulties involved in testing anti-inflammatory agents in acute sporting injuries, which may affect any part of the body, are considerably greater. Since a chronically inflamed joint in a patient with rheumatoid arthritis may remain in a similar condition for weeks on end, the effect of introduction and withdrawal of an effective anti-inflammatory agent on the level of inflammation of that joint should be seen fairly easily. A traumatic sporting injury should progressively heal over a fairly limited period without intervention. How then can you measure the efficacy of an anti-inflammatory drug superimposed on a naturally regressing inflammatory condition? The simple answer is with great difficulty!

The majority of clinical trials published on the efficacy of aspirin-like drugs in sports injury are organized with two groups of injured subjects. One group is treated with one example of a NSAID whilst the other group is treated with a different NSAID. The usual result of these trials is that no significant difference is established between the two drugs under test. Clinical trials using this protocol are usually used to establish that a new NSAID is effective. The trial protocol makes the assumption that the older, perhaps more established drug is, itself, effective. This assumption may not be valid and, if it is not, then the trial does not produce reliable results.

Whilst NSAIDs are clearly effective in the treatment of chronic disease, evidence that they do have a role to play in acute traumatic injury treatment is much more limited. To establish definitively that drugs can treat a sports injury effectively a number of criteria have to be met. First, suitable injuries, preferably all of a certain type, would be needed in reasonable numbers. Second, some measure of effectiveness would be required which is meaningful. Third, a comparison would have to be made with a group of similar patients receiving no active treatment, that is, a control group. Because many individuals are responsive to suggestion, subjects in the control group would have to receive what appears to be the same treatment as the test group but, of course, without the active drug. In other words one group would be given tablets containing the drug whilst the other group would be given identical-looking tablets but with no drug in them, so-called placebos.

Now with regard to the first two criteria, perhaps a good place to look for a plentiful supply of similar sports injuries would be in a club where members are involved in the same sport with, therefore, the same injury tendencies. A measurement of the period of time following injury until the injured person is fit for competition or full training again could serve as the key to assess effectiveness. If this time is reduced in the drug-treated group then it could be concluded that the drug is a successful therapy. With regard to the third criterion, however, there is a substantial ethical and moral problem. If the drug works or even if it is thought to work, it is difficult to justify the withholding of that treatment for the purpose of a trial since this action might unnecessarily prolong the period of absence from the sport. In many professional clubs such an action would be unacceptable.

The mechanism of action of anti-inflammatory drugs

Despite the relative paucity of convincing trials that demonstrate the effectiveness of these anti-inflammatory drugs, their use in the treatment of sports injuries is very widespread. The commencement of a course of NSAIDs immediately after the injury occurs appears to be an effective way to reduce the recovery time. The most commonly used drugs in this class are aspirin, diclofenac, ibuprofen, indomethacin, naproxen and piroxicam. The use of these drugs, though widespread, remains largely empirical, as there is no universally accepted explanation of how they reduce inflammation. Indeed our understanding of the processes involved in soft tissue injury is far from complete. Several suggestions have been made, however, to explain the anti-inflammatory activity of the aspirin-like drugs. Considerable attention has been focused on the possible interaction of these drugs with various factors involved in this inflammatory process. For example, many early attempts to explain the anti-inflammatory activity of these drugs considered their ability to interfere with proteolytic enzymes. These enzymes are involved both in the early stages of inflammation and in the later stages when the process is well established. An inhibition of proteolytic enzyme activity either at the start of the reaction, preventing the activation of the complement, kinin, fibrin or plasmin systems, or during the later, autocatabolic stage of inflammation could be the mechanism of action. Certainly many anti-inflammatory drugs have been shown to have some measure of anti-protease activity, but the general correlation between enzyme inhibition and anti-inflammatory activity is not impressive. Aspirin derivatives are known to inhibit a large number of enzyme systems, but inhibition is generally seen only at drug concentrations that exceed the normal therapeutic level. Another explanation that has been proposed which is closely related to this idea is that the anti-inflammatory drugs reduce inflammation by preventing the release of enzymes from lysosomes during the more established phase of the reaction. Again, whilst there is some experimental evidence available to support this idea, overall, it is not a convincing explanation.

With an improved understanding of the mediation of inflammation came the idea that the action of anti-inflammatory drugs might be due to an interference with the activities of one or more of the proposed chemical mediators of inflammation. It was not, however, until 1971 that any major headway was made in this area of our understanding. In a series of three papers published in *Nature* (Vane, 1971; Ferreira *et al.*, 1971; and Smith and

Willis, 1971) John Vane and his colleagues outlined the hypothesis that the action of the aspirin-like drugs could be attributed to their ability to suppress the synthesis of prostaglandins. Virtually all NSAIDs have been shown to inhibit the synthesis of prostaglandins and they generally exhibit this property at concentrations that are low enough to be achieved with normal therapeutic doses of the drugs.

The predictable consequences of the inhibition of prostaglandin synthesis on an inflammatory process (based on the known pro-inflammatory activities of the prostaglandins) easily lead us to the conclusion that this property of NSAIDs provides an explanation for their mechanisms of action. A reduction in the level of prostaglandins at an inflammatory site should result in a reduction in the symptoms of heat and redness since prostaglandins would normally promote an increased blood flow to the area by virtue of their ability to cause profound erythema. A reduction in the pain associated with the reaction could also be anticipated, since, in the absence of prostaglandins, there would be no state of hyperalgesia. In other words the tissue would not exhibit a greater sensitivity to painful stimuli than normal. Oedema would also be reduced in severity as the permeability-increasing effect of chemical agents on blood vessel walls would not be subject to the normal exaggerating action of the prostaglandins.

Thus we can see that the reduction in synthesis of the prostaglandins that can be demonstrated when using NSAIDs could account for the reduction of all the cardinal signs of inflammation. As additional support for this idea of a single, common mechanism of action for NSAIDs, other properties exhibited by this group of drugs can also be explained by an inhibition of prostaglandin synthesis. For example, as well as being analgesic, anti-inflammatory drugs, these compounds are invariably anti-pyretic agents as well, that is they have the ability to reduce elevated body temperature. During fever prostaglandins are detectable in increased quantities in the cerebrospinal fluid which fills the cavities of the brain, and it has been shown in animals that the injection of prostaglandins into the anterior hypothalamus evokes a pyrexic response. The inhibition of prostaglandin synthesis, therefore, offers an explanation for this property of these drugs, in addition to their anti-inflammatory action.

Another property, which is common to most of these agents, is that they inhibit platelet aggregation. To repair damaged blood vessels, platelets come together to form a plug to fill the gap and prevent bleeding. This activity is in part mediated via the synthesis of thromboxanes by the platelets. Drugs such as aspirin, which inhibits the cyclo-oxygenase enzyme, will prevent the synthesis, not only of prostaglandins but of thromboxanes as well, preventing normal platelet function. In some circumstances, notably when there is already some impairment to normal platelet function, this activity of these drugs may represent a hazard. There is, however, much interest in the use of this anti-platelet activity to prevent the development of thrombosis. Small blood clot fragments may lodge in the vascular beds of the brain or heart and a very small regular dose of aspirin may protect a subject from a stroke or a heart attack.

Another common feature of NSAIDs is their tendency to cause gastric irritation and this, too, can be explained by a mechanism of prostaglandin synthesis inhibition. Prostaglandins normally limit the amount of hydrochloric acid secreted by the parietal cells in the main gastric glands, probably by an action on the enzyme adenylate cyclase. In addition, prostaglandins may promote the functional vasodilatation necessary for the parietal cells in their secretory mode. If the levels of prostaglandins in the stomach are reduced then a greater amount of acid will be secreted and this acid will be produced by cells that have been forced into this synthetic activity without the usual increased provision of oxygen. This situation may thus result in a gastritis in which some mucosal tissue may be damaged by the ischaemia that can result from the increased metabolic activity occurring without increased blood flow.

We do, therefore, have a proposed mechanism of action for NSAIDs that can be invoked to explain not only their anti-inflammatory activity, but also their anti-pyretic and anti-platelet activities. The proposition even serves to explain their most common side-effect. This brief account of mechanism would be less than complete, however, if it did not at least indicate one or two of the many observations that have been reported which do not easily fit within this explanation. First, sodium salicylate is some 100 times less effective than acetylsalicylate (aspirin) as an inhibitor of prostaglandin synthesis whereas they are of similar anti-inflammatory activity. Secondly, in experiments in which inflammation has been induced in essential fatty acid-deficient animals (i.e. animals rendered incapable of generating prostaglandins) aspirin has been shown to be as effective at reducing inflammation as it is in normal animals (Bonta et al., 1977). As a final example of the type of observation that is not compatible with this theory it has been shown that even small sub-anti-inflammatory doses of aspirin render the inflamed synovial tissue of arthritic joints incapable of producing prostaglandins for several days (Crook et al., 1976). Clearly, however compelling the idea that inhibition of prostaglandin synthesis is the explanation for the mechanism of action of aspirin, an explanation is required as to why regular high doses of the drug are needed to achieve an anti-inflammatory action when two or three tablets, two or three times a week would seem to be all that is necessary to induce effective inhibition of prostaglandin synthesis.

The relationship between prostaglandin synthesis and the NSAIDs is, thus, confused. On the one hand we have a convincing and attractive hypothesis which explains the many and varied activities and even side-effects of this group of drugs by one, simple and elegant mechanism. On the other hand we have evidence that not all anti-inflammatory drugs are good inhibitors of prostaglandin synthesis, that aspirin can exert an anti-inflammatory effect in the absence of any prostaglandin synthesis and that it is too good at inhibiting prostaglandin synthesis in rheumatic patients to explain why such large amounts of the drug are needed in clinical practice.

NSAIDs in sports injury

Whatever the mechanism by which these drugs exert their effect, their use in the treatment of chronic inflammatory disease is well established and their efficacy beyond question. Similarly in the treatment of acute traumatic injury their use has become commonplace and although far too many clinical trails have failed to furnish proof of their efficacy, clear evidence that these drugs are of benefit in sports injury has been produced. These drugs represent a simple and relatively safe means of reducing the inflammatory response to an injury. They may also help to return an injured sports participant to competitive fitness more rapidly. Many clinical trials compare the use of two different anti-inflammatory drugs but the most common finding is that there is no significant difference between the two. Where differences are reported they are not consistent. It would therefore be difficult to indicate a rank order of efficacy for these drugs.

Sprains (rupture of ligaments, which may be partial) strains (partial tearing of muscles) and bruises are all painful examples of sports injuries. Commonly they may warrant the use of painkilling (analgesic) drugs such as paracetamol or even in severe cases a narcotic analgesic compound such as dihydrocodeine. Since, however, these conditions are generally associated with an inflammatory component the use of an analgesic drug with anti-inflammatory activity would seem to be a more logical choice.

About twenty different NSAIDs are available which could be used to treat sports injuries and some details are given here of a small selection of them.

Aspirin

Aspirin is a very effective analgesic drug at a dose of 2–3 g per day. (In the UK aspirin tablets generally contain 300 mg). At higher doses, that is in excess of 4 g per day, aspirin will reduce the swelling of an inflamed joint, a property not shown at the lower, analgesic level. Whilst anti-inflammatory activity is seen only at higher doses it is inadvisable to exceed the normal recommended doses without qualified medical supervision. Despite the antiquity of this preparation, unequivocal evidence that any of the newer challengers offers an all-round superior performance is lacking. The general availability, and low cost of aspirin make it an ideal candidate for self-treatment following sports injury. Aspirin use is, however, not devoid of side-effects, although the risks involved with the use of the drug are probably generally overstated.

Given that the injured athlete is an otherwise normal, healthy adult, the major problem liable to be encountered following the use of aspirin (or indeed, for that matter, any of the NSAIDs) is gastric irritation which may be experienced as a form of dyspepsia. Attempts to reduce this problem by modifying the tablets in a variety of ways have not been particularly successful. It is now generally recognized that the effect of these drugs on the stomach is due not so much to the unabsorbed drug in contact with the gastric mucosa as to the effect of the drug after its absorption. The most effective way to minimize this problem is to avoid the use of these drugs when the stomach is empty. If the drugs are taken following a meal then any increased acid production that ensues can be utilized in the digestive process rather than being free to attack the lining of the stomach itself.

In 1984 Anderson and Gotzsche compared the use of aspirin and another NSAID, naproxen, in patients with sports injuries. Perhaps not surprisingly, they found no significant differences between the two drugs. Whilst this type of trial is common and the finding typical, the authors did highlight a phenomenon very relevant to the treatment of this type of traumatic injury. They demonstrated that significantly better results were obtained when the interval between injury and the start of treatment was shorter. This effect is widely appreciated now and is exactly what would be predicted from experimental inflammation studies in animals. In laboratory tests of the type used to screen for anti-inflammatory activity of new drugs for the treatment of arthritis it can be shown clearly that NSAIDs are much more effective against developing inflammation than they are against established inflammation.

The implications of this are clear. If it is deemed necessary to use an anti-inflammatory drug to treat a sports injury, it should be given as early as possible after the damage is sustained and certainly before the inflammation becomes established. The principal reason for this probably lies in the realm of the intravascular/extravascular fluid equilibrium. The role of permeability changes has already been highlighted. Protein moves through the blood vessel wall during the development of the inflammatory reaction and draws water with it resulting in the oedematous swelling. Once this oedema is formed, its resolution is dependent on the removal of the extravascular protein. NSAIDs do not appear to have any effect on the extravascular protein. It is an inevitable conclusion, therefore, that preventing oedema development is easier than resolving established oedema as there is no mechanism for the rapid removal of this protein for the resolution of an established reaction.

Naproxen

Naproxen is one of the mainstays of treatment for chronic inflammatory conditions. Its efficacy and safety record are excellent and it is one of the most frequently prescribed drugs for the treatment of arthritis. Since its introduction in the early 1970s naproxen has been the subject of a large number of trials in the treatment of soft tissue injuries. Whilst many of these compare naproxen with another NSAID and find no difference in activity, several trials have shown naproxen to be better than the other drug in some respects and naproxen has been shown to be superior to placebo. In view of the popularity of this drug and the generally good reports of its efficacy in the literature, naproxen must rank high amongst the most suitable drugs for the treatment of sporting injuries. The drug is given at a dose of 0.75–1.25 g per day in 3 or 4 divided doses. Initially a high loading dose of 500 mg may be given to aid the rapid attainment of suitable plasma levels of the drug (750 µg/ml). The drug may be taken at meal times to help combat any gastric discomfort felt, although in the presence of food the drug is absorbed more slowly. More rapid absorption occurs with the use of naproxen sodium. A 500 mg naproxen suppository preparation is available, principally for use at night.

Ibuprofen

Ibuprofen is another NSAID with a similar structure to naproxen. It is the oldest propionic acid derivative anti-inflammatory agent in use and considerable experience has, therefore, been obtained with it. This drug is also one of the few drugs of this class available in the UK without prescription. It has a reputation for being well tolerated. In other words, it is widely felt that this particular anti-inflammatory agent does not induce the same degree of dyspepsia as many of its rivals. In the UK, the Committee on Safety of Medicines (CSM) advises that ibuprofen is associated with the lowest risk of serious upper gastrointestinal side-effects of seven oral NSAIDs reviewed. The other NSAIDs considered by the CSM were piroxicam, ketoprofen, indomethacin, naproxen and diclofenac which were considered to be associated with intermediate risk and azapropazone which was considered to be associated with the highest risk.

Ibuprofen has always been perceived to be a well-tolerated drug. It is possible, however, that much of its reputation is based on early experiences with the drug when it was used at relatively low dose levels. To improve the often disappointing activity of ibuprofen the doses used have been increased and whilst the drug is still generally well tolerated it is certainly not without gastric irritant activity at these higher levels. Trials using ibuprofen at doses as low as 1200 mg per day have been shown to reduce pain and recovery time of soft-tissue sports injuries. Trials have, however, tended to use higher doses than this. Hutson (1986) found no significant differences between the activity of ibuprofen given at doses of 1.8 or 2.4 g daily amongst 46 patients with sporting injuries to the knee. The normal recommended dose range for ibuprofen for musculoskeletal disorders is 1.2–1.8 g daily in 3 or 4 divided doses, preferably after food. This may be increased if necessary to the maximum recommended daily dose of 2.4 g.

Indomethacin

Indomethacin has been used for treating inflammatory conditions since the mid-1960s and remains a very frequently prescribed drug. Whilst being an effective anti-inflammatory drug it does suffer, apart from the gastric irrit- ant activity somewhat typical of this type of drug, from a number of central nervous system side-effects such as headaches, dizziness and light-headedness. Generally, indomethacin is found to be of similar efficacy to other NSAIDs, such as naproxen, in the treatment of soft-tissue sports injuries. As might be expected, the drop-out rate due to side-effects of this drug is generally higher than for other members of this group of drugs with normal therapeutic doses of indomethacin (50–200 mg daily). The drug is normally initiated as 25 mg 2 or 3 times daily and gradually increased if necessary. Edwards *et al.* (1984) found it necessary to withdraw only one patient from a group of 53 who were receiving 75 mg of indomethacin daily for acute soft-tissue sports injuries. It is possible that at this low starting dose toxicity is less of a problem.

Indomethacin is also available in 100 mg suppositories for night-time use and these may be of benefit in some individuals. It should be remembered that the combined rectal and oral doses should not amount to more than 200 mg in a 24-hour period.

Piroxicam

Piroxicam appears to be comparable with indomethacin or naproxen in treating acute musculoskeletal injuries and it is generally well tolerated. One particular advantage of piroxicam is that it has a long half-life, which per- mits its use as a single daily dose, usually of 20 mg. An initial, loading dose of 40 mg on each of the first 2 days of treatment, reducing to 20 mg for subsequent days may be used for acute musculoskeletal disorders. In a large study of acute sports injuries in Norway the authors concluded that piroxicam at 40 mg daily for the first 2 days and 20 mg daily for a further 5 days resulted in significant improvements in mobility and reductions in pain when compared with placebo (Lereim and Gabor, 1988). This treatment gave a marginally superior response when compared with naproxen at 500 mg twice daily, and both drugs were well tolerated.

Piroxicam may also be given as a deep intramuscular injection for the initial dose. Effective concentrations of drugs are usually achieved earlier in this way than when they are administered orally.

Diclofenac

Diclofenac is another useful drug of this class. Available in both 75 and 100 mg tablets, daily doses of 75–150 mg are recommended. In a trial involving subjects with severely sprained ankles, diclofenac at 150 mg daily was shown to be superior to both placebo and piroxicam at 20 mg daily (Bahamonde and Saavedra, 1990). Both drugs were well tolerated. One possible advantage of this drug is that it is available in a slow-release form that is administered once daily, although this may be less of an advantage in the acute situation. In general, therapeutic levels are not achieved as rapidly with drugs that have a long half-life. Drugs with a short duration of action will normally give therapeutic levels in a very short period of time.

Phenylbutazone

Phenylbutazone was introduced into clinical medicine in 1949 to take its place alongside the salicylates for the treatment of arthritic conditions. It is a powerful anti-inflammatory drug and is capable of treating acute exacerbations of rheumatoid arthritis and severe ankylosing spondylitis (an inflammatory condition of the spine). Compared with the many, newer anti-inflammatory agents now available it is subject to a large number of toxic side-effects, some of which have led to fatal outcomes. Whilst many physicians believe this to be an extraordinarily useful anti-inflammatory agent, others have argued that it is too dangerous to use. The most serious side-effects are undoubtedly the retention of fluid which in predisposed individuals may precipitate cardiac failure, and the interference with normal blood cell production, most commonly resulting in aplastic anaemia and agranulocytosis which can occur within the first few days of treatment. Its use, therefore, in self-limiting musculoskeletal disorders is difficult to justify. In the UK phenylbutazone is now only indicated for the treatment of ankylosing spondylitis in hospital situations.

Its inclusion in this chapter is because of its historical use in sports injuries and its use in equestrian sport. In the past it has been somewhat abused, particularly in the United States. A report by Marshall (1979) indicates that in the National Football League, for example, an average of 24–40 unit doses of phenylbutazone was used per player per season.

Whatever the role of phenylbutazone in injuries in sportsmen and women, there is no doubt that this drug has been used considerably in the field of equestrian sports. In show jumping the horses' feet are subjected to constant concussion. By the age of 10 many show-jumping horses will have suffered pathological changes in their feet but in many cases will be at their peak. Similarly 3-day event horses are subject to considerable physical stress, with strain of a tendon or the suspensory ligament being common injuries. Even without jumping-related competition, the regular galloping activity, as in for example, flat racing or polo, may result in substantial changes in bones, joints and ligaments of a horse. When pushed too hard or for too long lameness may develop due to the pain and inflammation caused. The time-honoured remedy for reducing the pain and inflammation of these injuries in horses is to administer an anti-inflammatory drug, the most frequently used example being phenylbutazone.

Horses generally tolerate phenylbutazone very well and may be treated with the drug to improve their comfort. Whilst there are many indications for the use of phenylbutazone in horses, dilemmas do arise as to whether their use may mask an injury and lead to a complete breakdown of an affected limb. The governing bodies of equestrian sports generally recognize the usefulness of this drug but exclude the use of the drug on, or immediately before, competition days in order that no unfair advantage may be gained by improving performance and also to protect unfit horses from being used competitively.

Cyclo-oxygenase 2 inhibitors

These newer NSAIDs are notable for their selective inhibition of the inducible cyclo-oxygenase 2. If the ability to inhibit the cyclo-oxygenase enzyme selectively is advantageous for the treatment of acute inflammatory problems then these drugs may prove to be valuable in the future. In 2004, one member of this group of drugs, Rofecoxib, was withdrawn from the market after reports of cardiotoxic side-effects.

Duration of NSAID treatment

There are obvious advantages to the early treatment of inflammatory responses to injury. How long treatment should continue is less clear. Studies of NSAID treatment of soft tissue injuries in animals have generally demonstrated the advantage of treatment in the early, post-injury stage. The effectiveness of treatment over longer periods is less apparent. Some sports injuries studies have also reported no differences between treated and untreated groups at later stages of the inflammatory and healing processes.

In self-limiting injuries healing will generally occur without treatment. It is perhaps inevitable that differences between treated and non-treated groups will diminish with time. Whilst treatment may result in earlier return to normality, untreated subjects are likely to 'catch up'. There is, however, an alternative interpretation, which is that NSAIDs may actually slow down the healing process. Inhibiting the influx of inflammatory cells, particularly polymorphonuclear leucocytes, may limit the amount of local tissue injury that occurs following trauma. It is possible that this may lead to the slower removal of damaged tissue and a consequent delay in the resolution of the injury. The production of scar tissue may be impaired if fibroblast activity is reduced and this could, indeed, reduce the speed at which fully functional tissues are reformed (see Almekinders, 1999).

There is no consistent evidence that NSAIDs delay healing and, in consequence, explanations of possible mechanisms are largely speculative. Whilst

Table 8.1 Commonly available topical preparations in the UK

Piroxicam	Feldene
Ibuprofen	Fenbid Forte Gel, Ibugel, Ibumousse, Ibuspray, Proflex
Ketoprofen	Oruvail, Powergel
Felbinac	Traxam
Diclofenac	Voltarol

sports injuries studies with NSAIDs do not universally demonstrate their efficacy, the majority do. It would, therefore, seem to be a reasonable approach to treat acute traumatic sporting injuries immediately with NSAIDs but to discontinue treatment as soon as it is apparent that the acute inflammatory problem is resolving.

Topical NSAIDs in sports injury

Several pharmaceutical companies produce topical preparations of NSAIDs for the relief of musculoskeletal pain. Topical preparations of salicylates, piroxicam, ibuprofen, ketoprofen, felbinac (the active metabolite of fenbufen) and diclofenac are currently available in the UK (see Table 8.1). The concept of applying a NSAID locally in an effort to maximize the level of the drug at the site of injury whilst minimizing the systemic level of the drug is an interesting one. In theory this technique may achieve a good therapeutic effect without the troublesome gastrointestinal side-effects sometimes encountered with systemic therapy. There is good evidence that these preparations afford good penetration of the drug through the skin and that high levels of the active drug are achieved in the underlying tissues. Clinical trials with these preparations generally demonstrate that active drug formulations are more effective than placebo, but the differences are generally slight. In one celebrated double-blind study patients suffering bilateral inflammatory knee joint effusions were treated with diclofenac gel to one knee and a placebo gel to the other (Radermacher *et al.*, 1991). It was found that there were small reductions in swelling in both knees and no significant difference between the drug-treated and placebo-treated knees could be detected. In other words it did not seem to matter which knee the NSAID was applied to!

It has been suggested that the massage of an affected area with a gel or cream may in itself be beneficial irrespective of the presence of a NSAID. A significant point which should be considered here is whether these compounds actually exert their anti-inflammatory action at the inflamed site or elsewhere. If, for example, the reality of the situation is that the drugs reduce inflammation by interacting in some way with components in the bloodstream, then the concept of local application would be flawed. The statement found in the British National Formulary (2001) that these preparations 'may provide some slight relief of pain in musculoskeletal conditions' would seem to be a reasonable conclusion to this section.

Proteolytic enzymes as anti-inflammatory agents

Several reports have been published suggesting that proteolytic enzyme preparations are useful for the treatment of soft-tissue sports injuries. Hyaluronidase, which splits the glucosaminidic bonds of hyaluronic acid, reduces the viscosity of the cellular cement. Local injections of this enzyme have been shown to reduce healing time of sprained ankles. Chymotrypsin preparations, which are available in tablet form, have also been found to be useful in sporting injuries. Whilst these enzymes are obviously vulnerable to gastrointestinal breakdown, there is evidence that some active enzyme is absorbed. A number of clinical trials have been conducted amongst professional soccer players and whilst not all have shown favourable results, some trials have found significant reductions in the recovery time to match fitness. This is particularly the case when a haematoma or sprain is the major feature of the injury. In one notable trial an enzyme preparation was compared with placebo in injured footballers of a London club. The physicians monitoring the trial were so impressed by the apparent efficacy of the enzyme that the trial was abandoned since it was considered unjustifiable to withhold the enzyme from the placebo group (Boyne and Medhurst, 1967). This was deemed especially so since the club was in the running for major honours in that season!

Here though we have an enigma. On the one hand we have apparently convincing reports that proteolytic enzyme preparations aid recovery from sports injury. On the other hand we are faced with the fact that the bulk of these reports are over 30 years old. If these preparations could significantly reduce recovery time and return players to match fitness in perhaps only 70 per cent of the normal time it should take, why are they not in use? Perhaps the optimistic initial findings have not been reproducible on subsequent occasions or perhaps toxicity has limited their use; it is true that occasionally serious hypersensitivity reactions do occur when administering high molecular weight substances such as enzymes. Whilst they are not used now for treating mechanically induced trauma, these preparations are regularly used in a variety of post-surgical situations to reduce oedema.

Anti-inflammatory steroids

Many of the body's natural hormones are based on the four-ring steroid structure. The precise activity of a steroid depends on which of a small number of substitutions are made to the structure (Figure 8.1). Some steroids (oestrogens, progesterones and testosterones) have powerful effects on

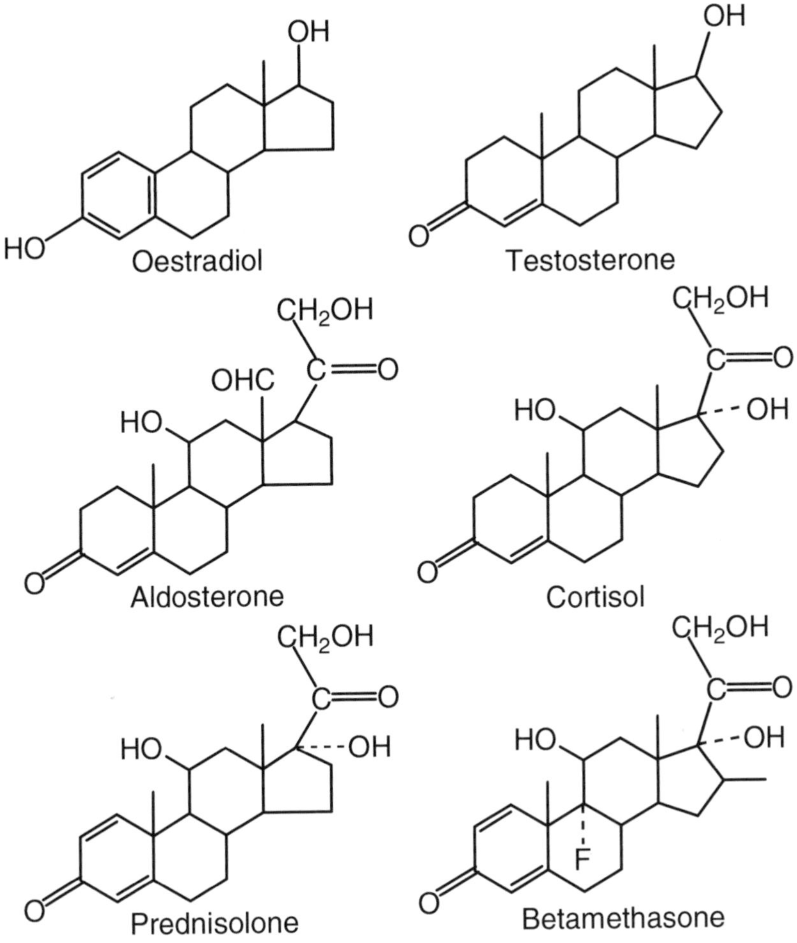

Figure 8.1 Structures of some steroids.

sex-related attributes and activities. Others, such as the glucocorticoids or mineralocorticoids, influence the metabolic activities or fluid balance of the body. The activities of steroids are seldom completely specific and often overlap each other. Of interest here are the most powerful anti-inflammatory agents known to humankind, the glucocorticoids. These are drugs that are based on the chemical structure of the steroids produced by the cortex of the adrenal gland and are generally referred to as corticosteroids. These corticosteroids were first used to treat inflammatory conditions in the late 1940s (Hench *et al.*, 1949). They represented an exciting and, possibly, fundamental new approach to the treatment of inflammatory disease. Initial optimism waned rapidly, however, as it quickly became apparent that these substances were not curative and that they were subject to considerable numbers of side-effects. The anti-inflammatory activity of these steroid hormones appears to be secondary to their glucocorticoid function, as despite the severe metabolic derangement which accompanies adrenal gland insufficiency (Addison's disease) there is no general precipitation of inflammatory reactions.

Many attempts have been made to increase the anti-inflammatory activity of these steroids. A large number of anti-inflammatory steroids are now available, many of which are an order of magnitude more potent than cortisol. All of these steroids have significant glucocorticoid activity. Inevitably, long-term use of these drugs will affect the general metabolic activity of the body and is likely to provoke symptoms similar to those seen when the adrenal cortex is hyperactive (Cushing's syndrome). It is, therefore, important that a distinction is made between the long-term use of anti-inflammatory steroids and their use in acute situations. The long-term use of these drugs may lead to a number of side-effects, some of which may be particularly unfortunate for an athlete. Osteoporosis is frequently encountered during corticosteroid therapy. This serious weakening of the skeletal structure affects principally those bones with the most trabecular structure such as the ribs and vertebrae and vertebral compression fractures are a frequent complication of steroid therapy. Long-term use of a drug which may weaken the bone structure of an individual (whose sporting activities may subject that structure to greater than normal stress) should not be contemplated lightly.

Perhaps an even more significant problem, however, is the catabolic effect of glucocorticoids on skeletal muscle. Weakness of muscles in the arms and legs can occur soon after treatment is started, even with quite modest doses of these anti-inflammatory drugs. Experiments with rats have shown that very significant reductions in muscle weight can occur within 7 days of treatment (Bullock et al., 1971). If long-term systemic steroid treatment is initiated, it must be realized that as well as the anti-inflammatory effect which will be achieved, the administered drug will largely take over the glucocorticoid role of the natural adrenal hormone. Due to negative feedback mechanisms operating in both the hypothalamus and the anterior pituitary, the release of corticotrophin-releasing factor and adrenocorticotrophic hormone is inhibited and so the adrenal cortex is not stimulated to produce its own glucocorticoids normally. Over a period of time the adrenal cortex regresses to a state such that the adrenal gland can no longer produce sufficient quantities of glucocorticoid to support the body if the drug treatment is stopped suddenly. It is important, therefore, that following long-term treatment with a steroid, the drug must be withdrawn gradually by progressively lowering the daily dose.

Steroids are double-edged weapons in the armoury of anti-inflammatory therapy. They are powerful, anti-inflammatory drugs but they are, unfortunately, subject to a great many side-effects. The direct application of these drugs to an affected site such that a high concentration of the steroid is achieved locally but without the attainment of significant systemic levels offers the possibility of gaining the maximum usefulness of steroids with minimal toxicity. Direct application of steroids to the skin is not an entirely satisfactory method as, although they are generally well absorbed, large proportions of the active drug will be transported away by the blood and, therefore, accumulation in affected muscle or connective tissue is limited. Additionally, topical application of steroids tends to cause thinning of the skin and a slowing down of wound healing.

The local injection of a corticosteroid preparation does offer considerable advantages in the treatment of an inflammatory condition restricted to a small area of the body. Early attempts to inject steroids locally were not particularly successful as these highly soluble drugs were rapidly redistributed from the site. The development of less soluble esters of hydrocortisone and prednisolone to give fairly insoluble microcrystalline preparations which are injected as suspensions has markedly improved the successfulness of this particular technique. A single dose of an insoluble steroid preparation will provide relief for several days or even several weeks. If necessary, these local injections can be repeated to extend the period of effectiveness. Great care must be taken when injections of steroids are given that aseptic precautions are taken to minimize the risk of the introduction of infective agents. This is especially the case where injections have to be administered intra-articularly to improve mobility and restrict damage of an affected joint. In the case of intra-articular injection, the use of a long-acting preparation such as triamcinolone hexacetonide is indicated so that repeated injections are less necessary, or at least, less frequent.

Local injection of steroids is also valuable for the treatment of soft tissue injuries. They may be injected into the interior of a bursa (the fibrous sac, filled with synovial fluid which may be found between muscles or between a tendon and bone, and which facilitates frictionless movement between the surfaces that it separates), into a tendon sheath to reduce the inflammation of an affected tendon or infiltrated around the area of an inflamed ligament. Tendinitis of the elbow (tennis elbow) is a classic example of the type of injury that responds well to local corticosteroid injection.

Steroids do have the property of delaying the wound healing process. Particular care should be taken when using them in situations where extensive new tissue will have to be produced (as may be the case, for example, where a collision on the sports field has led to an open wound). In this instance the use of steroids to reduce inflammation may not be appropriate.

Glucocorticoids are included in the WADA list of prohibited classes of substances. Dermatological administration is permitted, however, administration by other routes, such as orally, rectally and intravenous, intramuscular or intraarticular injection is permitted only when medically necessary and subject to a Therapeutic Use Exemption (TUE). Administration of corticosteroids by inhalation, for the treatment of asthma, is permitted subject to an Abbreviated TUE.

The means by which these steroids exert their anti-inflammatory effects is not clear. It is probable that they have a number of activities, all of which contribute to their anti-inflammatory effects. They have been shown to reduce the output of chemical mediators of inflammation and to inhibit the effects of mediators on the vascular endothelium, resulting in a reduction of oedema formation. They have also been shown to have a number of inhibitory actions on the responsiveness of white blood cells. They are, for example, particularly effective in reducing the activity of thymocytes, which are involved with delayed hypersensitivity reactions. Whatever their mechanism of action, and despite the potential hazards of long-term, high-dose therapy, glucocorticoids are profoundly effective in the reduction of inflammatory reactions and their place in the treatment of sporting injuries is assured.

8.5   Summary

Following a brief introduction putting sports injury in perspective, the nature of the inflammatory response is described. The role of chemical mediators of inflammation and the contribution of leucocytes to the inflammation is detailed.

The treatment of sporting injuries is then discussed with particular reference to the use of aerosol sprays, oral and topical NSAIDs, proteolytic enzymes and anti-inflammatory glucocorticoids. The place of each therapy is discussed and possible mechanisms of action of the drugs outlined.

8.6   References

Almekinders, L.C. (1999) Anti-inflammatory treatment of muscular injuries in sport. An update of recent studies. *Sports Med.*, **28**, 383–388.
Anderson, L.A. and Gotzsche, P.C. (1984) Naproxen and aspirin in acute musculoskeletal disorders: a double-blind, parallel study in patients with sports injuries. *Pharmacotherapeutica*, **3**, 531–537.
Bahamonde, L.A. and Saavedra, C. (1990) Comparison of the analgesic and anti-inflammatory effects of diclofenac potassium versus piroxicam versus placebo in ankle sprain patients. *J. Int. Med. Res.*, **18**, 104–111.
Bonta, I.L., Bult, H., Vincent, J.E. and Ziglstra, F.J. (1977) Acute anti-inflammatory effects of aspirin and dexamethasone in rats deprived of endogenous prostaglandin precursors. *J. Pharm. Pharmacol.*, **29**, 1–7.
Boyne, P.S. and Medhurst, H. (1967) Oral anti-inflammatory enzyme therapy in injuries in professional footballers. *The Practitioner*, **198**, 543–546.
British National Formulary (2001) British Medical Association and Royal Pharmaceutical Society of Great Britain, London.
Bullock, G.J., Carter, E.E., Elliott P., Peters R.F., Simpson, P. and White, A.M. (1971) Relative changes in the function of muscle ribosomes, and mitochondria during the early phase of steroid-induced catabolism. *Biochem. J.*, **127**, 881–892.

Crook, D., Collins, A.J., Bacon, P.A. and Chan, R. (1976) Prostaglandin synthetase activity from human rheumatoid synovial microsomes. *Ann. Rheum. Dis.*, **35**, 327–332.

Edwards, V., Wilson, A.A., Harwood, H.F. *et al.* (1984) A multicentre comparison of piroxicam and indomethacin in acute soft tissue sports injuries. *J. Int. Med. Res.*, **12**, 46–50.

Ferreira, S.H., Moncada, S. and Vane, J.R. (1971) Indomethacin and aspirin abolish prostaglandin release from the spleen. *Nature, New Biol.*, **231**, 237–239.

Hench, P.S., Kendall, E.C., Slocumb, C.H. and Polley, H.F. (1949) The effect of a hormone of the adrenal cortex (17-hydroxy-11-dehydrocorticosterone: compound E) and of pituitary adrenocorticotropic hormone on rheumatoid arthritis. *Proc. Staff Meet. Mayo Clinic*, **24**, 181–197.

Hutson, M.A. (1986) A double-blind study comparing ibuprofen 1800 mg or 2400 mg daily and placebo in sports injuries. *J. Int. Med. Res.*, **4**, 142–147.

Lewis, T. (1927) *The blood vessels of the human skin and their responses.* Shaw and Sons, London.

Lereim, P. and Gabor, I. (1988) Piroxicam and naproxen in acute sports injuries. *Am. J. Med.*, **84** (Suppl. 5A), 45–49.

MacLagan, T. (1876) The treatment of acute rheumatism by salacin. *Lancet*, **i**, 342–346.

Marshall, E. (1979) Drugging of football players curbed by central monitoring plan, NFL claims. *Science*, **203**, 626–628.

Radermacher, J., Jentsch, D., Scholl, M.A., Lustinetz, T. and Frolich, C. (1991) Diclofenac concentrations in synovial fluid and plasma after cutaneous application in inflammatory and degenerative joint disease. *Br. J. Clin. Pharmacol.*, **31**, 537–541.

Smith, J.B. and Willis, A.L. (1971) Aspirin selectively inhibits prostaglandin production in human platelets. *Nature, New Biol.*, **231**, 235–237.

Vane, J.R. (1971) Inhibition of prostaglandin synthesis as a mechanism of action for aspirin-like drugs. *Nature, New Biol.*, **231**, 232–235.

Virchow, R. (1858) *Cellular Pathology.*

Chapter 9

Alcohol, anti-anxiety drugs and sport

Thomas Reilly

9.1 Introduction

Throughout civilization and up to the present day human ingenuity has found various ways of coping with the stresses that life brings. Sometimes these entail a form of escapism into a drug-induced illusory world to eschew temporary troubles. A resort to alcohol, for example, can bring a transient euphoric uplift from pressing matters of the day. These strategies are perhaps truer today than they were in Dionysian cultures, exceptions being those countries where alcohol is taboo for religious reasons. It is generally believed that stress-induced illness is a phenomenon of contemporary urban civilization. The widespread prescription of tranquillizers and the high incidence of alcohol addiction support this view. Their impact on fitness and well-being has received scant attention.

Amongst athletes, participation in sports brings its own unique form of stress, usually before the more important contests. Though a certain amount of pre-competition anxiety is inevitable, the anxiety response varies enormously between individuals, with some people coping extremely poorly. Many find their own solutions to attenuate anxiety levels, albeit sometimes with exogenous aids. Anxiety may adversely affect performance, especially in activities highly demanding of mental concentration and steadiness of limbs. This has prompted the use of anti-anxiety drugs, although some are not permitted in many sports.

In this chapter the relationship between anxiety and sport performance is first explored. The next section concentrates on alcohol, its metabolism in the body and its effect on the central nervous system. The interactions between alcohol and health are then considered. Its impact on physiological responses to exercise and the uses in sport are examined next. The main 'minor' tranquillizers, the benzodiazepines and melatonin, are discussed before, finally, the uses and abuses of other anti-anxiety drugs are described.

9.2   Anxiety and performance

The psychological reaction to impending sports competition is variously referred to as anxiety, arousal, stress or activation. Though these concepts are not synonymous, their relationships to performance have sufficient similarities to group them together for the present purposes. Anxiety denotes worry or emotional tension, arousal denotes a continuum from sleep to high excitement, stress implies an agent that induces strain in the organism and activation refers to the metabolic state in the 'flight or fight' reaction. Irrespective of which concept is adopted, the effects of the biological responses on performance are generally assumed to fit an inverted-U curve. A moderate level of 'anxiety' about the forthcoming activity is deemed desirable to induce the right levels of harnessed motivation for action. The simpler the task the higher will be the level of anxiety that can be tolerated before performance efficiency begins to fall (Figure 9.1).

Although the inverted-U model is somewhat simplistic, it does illustrate that over-anxiety has a detrimental effect on the physical and psychomotor elements that comprise sports performance. In such instances anxiety-reducing strategies will have an ergogenic effect. The athlete or mentor may have to choose between mental relaxation techniques or drugs to alleviate anxiety.

There are various indices which the behavioural scientist employs in measuring anxiety in field conditions, such as sport, especially prior to competition. These include hand tremor, restlessness or other subjective estimates of 'tension', paper and pencil tests and so on. Linked to these are physiological indices which demonstrate increased sympathetic tone. These measures include muscular tension as indicated by electromyography, galvanic skin response or skin conductance and elevated concentrations of stress hormones or their metabolites in blood or in urine. These variables may be important

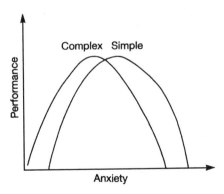

Figure 9.1 The relationship between level of anxiety and performance efficiency for simple and complex tasks.

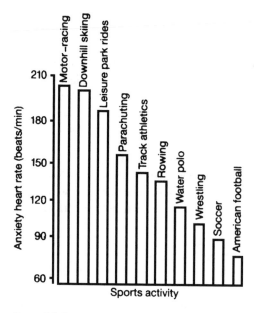

Figure 9.2 Pre-activity heart rate for various sports and recreations.

to consider if the mechanisms by which the ergogenic or adverse effects of anxiety-reducing drugs operate are to be understood.

High levels of anxiety generally militate against performance and so favour attempts to reduce anxiety. Anxiety level depends very much on the nature of the sport as well as on the individual concerned. Generally, high anxiety is associated with brief and high-risk activities. A league table of anxiety responses pre-start (Figure 9.2), as reflected in emotional tachycardia, shows motor-racing and downhill skiing to be top of the list. Activities like parachuting and high acceleration rides in leisure parks induce strong anxiety reactions albeit mingled with a feeling of exhilaration. In these cases heart rates have been found to correlate highly with adrenaline levels in blood and in urine (Reilly *et al.*, 1985). American football is lowest in the table, possibly because of the practice of relaxation techniques in this group and the long duration of such games.

Professional athletes regularly subjected to situations of high psychological stress tend to adapt. At this elite level highly anxious personalities are rare. The anxiety reaction of professional soccer players, for example, is highly reproducible although there are noticeable trends. Resting heart rates in the dressing-room tend to be higher when playing at home rather than away, because players are subject to more critical scrutiny by a home audience. Anxiety is highest in goalkeepers, for whose mistakes the team is usually punished. Players returning to the team after a spell of injury or making an initial appearance in the premier team show higher heart rates than their normal pre-match values. It is hardly surprising to find that goalkeepers are the most vulnerable members of the team to stress-related illnesses such as stomach ulcers.

Avoiding over-anxiety may be important in game players for reasons of safety. Anxiety has been found to correlate with joint and muscle injuries in soccer, the more anxious players tending to get injured most often. This supports the notion of injury proneness: the mechanism is probably lack of commitment or hesitancy in critical events (such as tackling) that might promote injury (Sanderson, 1981). Traditionally, some soccer players used to take a nip of whisky immediately prior to going on to the pitch, the communal bottle being euphemistically referred to as 'team spirit'. The inhibiting effects of alcohol used to be exploited by tournament rugby players, who were not averse to drinking beer in between rounds of 'rugby sevens' competitions for example.

Obviously there is a thin line to tread between, on the one hand, reducing anxiety to enhance well-being and mental states prior to competing in sport and, on the other hand, impairing performance because of a disruption in motor co-ordination accompanying the treatment. The outcome depends on the concentrations of the drug, the timing of ingestion and the individual susceptibility to it. There are also possibilities of tolerance to the drug with chronic use or of drug dependence developing. Residual effects may carry over to the following day, affecting training or subsequent competitive performance. These aspects are now considered in the context of alcohol in sports and exercise.

9.3 Alcohol

Metabolism of alcohol

The alcohols are a group of chemicals, most of which are toxic. The most common is ethanol or ethyl alcohol which is obtained by the fermentation of sugar. It is non-toxic, except in large and chronic doses, and has been enjoyed as a beverage for many centuries.

Ethyl alcohol is both a drug and a food, accounting for about 100 kcal (420 kJ) of energy per adult of the UK population each day. Its energy value per unit weight (kcal/g), the Atwater factor, is 7 compared with a value of 9 for fat, but this is higher than the value of 4 for both carbohydrate and protein. Wine contains about 12 per cent alcohol, and so a litre bottle will contain about 120 g with a calorific content of 840 kcal (3516 kJ). The value of alcohol as a food stuff is limited, as it is metabolized mainly in the liver and at a fixed rate of about 100 mg/kg body weight per hour. For a 70-kg individual this amounts to 7 g of alcohol hourly. The energy is not available to active skeletal muscle and consequently it is not possible to exercise oneself to sobriety. Beer contains some electrolytes but its subsequent diuretic effect makes it less than the ideal agent of rehydration after hard physical training.

Alcohol is a polar substance which is freely miscible in water. This is due to the fact that alcohol molecules are held together by the same sort of intermolecular forces as water, namely hydrogen bonds. The alcohol molecule is also soluble in fat, it is small and has a weak charge. (As the lipophilic alkyl group becomes larger and the hydrophilic group smaller, the alcohol molecules associate preferentially with other alcohol, hydrocarbon or lipid molecules rather than water.) It easily penetrates biological membranes and can be absorbed unaltered from the stomach and more quickly from the small intestine. The rate of absorption is influenced by the amount of food in the stomach, whether there are gas molecules in the drink and the concentration of alcohol in the drink. Absorption is quickest if alcohol is drunk on an empty stomach, if gas molecules are present in the drink and the alcohol content is high. Intense mental concentration, lowered body temperature or physical exercise tend to slow the rate of absorption.

From the gastrointestinal tract the alcohol is transported to the liver by means of the hepatic circulation. The activity of the enzyme alcohol dehydrogenase, present chiefly in the liver, governs the disappearance of alcohol from the body. In the liver, alcohol dehydrogenase converts the alcohol to acetaldehyde; it is then converted to acetic acid or acetate by aldehyde dehydrogenase. About 75 per cent of the alcohol taken up by the blood is released as acetate into the circulation. The acetate is then oxidized to carbon dioxide and water within the Krebs (or citric acid) cycle. An alternative metabolic route for acetate is its activation to acetyl co-enzyme A and further reactions to form fatty acids, ketone bodies, amino acids and steroids.

Ethyl alcohol is distributed throughout the body by means of the circulatory system and enters all the body water pools and tissues, including the central nervous system. Its distribution amongst the body fluids and tissues depends on several factors, such as blood flow, mass and permeability of the tissue. Organs such as the brain, lungs, liver and kidneys reach equilibrium quickly, whilst skeletal muscle with its relatively poorer blood supply attains its peak alcohol concentration more slowly. Initially, alcohol moves rapidly from blood into the tissues. When absorption is complete, arterial alcohol concentration falls and alcohol diffuses from the tissues into the capillary bed. This means that alcohol concentrations remain high in the peripheral venous blood due to the slower rates of metabolism and excretion.

The metabolism of alcohol in the liver is unaffected by its concentration in the blood. Some alcohol is eliminated in the breath, but this is usually less than 5 per cent of the total amount metabolized. This route is utilized in assessing safe levels for driving, forming the basis of the breathalyser tests. Small amounts of alcohol are excreted in urine and also in sweat if exercise is performed whilst drunk. Higher excretion rates through the lungs, urine and sweat are produced at high environmental temperatures and at high blood alcohol levels.

With a single drink the blood alcohol level usually peaks about 45 minutes after ingestion. This is the point where any influence on performance will be most evident. Effects on performance will generally be greater on the ascending limb than for a corresponding value on the descending limb of the blood alcohol curve; the rate of change and the direction of change of the blood alcohol concentration are more crucial factors than is the length of time alcohol is in the bloodstream. The peak is delayed about 15 minutes if strenuous exercise precedes the ingestion. This delay may be due to the reduction in blood flow to the gut that accompanies exercise, the increased blood flow to skeletal muscle and the needs of the thermoregulatory system post-exercise.

Besides the exogenous ethanol in body fluids, trace amounts of ethanol are synthesized endogenously. This endogenous ethanol is thought to arise both from bacterial fermentation in the gut and from the action of alcohol dehydrogenase on acetaldehyde derived from pyruvate. Blood levels of endogenous alcohol in the human are very low, ranging only up to about 7.5 mg in total.

Studies on alcohol and exercise are notoriously difficult to control, as most subjects will recognize the taste of the experimental treatment. Most experimenters use vodka in orange juice as the alcohol beverage: the placebo can include enough vodka to taste but not enough to produce a measurable blood alcohol concentration. Another strategy is to put a nose clip on the subject, who is then given anaesthetic throat lozenges. Subjects vary in their responses to alcohol, as does the same subject from day to day, making inferences from laboratory studies difficult. As the effects of alcohol differ with body size, dosage is usually administered according to body weight. Effects also vary with the level of blood alcohol induced, but there is not general international agreement on acceptable maximum levels for day-to-day activities such as driving. Alcohol doses that render subjects intoxicated or drunk have little practical relevance in exercise studies and so experimental levels are usually low to moderate. Additionally, experiments that entail alcohol ingestion should be approved by the local human ethics committee, and high alcohol dosages are unlikely to gain acceptance in experimental protocols.

Action of alcohol on the nervous system

The effects of ethanol administration on central nervous tissue are due to direct action rather than to acetaldehyde, its first breakdown product. Following ethanol ingestion, very little acetaldehyde crosses the blood–brain barrier, despite elevated levels in the blood. Alcohol has a general effect on neural transmission by influencing axonal membranes and slowing nerve conductance] The permeability of the axonal membrane to potassium and sodium is altered by the lowering of central calcium levels that results from ingesting alcohol (Wesnes and Warburton, 1983). Alcohol has differential effects on the central neurotransmitters, acetylcholine, serotonin, noradrenaline and dopamine.

Alcohol blocks the release of acetylcholine and disrupts its synthesis. As a result, transmission in the central cholinergic pathways will be lowered. The ascending reticular cholinergic pathway determines the level of cortical arousal and the flow of sensory information to be evaluated by the cortex. The lowering of electro-cortical arousal reduces the awareness of stressful information and the ability of the individual to attend to specific stimuli. These de-arousing changes are reflected in alterations in the electroencephalogram with moderate to large doses of alcohol. [The obvious results are impairments in concentration, attention, simple and complex reaction times, skilled performance and, eventually, short-term memory].

Alcohol decreases serotonin turnover in the central nervous system by inhibiting tryptophan hydroxylase, the enzyme essential for serotonin's biosynthesis. Activity in the neurones of serotonergic pathways is important for the experience of anxiety; output of corticosteroid hormones from the adrenal cortex increases the activity in these neurones. Alcohol has an opposing action and so may reduce the tension that is felt by the individual in a stressful situation.

An effect of alcohol is to increase activity in central noradrenergic pathways. This is transient and is followed, some hours later, by a decrease in activity. Catecholaminergic pathways are implicated in the control of mood states, activation of these pathways promoting happy and merry states. The fall in noradrenaline turnover as the blood alcohol concentration drops ties in with the reversal of mood that follows the initial drunken euphoric state. This is exacerbated by large doses of alcohol as these tend to give rise to depression.

The small alcohol molecules penetrating the blood–brain barrier stimulate the brain to release dopamine. Dopamine is regarded as a 'pleasure-related' hormone and its release is triggered in the limbic system. Stimulation of sweat glands also affects the limbic system whilst cerebral cortical activity is depressed. Pain sensors are numbed and later the cerebellum is affected, causing difficulty with balance.

Alcohol also has an effect on cerebral energy metabolism: the drug increases glucose utilization in the brain. As glucose is the main substrate furnishing energy for nerve cells, the result is that the lowered glucose level may induce mental fatigue. This will be reflected in failing cognitive functions, a decline in mental concentration and in information processing. It is unlikely that exercise, *per se*, will offset these effects.

The disruption of acetylcholine synthesis and release means that alcohol acts as a depressant, exerting its effect on the reticular activating system, whose activity represents the level of physiological arousal. It also has a depressant effect on the cortex: it first affects the frontal centres of the cortex before affecting the cerebellum. In large quantities it will interfere with speech and muscular co-ordination, eventually inducing sedation. In smaller doses it inhibits cerebral control mechanisms, freeing the brain from its normal inhibition. This release of inhibition has been blamed for aggressive and violent conduct of individuals behaving out of character when under the influence of alcohol. Undoubtedly, alcohol has been a factor in crowd violence and football hooliganism on the terraces. The belief led to the banning of alcohol at football and cricket grounds in Britain in the mid-1980s. These restrictions were extended to other sporting events in the years that followed.

Clearly, alcohol will have deleterious effects on performance in sports that require fast reactions, complex decision making and highly skilled actions. It will also have an impact on hand–eye co-ordination, on tracking tasks, such as driving, and on vigilance tasks such as long-distance sailing. An effect on tracking tasks is that control movements lose their normal smoothness and precision and become more abrupt or jerky. In vigilance tasks, some studies have shown a deterioration in performance with time on task (Tong et al., 1980). At high doses of alcohol, meaningful sport becomes impractical or even dangerous. Progressive effects of alcohol at different blood alcohol concentrations are summarized in Table 9.1. An important effect of alcohol, not listed, is that it diminishes the ability to process

Table 9.1 Demonstrable effects of alcohol at different blood alcohol concentrations

Concentration level (mg/100 ml blood)	Effects
30	Enhanced sense of well-being; retarded simple reaction time; impaired hand–eye co-ordination
60	Mild loss of social inhibition; impaired judgement
90	Marked loss of social inhibition; co-ordination reduced; noticeably 'under the influence'
120	Apparent clumsiness; loss of physical control; tendency towards extreme responses; definite drunkenness is noted
150	Erratic behaviour; slurred speech; staggering gait
180	Loss of control of voluntary activity; impaired vision

appreciable amounts of information arriving simultaneously from two different sources.

The most frequently cited study that reported facilitatory effects of alcohol on human performance was the classic experiment of Ikai and Steinhaus (1961). They showed that in some cases moderate alcohol doses could improve isometric muscular strength. This result was similar to that obtained by cheering and loud vocal encouragement. They explained the effect on the basis of central inhibition of the impulse traffic in the nerve fibres of the skeletal muscles during maximal effort. This depression of the inhibitory effect of certain centres in the central nervous system may allow routine practices to proceed normally without any disturbing effects. This finding has not generally been replicated when other aspects of muscular performance are considered. These are reviewed in a later section.

Alcohol and health

The effects of alcohol on health are usually viewed in terms of chronic alcoholism. Persistent drinking leads to a dependence on alcohol so that it becomes addictive. Most physicians emphasize that alcoholism is a disease rather than a vice and devise therapy accordingly. The result of excessive drinking is ultimately manifested in liver disease: cirrhosis, a serious hardening and degeneration of liver tissue, is fatal for many heavy drinkers. Cancer is also more likely to develop in a cirrhotic liver. There is evidence of increased susceptibility to breast cancer in women who drink alcohol regularly (Willett et al., 1987). Cardiomyopathy or damage to the heart muscle can result from years of heavy drinking. Other pathological conditions associated with alcohol abuse include generalized skeletal myopathy, pancreatitis and cancers of the pharynx and larynx. Impairment of brain function also occurs, alcoholic psychoses being a common cause of hospitalization in psychiatric wards.

Alcohol was formerly used as an anaesthetic until it was realized that it was too dangerous to supply in large quantities for that purpose. The result of applying alcohol to living cells is that the protoplasm of the cells precipitates as a consequence of dehydration. Long-term damage to tissue in the central nervous system may be an unwanted outcome of habitual heavy drinking.

Heavy drinking is not compatible with serious athletics. For the athlete, drinking is usually done only in moderation, an infrequent respite from the ascetic regimens of physical training, though the odd end of season binge is customary. Nevertheless, drinking is a social convention in many sports, such as rugby, squash and water-polo, where there may be peer-group pressure to take alcohol following training or competition or at club functions. Indeed, a few high-profile footballers in the English Premier League in the late 1990s admitted to an alcohol addiction and to referral to a rehabilitation clinic for alcoholics. The sensible athlete drinks moderately and occasionally, avoiding alcohol for at least 24 hours before competing. Hangovers may persist for a day and disturb concentration in sports involving complex skills. The attitude of the retired athlete may be very different. If his active career is terminated abruptly and the free time that retirement releases is taken up by social drinking, the result may well be a gradual deterioration in physical condition, with body weight increasing and fitness declining. In this context, the effect of alcohol on the ex-athlete may be quite harmful.

Various institutions within sports medicine have addressed the problems of alcohol and exercise. In 1982 the American College of Sports Medicine set out a position statement on alcohol which was unequivocally against any indulgence. It underlined the adverse effects of alcohol on health and condemned the resort to alcohol by athletes. Its estimate was that there were 10 million adult problem drinkers in the United States and an additional 3.3 million in the 14–17 year age range. No evidence for any of the beneficial aspects of alcohol was mentioned.

There is a belief that moderate drinking has some positive benefits for health. Small amounts increase the flow of gastric juices and thereby stimulate digestion: in large doses, alcohol irritates the stomach lining, causing gastritis and even vomiting of blood. A national survey of lifestyles in England and Wales provided support for the view that healthy people tended to drink a little. Amongst men under 60, the likelihood of high blood pressure was found to increase with the amount of alcohol consumed. For older men and for women, light drinking was associated with lower blood pressure, even when effects due to body weight were taken into account (Stepney, 1987).

It is thought also that moderate drinking provides a degree of protection against coronary heart disease. This belief may have been nurtured originally in the vineyards of France where a habitually modest consumption of wine is associated with a low incidence of heart disease. One report claimed that myocardial infarction rates were lower in moderate drinkers than in non-drinkers (Willett et al., 1980). A possible mechanism is the reduction in hypertension and the relaxation from business cares that drinking can bring. Moderate alcohol consumption may help haemostasis, in balancing the processes of coagulation and fibrinolysis. A link has also been shown by an increase in high-density lipoprotein cholesterol levels with moderate levels of drinking alcohol. High-density lipoprotein particles remove cholesterol from the tissues and transfer it into other particles in the blood; low-density lipoprotein, on the other hand, obtains its cholesterol from these other particles and transfers it to the tissues. A high ratio of high-density to low-density lipoprotein fractions is generally found in well-trained endurance athletes, a low ratio being indicative of poor cardiovascular health. The effect is apparent in autopsies of alcoholics whose blood vessels are in good condition despite pathological changes in other tissues. The mechanism by which alcohol would raise the high-density lipoprotein cholesterol has not been fully explained.

It seems that for a healthy athlete in a good state of training, occasional drinking of alcohol in moderation will have little adverse effect. It is important to emphasize that any such occasional bouts of drinking should be restrained and should follow rather than precede training sessions, whose training stimulus is likely to be lowered by the soporific influence of drinking alcohol before strenuous exercise.

Alcohol and physiological responses to exercise

Alcohol ingestion has been shown to lower muscle glycogen at rest compared with control conditions. As pre-start glycogen levels are important for sustained exercise at an intensity of about 70–80 per cent VO_{2max}, such as marathon running, taking alcohol in the 24 hours before such endurance activities is ill-advised. Effects of alcohol on the metabolic responses to submaximal exercise seem to be small. Juhlin-Dannfelt and co-workers (1977) reported that alcohol does not impair lipolysis or free fatty acid utilization during exercise. It may decrease splanchnic glucose output, decrease the potential contribution of energy from liver gluconeogenesis, cause a more pronounced decline in blood glucose levels and decrease the leg muscle uptake of glucose towards the end of a prolonged (up to 3-hour) run. The impairment in glucose production by the liver would lead to an increased likelihood of hypoglycaemia developing during prolonged exercise.

Some studies have shown an increase in oxygen uptake (VO_2) at a fixed submaximal exercise intensity after alcohol ingestion. This may be due to a poorer co-ordination of the active muscles as the decrease in mechanical efficiency, implied by the elevation in VO_2, is not a consistent finding. Related to this is an increase in blood lactate levels with alcohol; metabolism of alcohol shunts lactate away from the gluconeogenic pathway and leads to an increase in the ratio of lactate to pyruvate. It is possible that elevated blood lactate concentrations during exercise, after taking alcohol, may reflect impairment in clearance of lactate rather than an increase in production by the exercising muscles. A failure to clear lactate would militate against performance of strenuous exercise.

Alcohol does not seem to have adverse effects on maximum oxygen consumption (VO_{2max}) or on metabolic responses to high-intensity exercises approaching VO_{2max} levels. At high doses (up to 200 mg per cent, i.e. 0.20 per cent blood alcohol level) it is understandable that athletes may feel disinclined towards maximal efforts that elicit VO_{2max} values and a reduction in peak VE (minute ventilation) is usually observed (Blomqvist et al., 1970). Similarly, they may be poorly motivated to sustain high-intensity exercise for as long as they would normally do. In middle-distance running events with an appreciable aerobic component, performance was found to be detrimentally affected in a dose-related manner, with increasing blood alcohol concentration (BAC) levels from 0.01 to 0.10 per cent (McNaughton and Preece, 1986).

Although it has not been shown conclusively that alcohol alters VE, stroke volume or muscle blood flow at submaximal exercise levels, it does decrease peripheral vascular resistance. This is because of the vasodilatory effect of alcohol on the peripheral blood vessels, which would increase heat loss from the surface of the skin and cause a drop in body temperature. This consequence would be dangerous if alcohol is taken in conjunction with exercise in cold conditions. Sampling from a hip-flask of whisky on the ski slopes may bring an immediate feeling of warmth but its disturbance of normal thermoregulation may put the recreational skier at risk of hypothermia. Frost-bitten mountaineers especially should avoid drinking alcohol as the peripheral vasodilation it induces would cause the body temperature to fall further. In hot conditions, alcohol is also inadvisable as it acts as a diuretic and would exacerbate problems of dehydration.

Studies of maximum muscular strength, in the main, show no influence of moderate to medium doses of alcohol on maximum isometric tension. Similar results apply to dynamic functions, such as peak torque measured on isokinetic dynamometers. Muscular endurance is generally assessed by requiring the subject to hold a fixed percentage of maximum for as long as possible. Here, too, the influences of moderate alcohol doses are generally found to be non-significant. This may be because the tests represent gross aspects of muscular function and, as such, are insensitive to the effects of the drug.

Alcohol in aiming sports

In aiming sports, a steady limb is needed to provide a firm platform for launching the missile at its target or to keep the weapon still. Examples of such sports are archery, billiards, darts, pistol shooting and snooker. Two pistol shooters were disqualified during the 1980 Olympics due to taking alcohol in an attempt to improve their performance. There are also aiming components in sports such as fencing and modern pentathlon, especially in the rifle-shooting discipline of the latter. In some of these sports alcohol levels are now officially monitored, whilst in others, notably darts, drinking is a conventional complement of the sport itself.

To understand how alcohol might affect the archer, it is useful to look at the task *in toto*. The competitive player has to shoot three dozen arrows at each of four targets – 90, 70, 60 and 50 m away – to complete a FITA (the world governing body) round. Technological improvements in bow design have helped to produce outstanding scores, leaving the gap to perfection solely due to human factors. The modern bow has two slot-in limbs which insert into a magnesium handle section and stabilizers which help to minimize vibration and turning of the bow. Muscle strength is needed to draw the bow, whilst muscle endurance is required to hold it steady, usually for about 8 seconds for each shot while the sight is aligned with the target. Deflection of the arrow tip by 0.02 mm at 90 m causes the arrow to miss the target, which gives some idea of the hand steadiness required. The archer, before release or loose, pulls the arrow towards and through the clicker (a blade on the side of the bow which aids in measuring draw length). The archer reacts to the sound of the clicker hitting the side of the bow handle by releasing the string which, in effect, shoots the arrow. Archers are coached to react to the clicker by allowing the muscles to relax; a slow reaction to the clicker is generally recognized as hesitation. This affects the smoothness of the loose and is reflected in muscle tremor causing a 'snatched loose'. For these reasons, the effects of alcohol on reaction time, arm steadiness, muscle strength and endurance, and the electromyogram of one of the arm muscles were selected as appropriate parameters to isolate and study under experimental conditions (Reilly and Halliday, 1985).

In the experiment, nine subjects underwent a battery of tests under four conditions: sober, placebo, 0.02 per cent blood alcohol level and 0.05 per cent blood alcohol level. The alcohol doses were administered in three equal volumes to total 500 ml over 15 minutes, 45 minutes being allowed for peak blood alcohol levels to be attained. The doses to elicit the desirable blood alcohol levels were calculated according to the formula of Hicks (1976) which was shown to be effective:

$$A = \frac{(454)(W)(R)(BAC + 0.0002)}{(0.8)(0.95)}$$

where A = ml 95 per cent ethanol, W = body weight (lb), R = distribution coefficient of 0.765, and BAC = desired blood alcohol concentration (0.05 per cent = 0.0005).

A summary of the results for the performance measurement appears in Table 9.2. There was no effect of alcohol on the muscular strength and muscular endurance measures; the holding time in the endurance test was about the same time as the archer normally holds the bow drawn before shooting, so that this test turned out to be reasonably realistic.

Reaction time was significantly slowed by the lower alcohol dose, a further small delay occurring at the higher blood alcohol dose. The more sensitive response of auditory reaction time to alcohol would mean, in practice, a slower reaction to the clicker and a faulty loose. Another adverse effect noted was the impairment in steadiness of the extended arm. Performance was degraded, especially at the 0.05 per cent blood alcohol level, and the variability in arm steadiness also increased with alcohol. This effect contradicts the conventional wisdom in archery and may have been due to the

Table 9.2 Effects of the alcohol treatments on four experimental tests (mean ± SD) (from Reilly and Halliday, 1985)

Variables	Sober	Placebo	0.02% BAC	0.05% BAC
Arm steadiness:				
Time-off-target(s)	2.64 + 0.89	3.05 ± 0.74	3.24 ± 1.01	8.17 + 1.49
Isometric strength (N)	546 ± 48	560 ± 37	541 ± 56	523 ± 78
Muscular endurance (s)	11.4 ± 2.1	12.0 ± 2.5	12.0 ± 2.0	10.8 ± 2.0
Reaction time (ms)	211 ± 6.5	209 ± 8.5	223 ± 9.6	226 ± 11.2

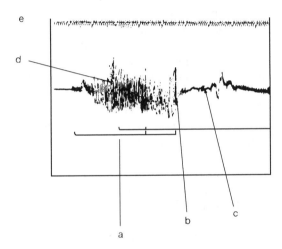

Figure 9.3 The electromyographic profile of an arm muscle whilst holding the bow down: (a) holding time; (b) the point of loose; (c) post-loose muscular activity; (d) tremor; (e) the time-scale of events marked in 100 ms.

high load on the arm muscles when holding the bow drawn. It is possible that alcohol only operates to advantage in steadying the limb in contexts more competitive than laboratory experiments.

Some benefits were noted in the electromyographic profile (Figure 9.3). A clearer loose was observed at the low alcohol levels which would be valuable in promoting a smoother release. This was supplemented by a tendency towards a reduced tremor in the muscle with both alcohol treatments. Together, these effects would indicate a greater muscle relaxation, the tremor being normally associated with a snatched loose. These factors were partly offset by the longer holding time prior to loose induced by the alcohol treatments. The overall conclusion was that alcohol has differential effects on tasks related to archery, depending on the concentrations, the components of the performance analysed and individual reactivity to the drug.

The deleterious effects of alcohol on some aspects of archery would not apply to other aiming sports, such as darts and pistol shooting. In these the loading on the arm muscles is light, so a greater arm steadiness is likely to be induced by the drug. Another consideration is that the timing of the release is at the discretion of the subject and also is unaffected by a retarded reaction time. Reactions will have importance where the target is moving: it is noteworthy that the discipline of clay-pigeon shooting, for example, is not steeped in a history of alcohol use.

The bar-room sports, such as snooker, billiards and darts, have the alcohol industry as an adjunct to their matches. At the highest level of competition these sports are popular television spectacles. Although it is widely thought that the top performers swig large quantities of alcohol, this is not the case. Imbibition is regular but in small doses so that a moderate blood alcohol level is continually maintained (needless to say, at high blood alcohol levels, 0.15 per cent or more, whole-body stability and mental concentration would be degraded and any possible ergogenic effect would be swamped). Alcohol is prohibited by the International Federation for Billiards.

A study of the effects of elevating blood alcohol levels on tasks related to dart throwing (Reilly and Scott, 1993) confirmed the finding in archery. Whilst there were negative effects from the light alcohol dose (BAC 0.02 per cent) on hand–eye coordination, effects were positive for balance and dart throwing score. A higher level of 0.05 per cent led to a fall-off in performance on all tasks. Results indicated some improvement with a light dose of alcohol for dart throwers, but performance deteriorated when BAC levels reached 0.05 per cent.

In those sports that discourage alcohol for competition there is a disharmony in standards for what constitutes legality. In addition to shooting events, archery and billiards, alcohol is banned in several other sports, for example automobile, karate, motor cycling, modern pentathlon and skiing. Each federation adopts its own threshold for alcohol.

Testing for alcohol is performed on competitors in the shooting event of the modern pentathlon. Here, participants are disadvantaged by any tremor in settling down to prepare for taking their shots. Although alcohol might help competitors to relax whilst taking aim, it has little ergogenic benefit in the other disciplines of the pentathlon. For various reasons, tranquillizers and beta-blocking agents have been preferred. These are considered in the sections that follow.

Alcohol and sports accidents

It has been recommended that alcohol should be outlawed prior to aquatic activities because of the potential for catastrophic accidents in the water. Alcohol is a significant factor in spinal injuries occurring in recreational water sports. In scuba diving the potential for fatal nitrogen narcosis increases at shallower depths when alcohol is consumed. Of 752 drowning victims studied in North Carolina, 53 per cent were positive for alcohol and 38 per cent had blood alcohol values of 0.10 per cent or greater (see Reilly, 1997).

Peak effects on motor performance following administration of alcohol are typically observed 45–60 min later, but impairment is evident for up to 3 hours after dosing (Kelly *et al.*, 1993). This could render the drinker susceptible to accidents if alcohol is imbibed after sports competitions before driving the journey home.

There is evidence also of impaired exercise performance the morning after a bout of nocturnal drinking, adverse effects being observed in aerobic performance (O'Brien, 1993). This finding has implications for the behaviour of players the night before competition or serious training.

9.4 Benzodiazepines

Benzodiazepines, derivatives of benzodiazepine, are widely employed as tranquillizers in the population at large and have been used for calming or sedative purposes in sports. They are included in the list of drugs that may be taken by sports competitors. There are now over two dozen benzodiazepine drugs and these form over 90 per cent of the tranquillizer market. More than 20 doses of these drugs per head of the USA population are prescribed annually, giving an idea of the vast scale of consumption.

The first benzodiazepine drug was synthesized in the mid-1950s, the best known of those that followed being Librium (chlordiazepoxide hydrochloride), introduced in the USA in 1960, and Valium (diazepam), introduced in 1963. The benzodiazepines have systematically replaced the barbiturates and the propranediol derivatives as drugs of clinical choice in treating stress and anxiety. There is little evidence that the barbiturates had a major use amongst active athletes as an ergogenic aid in the years when they were being widely prescribed, although they may have been used in more recent years.

Benzodiazepines decrease stress response indices, such as skin conductance and plasma corticosterone levels. They have been found to reduce anxiety in psychiatric and non-psychiatric patients and have demonstrated a superiority over barbiturates in clinical conditions. The drugs affect various neurotransmitters, the cholinergic and serotonergic effects having importance in reducing the stress response.

The benzodiazepines decrease the turnover in hemispheric cholinergic neurones by blocking the release of acetylcholine. By thus lowering the activity in cholinergic pathways, the drugs should have an adverse effect on human performance. Deterioration in the detection of sensory signals and in reaction time in a rapid information-processing task with nightly doses of flurazepam and temazepam have been found the morning after taking the drugs (Figure 9.4). The carry-over effects are due to the long half-lives of these particular drugs. Other types of performance which are affected

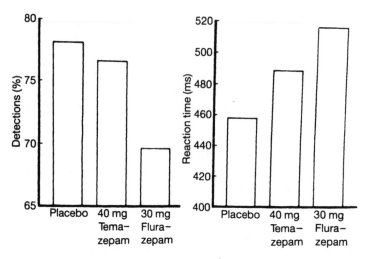

Figure 9.4 The effects of temazepam (40 mg) and flurazepam (30 mg) on the percentage of correct detections and the reaction time in a rapid information-processing task. The tasks were performed the morning after nightly administration of drugs. (From Wesnes and Warburton, 1983: reprinted with permission of John Wiley and Son Ltd.)

include the rate of tapping, motor manipulation and complex co-ordination tasks, as well as real and simulated driving.

The function of one particular cholinergic pathway is to trigger the release of corticotrophic-releasing factor from the hypothalamus into the pituitary blood vessels and produce a spurt of adrenocorticotrophic hormone (ACTH) from the anterior pituitary. The benzodiazepines would lower the emission of corticosteroid hormones from the adrenal cortex by affecting the ACTH release as a result of blocking cholinergic activity.

The benzodiazepines have been found to decelerate the turnover of noradrenaline. This effect is more apparent in conditions where the noradrenaline levels have been increased by stress. This change is not the basis of the drugs' anti-anxiety action, as repeated dosing with oxazepam results in a rapid tolerance to the decrease in noradrenaline turnover, whilst the drug maintains its anti-anxiety properties (Wesnes and Warburton, 1983). Similarly, dopamine turnover is retarded by benzodiazepines, but this effect is unrelated to the drugs' anti-anxiety properties.

The main anti-anxiety action of benzodiazepines seems to stem from the reduction in serotonergic activity which the drugs produce. Serotonergic neurones are important in the experience of anxiety, so that this feeling is attenuated by the drugs. The effects of the benzodiazepines on serotonergic neurones may be mediated by a primary action of the drugs on gamma-aminobutyric acid (GABA). (It is thought that administration of GABA has been tried by some sports competitors.) The GABA-releasing neurones are primarily inhibitory and it is possible that when these are stimulated by the benzodiazepines the release of serotonin is inhibited. The GABA system is recognized as playing a crucial role in anxiety: some anxiety-related states may be due to diminished transmission at the level of GABA receptors which are functionally linked to benzodiazepine recognition sites (Corda *et al.*, 1986).

The effects of benzodiazepines on components of human performance will depend on the dosage and on the particular drug. Oxazepam, diazepam, nitrazepam, flurazepam and chlordiazepoxide are all 1,4-derivatives. Clobazam, a 1,5-benzodiazepine derivative, does not seem to impair psychomotor performance but does retain its anti-anxiety properties (Wesnes and Warburton, 1983) and so may have more applications than the others in sport and exercise contexts.

Following the bans on alcohol overuse in the modern pentathlon, athletes at the 1972 Olympic Games in Munich were found to have used benzodiazepines and other tranquillizers, such as meprobamate, as anti-anxiety agents. They were thought preferable to alcohol as they might reduce anxiety without the potential adverse effects on judgement and co-ordination associated with alcohol. Meprobamate acts as a mild tranquillizer without producing drowsiness. It is highly addictive and reduces tolerance to alcohol. The benzodiazepines are relatively safe in that they have low toxicity and few side-effects. They can induce a dependence in chronic users and severe withdrawal symptoms are experienced when patients are taken off them abruptly. They are highly dangerous when used in overdoses combined with other central nervous system depressants, such as alcohol.

One of the primary effects of the GABA-mediated reaction to benzodiazepines is that the drugs act as muscle relaxants. For this reason, they can be beneficial in aiding recovery from spastic-type muscle injuries. The effect is associated with a feeling of freedom from 'nerves' and tension. There are repercussions for muscle function in both submaximal and extreme efforts. Spontaneous activity of animals is reduced under the influence of these drugs. A study of alprazolam by Cabri *et al.* (1990) demonstrated that the effects were dependent on the dose. Maximal torque on an isokinetic dynamometer was unaffected by a low dose (0.5 mg). Moderate doses of the drug (1.5 and 3.0 mg) caused a reduction in muscle performance during brief bouts of maximal effort, both 90 and 360 minutes after ingestion. The metabolic effects were reflected in a decrease in amplitude and integrated electromyogram, but these effects were reduced after 360 minutes. It was thought that GABA-ergic activity induced alterations both in central nervous system and in peripheral (neuromuscular) receptor sites for benzodiazepines. Different benzodiazepine drugs vary in their pharmacokinetic profiles and so their influence on muscle performance may also be variable. For this reason, Zinzen *et al.* (1994) compared the effects of therapeutic doses of flunitrazepam (plasma half-life of 31 hours) and triazolam (half-life of 8 hours) on performance, utilizing an isokinetic dynamometer. (Triazolam is banned from prescription in the UK and in other European countries due to its potential for dependence.) No hangover effects were noted after an 8-hour sleep with triazolam; in contrast, flunitrazepam was shown to impair muscle force production after the night's sleep and subjects were reported as having a 'sleepy impression' throughout the following day. Various stimulants, including caffeine, have been used to offset the depressant effects of benzodiazepines on psychomotor skills. Caffeine interacts with the GABA–benzodiazepine system and so may reverse some adverse effects of these tranquillizers. Collomp *et al.* (1993) showed that moderate benzodiazepine intake (1 mg of lorazepam) significantly impaired performance on an all-out exercise test over 30 seconds. Moderate caffeine intake (250 mg of caffeine in combination with 1 mg of lorazepam) antagonized the metabolic but not the performance effects of the tranquillizer.

Diazepam is frequently prescribed in the treatment of muscle spasm. As doses used for relaxation of skeletal muscle, the drug could cause drowsiness and impair intellectual as well as motor function. Diazepam would generally be used on a short-term basis for treating muscle spasm due to injury. Consequently it does not entail withdrawal symptoms when treatment is complete.

The effects of benzodiazepines on sustained exercise performance are poorly documented. In the resting normal human, coronary blood flow is increased by 22.5 per cent by diazepam but more so (73 per cent) in persons with coronary artery disease. Whether the drugs are of benefit in the treatment of angina associated with effort is unknown (Powles, 1981).

Barbiturates and sedatives have long been used in sleeping pills. Such a use, to facilitate the sleep of athletes the night before competition, is likely to be counterproductive because of a residual de-arousing effect the following day. The 'hangover' effect of benzodiazepines was found to be greater for flurazepam (30 mg) than for temazepam (40 mg). Although the former produced better sleep, it resulted in lowered clear-headedness on waking and impaired performance on a rapid visual information-processing task (Wesnes and Warburton, 1984).

The 'hangover' effect of sleeping tablets, including benzodiazepines, is likely to disturb complex skills more than simple motor tasks performed early the following day, and, depending on the sport, an increase in errors may promote a higher risk of injury. Alcohol can compound the adverse effects of other drugs on motor performance tasks (Kunsman *et al.*, 1992). Attention and reaction time tasks are impaired by a combination of temazepam and ethanol in doses which may not cause impairment when each is given alone. Subjects tend to be unaware of their reduced performance capabilities when taking these drugs in combination. There are likely to be increases also in injury risk. Of 402 victims of ski accidents, 20 per cent were positive for alcohol, 8.5 per cent had taken benzodiazepines and

2.5 per cent were positive for both drugs. Subjects positive for both tended to be older than the other persons examined (Barnas *et al.*, 1992).

Benzodiazepines have been thought to help in adjusting circadian rhythms following time-zone transitions because of their promotion of sleep. Reilly *et al.* (2001) found temazepam had no effect in combating jet-lag in British athletes travelling over five time-zones to the USA. There was no effect on the rate of adjustment to the new time-zone, either in core temperature, performance measures or subjective symptoms. The ease of sleeping following travelling westwards and arriving in the evening local time probably rendered any sleep elixir superfluous in these circumstances. Low doses of benzodiazepines may benefit shift workers who have difficulty in sleeping during the day after a nocturnal shift. In a study of simulated shift work, Wesnes and Warburton (1986) found that 10–20 mg doses of temazepam helped daytime sleep without detrimental residual effects on subsequent information processing.

The circadian or 24-hour rhythm in arousal may have implications for the pharmacological effects of anti-anxiety drugs. The optimum dosage of drugs affecting the nervous system differs with the time of day at which they are administered. The barbiturate dose that is safe in the evening may have exaggerated effects in early morning (Luce, 1973). The same is true for alcohol and this is reflected in social drinking habits: usually only alcoholics drink before breakfast and in the late morning. Alcohol taken at lunch time has a much more detrimental effect on psychomotor performance than if taken in the evening (Horne and Gibbons, 1991). The diurnal variation in responses to benzodiazepines and the implications this has for the dosage at different times of day for effective pre-contest tranquillization does not seem to have been the subject of any serious research attention.

9.5 Melatonin

Melatonin is a hormone produced by the pineal gland. The main claims for its use have been as a hypnotic to aid sleep and as a chronobiotic to counteract jet-lag. It has antioxidant properties and so has been promoted to combat free radicals which are produced during exercise. It is widely available in the USA but is not licensed for use in the UK and some other European countries. In countries where it is openly available, it has been used with the aim of reducing stress.

Melatonin has a lowering effect on body temperature, probably due to its vasodilatory effects on peripheral blood vessels. Its chronobiotic effect depends on the timing of the dose and whether the intention is to shift the timing of the body clock forwards or backwards, its so-called phase-response curve. Bright light opposes the action of melatonin, inhibiting its production. Secretion would normally start at about 21:00 hours or after onset of darkness and ends at around 08:00 hours. The normal circadian rhythm is disrupted on rapid time-zone transitions and has led to the use of melatonin to hasten the adjustment of the body clock to the new time-zone (Waterhouse *et al.*, 1997).

Like benzodiazepines, melatonin can have unpredictable side-effects. These include fuzzy head, sleepiness, disrupted concentration and increased feelings of fatigue. There are possible allergic reactions in some individuals. For these reasons the British Olympic Association has advised caution among its athletes and officials considering using melatonin. In promoting adjustment of the body clock following long-haul flights, behavioural and natural means – such as light, exercise, social activity, sleeping/waking – were preferred (Reilly *et al.*, 1998). In the typical circumstances which travellers experience, melatonin appears to be ineffective (Edwards *et al.*, 2000).

The hypnotic effects of melatonin are reflected in the advice not to drive after ingesting this substance. Auditory vigilance, reaction time and feelings of vigour have all been adversely affected after ingesting melatonin during the day (see Atkinson *et al.*, 1997). Atkinson *et al.* (2001) found no deterioration in muscle strength or performance in a 4-km cycle time-trial the morning after taking melatonin prior to going to bed. There was little evidence of an improvement in sleep quality among the athletes.

9.6 Marijuana

Marijuana is obtained from the hemp plant *Cannabis sativa*. It contains the compound tetrahydrocannabinol which accounts for its psychological effects. These include a sedating and euphoric feeling of well-being and relaxation, with a sensation of sleepiness. Balance may be disturbed; aggression and motivation to perform may be blunted. Maximum muscular strength is reduced, probably because of the reduced drive towards all-out effort.

Largely because of its promotion of happy and euphoric mood states, marijuana has been prominent amongst the drugs of abuse, notably by youngsters and college students in the USA and Europe. It was the main recreational drug used by late adolescents and young adults in the 1970s. A report of the US Department of Health and Human Services, *Student Drug Use in America 1975 to 1980*, claimed that nearly one-third of students had tried marijuana before entering high school. This background of experience with the drug might explain its popularity amongst young athletes as a mode of release from tension during the competitive season. Marijuana is banned in all sports by the World Anti-Doping Agency (WADA). However, cannabinoids are included on WADA's specified substances list. Therefore, athletes who test positive for cannabinoids may incur a reduced sanction provided the athlete can establish that its use was not intended to enhance sport performance.

Statistics from IOC-accredited laboratories indicated an increasing number of positive tests for marijuana since 1994 when 75 positive results were reported. Between 1996 and 1999 the figures rose in successive years from 154 to 164, 233 and 312, respectively. In 2003 WADA results revealed 378 cases which accounted for 13.9 per cent of all positive results for 2003. It is likely that this trend reflects an increased use of the drug in society as a whole. The positive result from Ross Rebagliati at the 1998 Winter Olympic Games in Nagano was attributed by the athlete to passive smoking. Clearly elite athletes are equally exposed to the leisure-drug culture as are non-athletic young members of society.

Persistent marijuana smoking is incompatible with serious athletic training. The single-mindedness of the athlete will be disturbed by the demotivating influence of the drug. A few cigarettes of marijuana may cause minor changes in personality, while high doses can induce hallucinations, delusions and psychotic-like symptoms. The major abuse of marijuana has been by collegiate games teams, playing basketball and football, in the USA. The practice of smoking marijuana is generally condemned by athletic trainers and coaches in that country.

The active ingredient in marijuana is 1–5–9-tetrahydrocannabinol (THC). About 60 to 65 per cent of the THC in a marijuana cigarette is absorbed through the lungs when it is smoked. Effects of drug action are noted within 15 minutes of smoking and last for 3 hours or so. The primary effects are produced by changes in central nervous system function. Motivation for physical effort is decreased and motor co-ordination, short-term memory and perception are impaired. Chronic marijuana abuse has been found to include decreased circulating testosterone levels amongst its toxic effects (Nuzzo and Waller, 1988). In addition to the psychological effects, marijuana induces tachycardia, bronchodilation and an increase in blood flow to the limbs. The bronchodilation effect does not lead to substantial alteration of the respiratory pattern during exercise. A pre-exercise increase of heart rate by 25 beats/minute is sustained during exercise up to about 80 per cent of maximal effort. This means that maximal heart rate is attained at a lower intensity during a graded exercise test and the maximal work capacity is decreased after marijuana smoking (Renaud and Cormier, 1986). In another study, a general decrement in standing steadiness, simple and complex reaction times, and psychomotor skills was observed following administration of 215 mg/kg of the active ingredient of marijuana (Bird *et al.*, 1980).

9.7 Nicotine

The tobacco leaf, *Nicotiana tabacum*, is the source of the cigarettes on which the massive tobacco industry is based. As the tobacco burns it generates about 4000 different compounds, including carbon monoxide (CO), ammonia, hydrogen cyanide, many carcinogens, DDT and tar. Carbon monoxide reduces the oxygen transport capacity of the blood by combining with haemoglobin (Hb) and so takes the place of oxygen in the bloodstream, adversely affecting aerobic exercise performance. The affinity of CO for Hb is 230 times that of oxygen. Tobacco smoke contains about 4 per cent CO; smoking 10–12 cigarettes a day results in a blood COHb level of 4.9 per cent, 15–25 a day raises the value to 6.3 per cent, whilst 30–40 each day takes the level to 9.3 per cent. Adverse effects are noticeable only during physical exertion, and after smoking it may take 24 hours or more for blood CO levels to return to normal. The smoke also paralyses the cilia in the respiratory passages so that their filtering becomes ineffective and the individual is more susceptible to respiratory tract infections.

The anti-smoking argument is centred around the links between smoking and cancer. Another strong link has been shown between smoking and hardening of the peripheral arteries and deterioration of the circulation to the limbs. The result can be a need for amputation of the affected limb. Other long-term health hazards associated with heavy smoking are acceleration of coronary atherosclerosis, pulmonary emphysema and cerebral vascular disease.

About 30 per cent of the adult population throughout the world smoke cigarettes and it is likely that double this number have sampled cigarettes at some time or another. As passive inhalation of smoke by non-users of tobacco – especially in crowded public places – has similar effects to those in smokers, smoking in public facilities is now restricted in many countries. About 20 per cent of the smoke exhaled can be recirculated in passive inhalation.

The psychological and addictive effects of smoking are attributable to nicotine. Smokers report that cigarettes help them to relax, and the intensity of smoking increases at times of stress. They also report that smoking has a tranquillizing effect when they are angry. These influences on subjective states do not tally with the neurochemical and physiological responses to nicotine.

Nicotine is a cholinergic agonist and so by acting as a brain stimulant is likely to enhance arousal. In this respect it differs from alcohol and the benzodiazepines. There is a secondary rise in plasma corticosteroids, and an increase in central release of noradrenaline and in urinary catecholamine output. These changes are normally associated with the stress response, so that the relaxing characteristics of nicotine present a paradox. A few theories attempting to resolve this conflict were reviewed by Wesnes and Warburton (1983), though none fitted all the experimental evidence satisfactorily. They argued that it is the action of nicotine on cholinergic pathways controlling attention that reduces stress by enabling individuals to concentrate more efficiently. Neurotic individuals, who comprise the majority of smokers, are helped by the drug to filter out distracting thoughts; this enables them to perform more effectively, increasing their self-confidence in the process.

Smokers tend to experience stress when trying to give up cigarettes. For this reason, games players and other athletes who smoke pre-competition need astute counselling in attempting to overcome the habit. This would be best done during non-critical periods of the week and the pre-match smoking could be replaced unobtrusively by behavioural techniques of relaxation. However, resort to smoking may be easily replaced by an increase in snacks between meals, leading to unwanted weight gain. This occurs because the appetite centre in the brain is released from the depressant effect that smoking has on it. This problem will be greatest in the casual recreationist whose energy expenditure during physical activity will generally be low.

Quite apart from the effects on health and on human performance, smoking may also have repercussions for sports injury, particularly under conditions of cold. An acute effect of smoking is peripheral vasoconstriction which decreases blood flow to the limbs. For this reason, the frost-bitten climber should avoid any temptation to smoke until after recovery through hospitalization where alternative therapies are ensured.

Clearly cigarette smoking has few advocates in sport and the sports sciences. Advertising of cigarettes is prohibited in some Scandinavian countries and top athletes are frequently prominent in anti-smoking campaigns. Sports associations that enjoy sponsorship from tobacco companies have come under pressure to find alternative benefactors. Smoking is rare amongst elite athletes, so that there are few models for youngsters taking up smoking to cite as examples. Those sports stars that do smoke might ultimately benefit from adopting alternative strategies to ease their troubled minds at times of emotional stress.

9.8 Beta blockers

Sympathetic adrenergic nerve fibres are classified according to their alpha and beta receptors. Effects of these receptors are sometimes contradictory. In the blood vessels of muscle and skin, α-adrenergic receptors cause vasoconstriction, whereas β-receptors induce vasodilation. The beta β-receptors are further divided into β_1- and β_2-categories according to the responses to sympathomimetic drugs. Functions of β_1-receptors include cardiac acceleration and increased myocardial contractility; β_2-receptors cause bronchodilation and glycogenesis. The action of these receptors is blocked by the activities of inhibitory drugs, the so-called beta blockers. These include, for example, atenolol, a cardioselective beta blocker with selectivity for β_1-adrenoceptors; propranolol, which blocks both types of β-receptors, and labetalol which is a combined alpha and beta blocker. A more detailed description of sympathomimetic amines and their antagonists is given in Chapter 4.

Besides decreasing heart rate and myocardial contractility, the beta-blocking agents also reduce cardiac output, stroke volume and mean systemic arterial blood pressure. These effects explain the use of beta blockade in hypertension and in individuals with poor coronary health. Because of the effects on the circulation, beta blockade in clinical doses reduces maximal oxygen uptake and endurance time in normal individuals, but increases maximal work capacity in patients with angina pectoris. At submaximal exercise levels a decrease in heart rate and contractility is balanced by a decrease in coronary blood flow and an increased duration of myocardial contraction. The fall in exercise heart rate is not matched by a corresponding drop in perceived exertion rating, so that the usual close correlation between these variables is dissociated by beta blockade.

The effects of beta blockers on metabolism have implications for the performance of submaximal exercise. By inhibiting the enzyme phosphorylase, beta blockade may decrease the rate of glycogenolysis in skeletal muscle. Breakdown of liver glycogen is also likely to be inhibited, so that in sustained exercise blood glucose levels may decline. This fall is noted with propranolol but is not so evident with atenolol or metoprolol, two cardio-selective beta blockers. Kaiser (1982) showed that jogging was markedly influenced only by propranolol at the low dose of 40 mg: at doses of 80 mg and above, atenolol had a similar adverse effect. Selective beta blockade inhibits lipolysis, which may reduce the availability of free fatty acids as a substrate for prolonged exercise and cause an earlier onset of fatigue.

The effect of beta blockade on short-term high-intensity performance was examined by Rusko et al. (1980). The subjects performed a range of anaerobic tasks after taking the beta blocker oxprenolol, and results were compared with performances after being given an inert placebo. The drug had no effect on isometric strength of leg extension, vertical jumping and stair running. Power output over 60 seconds on a cycle ergometer was reduced under the influence of the drug, whilst peak blood lactate and heart rates were also decreased. It seems that the beta blocker caused a reduction in anaerobic capacity as well as in heart rate.

Use of beta blockers has implications for thermoregulation if exercise is conducted in the heat. Gordon et al. (1987) showed that a non-selective beta blocker (propranolol) produced greater sweating than did a β_1-selective blocker (atenolol). In this study, both drugs produced equivalent reductions in exercise tachycardia, a similar decrease in skin blood flow and a similar rise in rectal temperature. The authors suggested that β_1-selective adrenoceptor blockers should be the preferred therapy during prolonged physical activity when adequate fluid replacement cannot be guaranteed. The findings indicated an increased need for persons treated with propranolol to stick to a strict fluid replacement regimen during sustained exercise.

Another consideration is whether the physiological adaptations to a fitness training programme are altered by the use of beta blockers. Propranolol, even in low doses of 80 mg daily, does blunt the effects of exercise training in normal individuals. At higher doses of 160–320 mg/day, this impairment is more pronounced. The apparent mechanism is a prevention of the normal peripheral circulatory and metabolic responses to exercise (Opie, 1986).

Although beta blockade permits patients with angina to exercise more easily, the chronic effects of physical training in patients with ischaemic heart disease may still be attenuated. Indeed, Powles (1981) considered that the many physiological effects of beta blockade meant that for each patient there may be an optimal dosage. This optimal point is that at which adverse effects on the functioning of the left ventricle, the myocardial perfusion and metabolism did not outweigh the benefits associated with decreased heart rate.

Beta blockers cross the blood–brain barrier to varying extents, depending on their lipid solubility; for example, propranolol does so to a greater degree than atenolol. Their anti-anxiety effect may not necessarily be centrally mediated. The suppression of cardiac activity which would result in a reduction in the afferent information from the heart may be the cause. Inhibition of the β-receptors, through which glycogenolysis is stimulated by adrenaline and lactic acid production is increased, is an alternative mechanism. Low levels of lactic acid tend to be associated with a state of relaxation, free from anxiety. On balance, however, the evidence favours the interpretation that the anti-anxiety effects of these drugs are due to direct action within the central nervous system.

As beta-blocking agents are not addictive they tend to be preferred over the benzodiazepines and alcohol in combating anxiety. They attenuate emotional tachycardia, limb tremor and unpleasant manifestations of anxiety, such as palmar sweating, pre-competition. These drugs have proved effective in reducing anxiety in students undergoing oral examinations, in public speakers and in musicians liable to 'stage-fright' (Orme, 1997). High-risk sports, such as ski-jumping, motor-racing and bobsleighing, provide especially suitable contexts for their use. Undesirable effects might be produced by beta blockers in athletes suffering from asthma and in individuals with reduced cardiac function.

The beta blockers have been banned by the International Shooting Union as they are believed to be of potential use to marksmen in reducing anxiety before competitions and enhancing performance. Nevertheless, they were repeatedly used by many competitors in shooting events at the 1984 Olympic Games (and to a lesser extent at the subsequent Games), being prescribed by team physicians for health reasons. Similar practices by top professional snooker players were disclosed at the 1987 World Championship. They are unlikely to be used in endurance events where the aerobic system is maximally or near-maximally taxed. They would have an ergogenic effect in the shooting discipline of the modern pentathlon, an event in which they have allegedly been used for a steadying influence before shooting.

The use of beta blockers in selected sports was reflected in the IOC Medical Commission's decision to test for beta blockers only in the biathlon, bob sled, figure-skating, luge and ski-jump competitions at the 1988 Winter Olympic Games in Calgary. In the 1988 Summer Olympic Games in Seoul, and the 1992 Summer Games in Barcelona, the IOC Medical Commission tested for beta blockers in the archery, diving, equestrian, fencing, gymnastics, modern pentathlon, sailing, shooting and synchronized swimming events only.

In the March 1993 revision of the IOC list of doping classes and methods, beta blockers were transferred from Section I, Doping Classes to Section II, Classes of Drugs Subject to Certain Restrictions, and in January 2004, WADA listed beta blockers under Substances Prohibited in Particular Sports, indicating that they should be tested for only in those sports where they are likely to enhance performance. In January 2005, WADA listed 18 sports for which beta blockers were prohibited (WADA, 2005). These included: archery, automobile, billiards, gymnastics, motorcycling, modern pentathlon (shooting events), sailing, skiing (ski jumping and free-style snow boarding) shooting and wrestling. In the majority of these sports beta blockers are prohibited in-competition only. However, archery and shooting also prohibit beta blockers out-of-competition. WADA statistics for 2003 indicate that beta blockers were identified on 297 occasions, which accounts for 10.9 per cent of all adverse analytical findings.

Studies of the effects of beta blockers on pistol shooters suggest that they are mainly of benefit to the less competent and less experienced shooters, as well as those most anxious prior to competition (Siitonen *et al.*, 1977). A study of the British national pistol squad found that significant improvement in shooting scores was restricted to slow-fire events, the ergogenic effect being slightly greater for an 80 mg dose than for 40 mg of oxprenolol (Antal and Good, 1980). The effect of a 40 mg dose of oxprenolol was matched by an effect of alcohol equivalent to a half pint (284 ml) of beer (S'Jongers *et al.*, 1978). There appeared to be a substantial placebo effect which applied equally to alcohol and beta blockers.

9.9   Overview

Stress and anxiety are inescapable corollaries of contemporary professional activities and participation in top-level sport. Indeed, a high degree of competitiveness seems to be a prerequisite for success in both spheres, and those without the essential coping mechanism fail to climb to the top of the ladder. The relationship between sport and anxiety is paradoxical in that sport, as a recreational activity, offers release from occupational cares, whilst at a highly competitive level it becomes a strong stressor. Indeed, exercise is effective therapy for highly anxious individuals, though this function was not central to the present topic. Neither has the role of behaviour modification strategies been considered here, either as a replacement for or complement to anti-anxiety drugs, although behavioural techniques are common in treating anxiety in competitive sports contexts.

In the past decade or so, sports officials and governing bodies in sport have assumed increasing responsibility for attempts to eliminate the use of drugs for ergogenic purposes. It is likely that the process of adding new pharmacological products to the list of banned substances will continue in spite of a running contest with those practitioners prepared to grasp at any means of improving their performances. The risks and benefits of anti-anxiety drugs, as described, demonstrate that regulations for their use in sport must be set down with care and circumspection. Legislation must ensure that, for the sport in question, participants especially prone to anxiety are not endangered by being deprived of their genuine prescriptions, whilst at the same time allowing fair competition to all entries.

9.10   References

Antal, L.C. and Good, C.S. (1980) Effects of oxprenolol on pistol shooting under stress. *Practitioner*, **224**, 755–760.

Atkinson, G., Reilly, T., Waterhouse, J. and Winterburn, S. (1997) Pharmacology and the travelling athlete, In: *The Clinical Pharmacology of Sport and Exercise* (eds T. Reilly and M. Orme). Elsevier, Amsterdam, pp. 293–304.

Atkinson, G., Buckley, P., Edwards, B., Reilly, T. and Waterhouse, J. (2001) Are there hangover-effects on physical performance when melatonin is ingested by athletes before nocturnal sleep? *Int. J. Sports Med.*, **22**, 232–234.

Barnas, L., Miller, G.H., Sperner, G. *et al.* (1992) The effects of alcohol and benzodiazepines on the severity of ski accidents. *Acta Psychiat. Scand.*, **86**, 296.

Bird, K.D., Boleyn, T., Chester, G.B. *et al.* (1980) Inter-cannabinoid and cannabinoid–ethanol interactions and their effects on human performance. *Psychopharmacology*, **71**, 181–188.

Blomqvist, G., Saltin, B. and Mitchell, J. (1970) Acute effects of ethanol ingestion on the response to submaximal and maximal exercise in man. *Circulation*, **62**, 463–470.

Cabri, J., Clarys, J.P., Vanderstappen, D.V. and Reilly, T. (1990) Les influences de différentes doses d'alprazolam sur l'activité musculaire dans des conditions de mouvements isocinétiques. *Arch. Int. Physiolog. Biochem.*, **98(4)**, c 48.

Collomp, K.R., Ahmaidi, S.B., Caillaud, C.F. *et al.* (1993) Effects of benzodiazepine during a Wingate test: interaction with caffeine. *Med. Sci. Sports Exerc.*, **25**, 1375–1380.

Corda, M.G., Concas, A. and Biggio, G. (1986) Stress and GABA receptors. In *Biochemical Aspects of Physical Exercise* (eds G. Benzi, L. Packer and N. Siliprandi). Elsevier, Amsterdam, pp. 399–409.

Edwards, B.J., Atkinson, G., Waterhouse, J., Reilly, T., Godfrey, R. and Budgett, R. (2000) Use of melatonin in recovery from jet-lag following an eastward flight across 10 time-zones. *Ergonomics*, **43**, 1501–1513.

Gordon, N.F., van Rensburg, T.P., Russell, H.M.S. *et al.* (1987) Effect of beta-adrenoceptor blockade and calcium antagonism, alone and in combination, on thermoregulation during prolonged exercise. *Int. J. Sports Med.*, **8**, 1–5.

Hicks, J.A. (1976) An evaluation of the effect of sign brightness and the sign reading behaviour of alcohol impaired drivers. *Hum. Factors*, **18**, 45–52.

Horne, J.A. and Gibbons, H. (1991) Effects on vigilance performance and sleepiness of alcohol given in the early afternoon (post lunch) vs. early evening. *Ergonomics*, **34**, 67–77.

Ikai, M. and Steinhaus, A.H. (1961) Some factors modifying the expression of human strength. *J. Appl. Physiol.*, **16**, 157–161.

Juhlin-Dannfelt, A., Ahlberg, G., Hagenfelt, L. *et al.* (1977) Influence of ethanol on splanchnic and skeletal muscle substrate turnover during prolonged exercise in man. *Am. J. Physiol.*, **233**, E195–202.

Kaiser, P. (1982) Running performance as a function of the dose–response relationship to beta-adrenoceptor blockade. *Int. J. Sports Med.*, **3**, 29–32.

Kelly, T.H., Fultin., R.W., Emurian, C.S. and Fischman, M.W. (1993) Performance based testing for drugs of abuse: dose and time profiles of marijuana, amphetamine, alcohol and diazepam. *J. Analyt. Toxicol.*, **17**, 264–272.

Kunsman, G.W., Manno, J.B., Przekop, M.A. *et al.* (1992) The effects of temazepam and ethanol on human psychomotor performance. *Eur. J. Clin. Pharmacol.*, **43**, 603.

Luce, G.G. (1973) *Body Time: The Natural Rhythms of the Body*. Paladin, St Albans.

McNaughton, L. and Preece, D. (1986) Alcohol and its effect on sprint and middle-distance running. *Br. J. Sports Med.*, **20**, 56–59.

Nuzzo, N.A. and Waller, W.D. (1988) Drug abuse in athletes. In: *Drugs, Athletics and Physical Performance* (ed. J.A. Thomas). Plenum Medical Book Co., New York, pp. 141–167.

O'Brien, C. (1993) Alcohol and sport: impact of social drinking on recreational and competitive sports performance. *Sports Med.*, **15**, 71–77.

Opie, L.H. (1986) Biochemical and metabolic responses to beta-adrenergic blockade at rest and during exercise. In: *Biochemical Aspects of Physical Exercise* (eds G. Benzi, L. Packer and N. Siliprandi). Elsevier, Amsterdam, pp. 423–433.

Orme, M. (1997) Health-related aspects of the use and abuse of beta-adrenoceptor blocking drugs. In: *The Clinical Pharmacology of Sport and Exercise* (eds T. Reilly and M. Orme). Elsevier, Amsterdam, pp. 61–69.

Powles, A.C.P. (1981) The effect of drugs on the cardiovascular response to exercise. *Med. Sci. Sports Exerc.*, **13**, 252–258.

Reilly, T. (1997) Alcohol: its influence in sport and exercise. In: *The Clinical Pharmacology of Sport and Exercise* (eds T. Reilly and M. Orme). Elsevier, Amsterdam, pp. 281–290.

Reilly, T. and Halliday, F. (1985) Influence of alcohol ingestion on tasks related to archery. *J. Hum. Ergol.*, **14**, 99–104.

Reilly, T. and Scott, J. (1993) Effects of elevating blood alcohol levels on tasks related to dart throwing. *Percept. Motor Skills*, **77**, 25–26.

Reilly, T., Lees, A., MacLaren, D. and Sanderson, F.H. (1985) Thrill and anxiety in adventure leisure parks. In: *Proceedings of the Ergonomics Society's Conference* (ed. D. Oborne). Taylor & Francis, London, pp. 210–214.

Reilly, T., Maughan, R. and Budgett, R. (1998) Melatonin: A position statement of the British Olympic Association. *Br. J. Sports Med.*, **32**, 99–100.

Reilly, T., Atkinson, G. and Budgett, R. (2001) Effects of low-dose temazepam on physiological variables and performance tests following a westerly flight across five time zones. *Int. J. Sports Med.*, **22**, 166–174.

Renaud, A.M. and Cormier, Y. (1986) Acute effects of marijuana smoking on maximal exercise performance. *Med. Sci. Sports Exerc.*, **18**, 685–689.

Rusko, H., Kantola, H., Luhtanen, R. *et al.* (1980) Effect of beta-blockade on performances requiring force, velocity, coordination and/or anaerobic metabolism. *J. Sports Med. Phys. Fit.*, **20**, 139–144.

Sanderson, F.H. (1981) The psychology of the injury-prone athlete. In: *Sport Fitness and Sports Injuries* (ed. T. Reilly). Wolfe, London, pp. 31–36.

Siitonen, L., Solnck, T. and Janne, J. (1977) Effect of beta-blockade on performance: use of beta-blockade in bowling and in shooting competitions. *J. Int. Med. Res.*, **5**, 359–366.

S'Jongers, J.J., Willain, P., Sierakowski, J., Vogelaere, P., Van Vlaenderen, G. and De Ruddel, M. (1978) Effet d'un placebo et de faibles doses d'un bêta-inhibiteur (oxprenolol) et d'alcool éthylique, sur la précision du tir sportif au pistolet. *Bruxelles-Medical*, **58**, 395–399.

Stepney, R. (1987) *Health and Lifestyle: A Review of a National Survey*. Health Promotion Research Trust, Cambridge.

Tong, J.E., Henderson, P.R. and Chipperfield, G.A. (1980) Effects of ethanol and tobacco on auditory vigilance performance. *Addict. Behav.*, **5**, 153–158.

WADA (2005) World Anti-Doping Code 2005 Prohibited List. Available at http://www.wada-ama.org (accessed 02/02/05).

Waterhouse, J., Reilly, T. and Atkinson, G. (1997) Jet-lag. *Lancet*, **350**, 1611–1616.

Wesnes, K. and Warburton, D.M. (1983) Stress and drugs. In: *Stress and Fatigue in Human Performance* (ed. R. Hockey). John Wiley, Chichester, pp. 203–243.

Wesnes, K. and Warburton, D.M. (1984) A comparison of temazepam and flurazepam in terms of sleep quality and residual changes in performance. *Neuropsychobiology*, **11**, 255–299.

Wesnes, K. and Warburton, D.M. (1986) Effects of temazepam on sleep quality and subsequent mental efficiency under normal sleeping conditions and following delayed sleep onset. *Neuropsychobiology*, **15**, 187–191.

Willett, W., Hennekens, C.H., Siegel, A.J. *et al.* (1980) Alcohol consumption and high-density lipoprotein cholesterol in marathon runners. *N. Eng. J. Med.*, **303**, 1159–1161.

Willett, W., Starnpfer, M.J., Colditz, G.A. *et al.* (1987) Moderate alcohol consumption and the risk of breast cancer. *N. Eng. J. Med.*, **316**, 1174–1179.

Zinzen, E., Clarys, J.P., Cabri, J. *et al.* (1994) The influence of triazolam and flunitrazepam on isokinetic and isometric muscle performance. *Ergonomics*, **37**, 69–77.

Chapter 10

Creatine

Don MacLaren

10.1 Introduction

Creatine has been known as a constituent of food for over 150 years having been discovered in 1832 by Chevreul who extracted it from meat. However, although phosphocreatine and its role in exercise was established in 1927, it was not until the early 1990s that significant levels of research were undertaken examining the effects of creatine supplementation on sports performance. This chapter briefly examines the synthesis and breakdown of creatine before considering its metabolic role in energy production within cells. Sections on the effectiveness on creatine loading regimens are also dealt with, as are explorations of enhanced muscle creatine on performance. Final sections relate to the health aspects and clinical implications of creatine supplementation.

10.2 Metabolism and storage of creatine

Creatine, or methyl guanidine-acetic acid, is a naturally occurring nitrogenous molecule (Figure 10.1) found mainly in the skeletal muscles of vertebrates. It is also found in smaller amounts in liver, kidney and brain. Although found mainly in skeletal muscle, creatine is metabolized in the liver and then transported to muscle. This is due to the fact that most tissues lack several of the enzymes involved in creatine synthesis.

Three amino acids are involved in the synthesis of creatine, these being arginine, glycine and methionine. Synthesis involves two stages, the first of

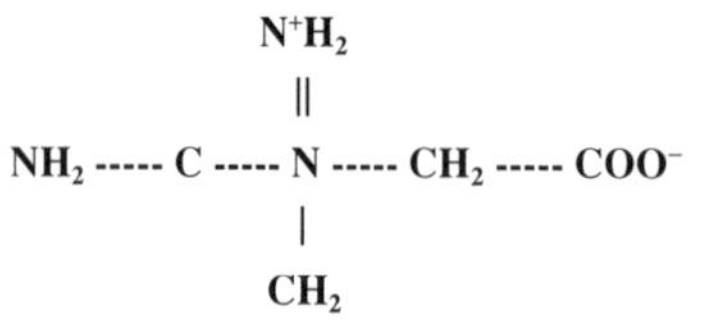

$$N^+H_2$$
$$\|$$
$$NH_2 \text{-----} C \text{-----} N \text{-----} CH_2 \text{-----} COO^-$$
$$|$$
$$CH_2$$

Figure 10.1 Structure of creatine.

arginine   +   glycine $\rightarrow$ ornithine   +   guanidinoacetate
$\uparrow$

arginine:glycine amidinotransferase (**AGAT**)

guanidinoacetate + S-adenosylmethionine $\rightarrow$ creatine + S-adenosylhomocysteine
$\uparrow$

guanidinoacetate methyltransferase (**GAMT**)

Figure 10.2 Reactions involved in the synthesis of creatine.

which is the transfer of the amidine group of arginine to glycine to produce guanidinoacetic acid (GAA) and ornithine, and is catalysed by the enzyme glycine amidinotransferase. The second reaction is the irreversible transfer of the methyl group from GAA to produce creatine (Figure 10.2).

De novo synthesized creatine is transported from the liver to skeletal muscle where it is taken up by active transport using a Na^+-dependent transporter. Once inside the muscle cell the creatine is 'trapped' by being converted to phosphocreatine, which is unable to pass through the membrane. It is also possible that creatine is bound to an intracellular component and/or that restrictive cellular membranes exist to stop efflux of creatine from muscle to blood (Fitch, 1977). Approximately 70 per cent of the creatine in muscle is in the phosphorylated form (phosphocreatine), the other 30 per cent being free creatine.

Creatine is constantly degraded to creatinine, which is its sole end product, via a non-enzymatic irreversible reaction. The creatinine diffuses through the muscle membrane and is taken to the kidney where it is excreted in a passive process before being voided in urine. The daily urine creatinine excretion is relatively constant, although it varies between individuals due to differences in muscle mass. For a more detailed examination of creatine and creatinine metabolism, the reader should consult Wyss and Kaddurah-Daouk (2000).

The daily turnover of creatine to creatinine in humans is about 2 g/day for a 70 kg person. This amount of creatine is replaced by endogenous synthesis and exogenous sources in the diet, with the synthesis being regulated by the exogenous intake through a feedback mechanism (Walker, 1960).

About 95 per cent of the creatine pool can be found in skeletal muscle. Significant amounts can also be found in heart, spermatozoa, brain, seminal vesicles, macrophages and photoreceptor cells of the retina, and low levels in kidney, liver, spleen and lungs. The stores of creatine exist in both the free and phosphorylated (phosphocreatine) forms. Free creatine constitutes 30 per cent of the total creatine pool whilst phosphocreatine constitutes the remaining 70 per cent and hence may be considered the 'trapped' form unable to leave the tissue. In a 70 kg male the store of creatine is approximately 120 g in total.

Muscle possesses two extreme types of fibres, these being slow oxidative and fast glycolytic fibres. The former are more readily recruited and are those fibres essentially used during prolonged, steady-state exercise. The slow oxidative fibres have a more plentiful supply of mitochondria and also possess more capillaries per fibre. The fast glycolytic fibres are recruited during more intense exercise and are able to generate greater power. They possess fewer mitochondria and have fewer capillaries per fibre. As such, the fast glycolytic fibres possess significantly higher concentrations of phosphocreatine than slow oxidative fibres. This has been established both in whole muscle biopsy (Edstrom et al., 1982) and single fibre studies (Soderlund et al., 1992). The difference between fibre types is about 30 per cent higher phosphocreatine in fast glycolytic than slow oxidative.

Muscle creatine concentration is expressed in millimoles per kilogram (mmol/kg) of dry mass. The total creatine concentration in muscle is approximately 30 mmol/kg when analysed from a biopsy sample which includes water. Since 1 mmol of creatine is equivalent to 131 mg, the creatine content of skeletal muscle is 4 g/kg of muscle. However, concentrations of metabolites are normally expressed in dry mass, thereby giving a total creatine concentration of 120 mmol/kg dry mass. Please note that this is the total creatine concentration, which includes the phosphorylated form.

Factors such as age, sex and diet influence muscle creatine concentration. Resting phosphocreatine levels have been shown to be lower in older (60 year) compared with younger (30 year) subjects (Smith et al., 1998b), although there is no significant difference in the total creatine concentration. In this instance it is possible that the degree of inactivity in the older subjects may have led to the attenuated phosphocreatine levels. To date, one study has shown that females have an elevated creatine concentration compared with males (Forsberg et al., 1991). Diet can significantly influence muscle creatine concentration as will be seen in the next section. However, it should be noted that since the exogenous source of creatine is via consuming foods containing meat and fish, vegetarians may have lower concentrations as their only source is de novo synthesis. Studies have shown that vegetarians do have marginally lower muscle creatine concentrations than those who eat meat and fish (Delanghe et al., 1989; Harris et al., 1992).

Another influence on muscle creatine is that of training. The results from training studies have been equivocal, although a recent study clearly established that sprint-trained athletes had elevated levels of phosphocreatine when compared with endurance athletes (Bernus et al., 1993). In this instance the differences could be due to the muscle fibre composition of the athletes, although the effect of training cannot be overlooked. Results from longitudinal training studies which have employed sprinting or resistance modes have failed to show elevated levels of phosphocreatine or creatine (Sharp et al., 1986; Nevill et al., 1989).

10.3   Energy metabolism

Energy is supplied by adenosine triphosphate (ATP) during any form of biological work. The hydrolysis of ATP to produce energy for muscle contraction is catalysed by the enzyme myosin ATPase, and the reaction is represented as follows:

$$ATP + H_2O \rightarrow ADP + P_i + Energy$$
$$\uparrow$$
myosin ATPase

However, the stores of ATP in muscle are small and need continuous replenishment if activity is to continue beyond a few seconds. Consequently, ATP is resynthesized by three energy systems:

1.   Phosphocreatine/creatine – **ADP + Phosphocreatine $\rightarrow$ ATP + Creatine**
2.   Glycolysis – **ADP + Glycogen $\rightarrow$ ATP + Lactic acid**
3.   Aerobic – **ADP + Glucose/Glycogen/Fatty Acids $\rightarrow$ ATP + CO_2 + H_2O**

The first two energy systems do not require the use of oxygen and so are deemed anaerobic. Furthermore, these sources of energy are rapidly promoted and are the major sources of ATP restoration during exercise of maximal intensity. Indeed the use of phosphocreatine is maximal in the first second of high intensity exercise and thereafter decreases over 30 seconds as first glycolysis and then aerobic sources predominate. It has been demonstrated that during a 6-second sprint on a cycle ergometer, phosphocreatine contributed approximately 50 per cent of the total ATP production (Boobis, 1987).

Creatine is reversibly phosphorylated by the enzyme creatine kinase (CK):

$$\textbf{phosphocreatine + ADP} \leftrightarrow \textbf{ATP + Creatine}$$
$$\uparrow$$
creatine kinase **(CK)**

Creatine kinase exists as four isoenzymes which are compartmentalized at a number of sites where energy is produced or utilized. Three of these isoenzymes have been labelled as MM-CK, MB-CK and BB-CK, all of which favour the above reaction from left to right and are found in the cytosol of either muscle (MM-CK) or muscle and brain (MB-CK) or brain (BB-CK). The fourth isoenzyme (Mi-CK) favours the reaction from right to left (i.e. formation of phosphocreatine from creatine) and is located on the outer side of the inner mitochondrial membrane (Clarke, 1997). The essential isoforms compartmentalized in skeletal muscle are MM-CK in the cytosol and Mi-CK in the mitochondria.

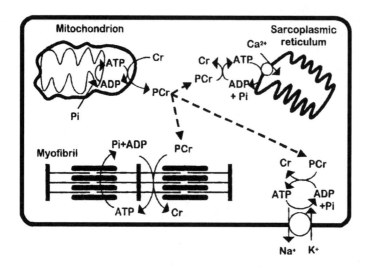

Figure 10.3 Schematic of creatine/phosphocreatine shuttling between sites of energy use and energy production (from Ruggeri, 2000 with permission).

Basal phosphocreatine concentrations as well as CK activity are higher in fast glycolytic than slow oxidative muscle fibres, and furthermore the rate of phosphocreatine degradation is higher in fast glycolytic than slow oxidative. On the other hand, the rate of resynthesis of phosphocreatine is faster in slow oxidative than fast glycolytic. This is because the resynthesis of phosphocreatine from creatine and ATP is dependent on the presence of oxygen and the hydrogen ion concentration, $[H^+]$. The better capillary supply to slow oxidative fibres and the lower $[H^+]$ leads to the enhanced rate of phosphocreatine resynthesis during recovery from maximal exercise. The rate of resynthesis of phosphocreatine following high-intensity exercise is rapid and biphasic (Harris *et al.*, 1976). Studies have concluded that 70 per cent of the phosphocreatine stores are replenished in the first 60 seconds of recovery, and that complete recovery is established in 5 minutes (Nevill *et al.*, 1997).

The creatine/phosphocreatine system has at least two major functions according to Ruggeri (2000), these being that of a 'temporal energy buffer' and that of a 'spatial energy buffer'. The former is concerned with the rephosphorylation of ATP from ADP involving the breakdown of phosphocreatine by MM-CK, whilst the latter is related to the shuttling of creatine and phosphocreatine between site of phosphocreatine hydrolysis and its resynthesis. Figure 10.3 illustrates the concept of 'spatial energy' in which phosphocreatine hydrolysis occurs at the myofibril, whereas the rephosphorylation of the creatine occurs at the mitochondria. At the mitochondrial site, newly synthesized ATP from oxidative phosphorylation enters the intermembrane space where some of it is used by Mi-CK to phosphorylate creatine and produce phosphocreatine. The phosphocreatine then diffuses out into the cytosol to the myofibrils. This shuttling system was initially proposed by Bessman and Geiger (1981), and provides a mechanism whereby sites of energy utilization (myofibril) are linked to sites of energy production (mitochondria). The creatine/phosphocreatine shuttling system is greater in slow oxidative and cardiac muscle fibres than fast glycolytic fibres, a factor demonstrated by the higher levels of mitochondrial CK than cytosolic CK in slow oxidative fibres compared with fast glycolytic fibres.

In addition to the two functions associated with energy use and production, creatine is also a metabolic buffer (Hochachka, 1994). Hydrolysis of ATP during muscle contraction together with the function of Ca^{2+} and Na^+ pumps results in the release of protons. Conversely, resynthesis of ATP utilizes protons. Since creatine/phosphocreatine are involved in ATP synthesis, the system acts as a buffer as follows:

$$ADP + Phosphocreatine + H^+ \leftrightarrow ATP + Creatine$$

Because the increase in hydrogen ions, H^+, and the concomitant decrease in pH has been associated with muscle fatigue, the ability to buffer H^+ may serve to attenuate the decrease in muscle pH and thereby delay fatigue.

A further point needs to be made in relation to the metabolic functions of creatine/phosphocreatine, and that is the fact that the increase in concentration of ADP is attenuated by the availability of phosphocreatine. It should be remembered that ADP is an allosteric effector in so far as elevated levels inhibit various enzymes involved in glycolysis and also the ATPases. In this respect, creatine/phosphocreatine acts as a cellular buffer.

It is now possible to consider the reasons for the numerous investigations into the use of creatine supplementation as an ergogenic aid for sports performance which involves high intensity activity. The fact that phosphocreatine is an important energy source during this type of activity, and that creatine/phosphocreatine acts as an H^+ buffer, make it an attractive potential nutritional support for athletes where either single bouts of intense activity lasting around 10 seconds or repeated bouts of sprint activity are involved. The latter makes the potential use of creatine supplementation of particular interest for most games players where the activity is intermittent.

In addition, it is recognized that creatine is an osmotically active substance, and consequently elevated levels lead to an increase in water retention in the tissues where it is taken up. The initial weight gain by athletes who supplement with creatine is probably due to enhanced water retention within muscle. A positive effect of increased muscle water is that it has been shown to stimulate protein synthesis (Ingwall, 1976; Bessman and Savabi, 1988). Clearly this is of benefit for athletes who need to increase lean body mass, power and strength.

10.4 Muscle creatine loading

Muscle creatine is restored at a rate of approximately 2 g/day by a combination of dietary creatine ingestion from sources such as meat and fish, and from endogenous synthesis using the amino acids arginine, glycine and methionine. The absence of creatine in the diet of vegetarians results not only in diminished levels in muscle, but also lower rates of creatine and creatinine excretion within urine. On the other hand, increased retention of creatine occurs in vegetarians supplemented with creatine, thereby demonstrating that endogenous synthesis of creatine does not match requirements in vegetarians.

It has only been possible since the advent of the muscle biopsy technique, and more recently that of phosphorus nuclear magnetic resonance spectroscopy (^{31}P-MRS), to determine the levels of creatine and phosphocreatine in muscle. One of the earliest reported studies to show elevated muscle creatine and phosphocreatine following ingestion was that by Harris et al. (1992), who found that ingestion of 5 g of creatine 4 to 6 times a day for 2 days resulted in an increase in total creatine from 127 to 149 mmol/kg, with an increase in phosphocreatine from 84 to 91 mmol/kg. These increases were individual responses, in which some subjects increased significantly and others less so. The term 'responders' and 'non-responders' applies in this instance, although there was a relationship between the initial resting level and the level of increase. The two vegetarians in the study possessed the lowest initial resting levels and responded with significant increases. Furthermore, Harris et al. (1992) were also able to demonstrate that whereas on the first 2 days the creatine storage was approximately 30 per cent of that ingested, the amount stored in the following 2 days diminished to around 15 per cent of the creatine ingested.

Some studies have shown that muscle creatine concentrations can be significantly enhanced using lower daily doses for a prolonged time period. For example, Hultman et al. (1996) reported that creatine ingestion of 3 g/day over a 4-week period produced muscle creatine concentrations similar to those found when 20 g/day were ingested over a 5-day period.

Most recent studies have employed a regimen in which 5 g of creatine is administered in a warm solution during 4 equally spaced time intervals through a day. Such a procedure results in a significant elevation in plasma creatine within 20 minutes of ingestion, and remains elevated for 3 hours. Since the Km value for muscle creatine transport is 20–100 µmol/l, the concentrations of plasma creatine following ingestion (approximately 1000 µmol/l) are unlikely to be limiting.

There is considerable variation between subjects to the extent muscle creatine concentrations are elevated following supplementation, although it appears that there is an upper limit of 160 mmol/kg dry muscle. It should also be recognized that 20 per cent of subjects investigated are non-responders, in that their levels of muscle creatine increase by less than 10 mmol/kg. As a consequence of the fact that there are non-responders, methods have been developed which increase the likelihood for such persons to augment their muscle creatine stores successfully. The result has been that total creatine accumulation in muscle has been enhanced by approximately 60 per cent when ingested in combination with at least 370 g of simple carbohydrates in a day (Green *et al.*, 1996a,b). This regimen promoted creatine stores to around 160 mmol/kg in the non-responders. Interestingly, the data from these studies showed that whereas previously there was an inverse relationship between initial muscle creatine and the level of loading when creatine alone was ingested, no such relationship existed when creatine was combined with carbohydrate.

It seems likely that the increase in muscle creatine stores when taken with carbohydrates is as a result of insulin action. Indeed, hyperinsulinaemia results in enhanced muscle creatine storage, probably by stimulating the Na^+-dependent muscle creatine transporter activity. A specific, saturable, Na^+-dependent transporter responsible for creatine uptake across the plasma membrane has been described for skeletal muscle, heart, brain, kidney, intestine and red blood cells, but not for liver. Quite how these transporters are regulated remains unclear, although β_2-adrenergic receptors that have cAMP as their intracellular signal have been strongly implicated. The role of insulin may be due to its stimulation of Na^+-ATPase and K^+-ATPase activity, which indirectly stimulates creatine transporter activity (Steenge *et al.*, 1998). Despite many investigations, the regulation of creatine uptake is not fully understood. It could be that there is a direct effect by modulation of the expression of the creatine transporter, or indirectly by alterations of the transmembrane electrochemical gradient of Na which depends on Na^+-ATPase and K^+-ATPase activity.

The most critical determinant for the regulation of creatine uptake is plasma creatine concentration. An elevated concentration of plasma creatine points either to an increase in *de novo* synthesis or an increase in dietary intake of creatine. The net effect is to spare the precursors of creatine, and possibly to downregulate the creatine transporter.

Following the creatine loading phase of 20 g/day for 5 days, recommended maintenance doses are considerably lower. Most studies have used doses ranging from 2 to 5 g/day during the maintenance phase. Hultman *et al.* (1996) recommend a maintenance dose of 0.03 g/kg body mass per day, which for a 70 kg person amounts to approximately 2 g/day. This level is suggested because it is at, or above, the daily turnover rate of creatine metabolism (i.e. 2 g/day), and hence maintains the enhanced muscle creatine concentrations produced during the loading phase.

When an athlete stops ingesting creatine, the muscle creatine diminish to normal levels, but over what period of time? By measuring creatinine excretion, Greenhaff (1997) estimated that the elevated muscle creatine stores would take 4 weeks to return to normal. Hultman *et al.* (1996) reported that muscle creatine levels returned to normal after 30 days from cessation of supplementation. The implications of this are such that studies involving creatine supplementation with a cross-over design need to be aware of the length of time for 'wash out' of elevated muscle creatine stores.

10.5   Creatine and performance

The theoretical benefits of creatine supplementation are related to the role of creatine and phosphocreatine in the energetics of muscle contraction, and also to the potential for buffering increases in [H⁺] as a consequence of raised intramuscular lactic acid concentrations. Specifically, mechanisms purported to provide an ergogenic effect of creatine include the fact that supplementation results in elevated phosphocreatine in muscle and hence a greater immediate source of generation of ATP, that increased levels of creatine facilitate an enhanced rate of phosphocreatine resynthesis in recovery bouts, and that there is enhanced buffering of H⁺.

Intramuscular stores of ATP and phosphocreatine are limited, and it has been estimated that these phosphagen stores could supply sufficient energy for high-intensity exercise for not more than 10 seconds (Balsom *et al.*, 1994). Furthermore, Sahlin (1998) has suggested that the maximum rate of phosphocreatine hydrolysis decreases as phosphocreatine content of muscle decreases, and that complete depletion is not necessary to cause a reduction in power production. In fact, a number of researchers have concluded that phosphocreatine availability is a limiting factor during high-intensity exercise (Hultman *et al.*, 1991; Greenhaff, 1997).

Creatine supplementation, by increasing both creatine and phosphocreatine, particularly in the fast glycolytic fibres, should prolong single bouts of high-intensity exercise and especially repeated bouts of high-intensity exercise. Probably the first two studies which reported on creatine supplementation and intense exercise were those of Greenhaff *et al.* (1993) and Balsom *et al.* (1993a). Greenhaff and colleagues (1993), using 12 active subjects, employed 5 bouts of 30 maximal isokinetic knee extensions with 1 minute recovery between the bouts. When subjects were loaded with 20 g/ day of creatine for 5 days, peak muscle torque was significantly enhanced in the final 10 contractions during the first bout, and during the whole of the next 4 bouts. The authors concluded that creatine supplementation accelerated phosphocreatine resynthesis and that the increased availability of phosphocreatine was responsible for the higher peak torque production.

The study by Balsom *et al.* (1993a) used 16 subjects who undertook ten 6-second bouts of high-intensity cycling with 30 seconds' recovery between the tests. Subjects were expected to maintain a pedal rate of 140 rpm with a resistance set so that they could complete 6 seconds. The test was undertaken by a placebo group and a creatine group in a random, double-blind design. Creatine loading entailed 6 days of 20 g/day of creatine. The creatine-loaded group were able to maintain 140 rpm in the last 2 seconds of each of the bouts, whereas those on placebo failed to do so after the 4th bout of cycling. Indeed, at the 9th and 10th bouts, the placebo group were averaging 125 rpm as opposed to 138 rpm for the creatine-loaded group.

Since these early reports, in excess of 200 studies have now been published in peer reviewed articles. The majority of these studies highlight the effectiveness of creatine supplementation for enhancing sports performance. These studies have examined the effects on high-intensity exercise (both single bouts and repeated bouts), strength and power, field based activities and endurance. Other studies have purely examined the effects of supplementation on lean body mass and body composition, although many of the other studies have also reported data on body mass changes. The reader is advised to examine Williams et al. (1999) for a broader exploration of approximately 150 studies published up to early 1999.

Creatine and single bouts of high-intensity exercise

In spite of the fact that creatine supplementation leads to increases in muscle creatine and phosphocreatine, it would be expected that single bouts of high-intensity exercise would produce enhanced performance. In general, this is not the case. A few studies have shown significant improvements in running 36.6 metres (Goldberg and Bechtel, 1997; Noonan et al., 1998) or 91.4 metres (Stout et al., 1999), or vertical jump performance (Stout et al., 1999). The majority of studies using single bouts of running, cycling, swimming and jumping have failed to show significant improvements. It appears that the possibility of elevated creatine stores in muscle being available to maintain a short, sharp burst of activity when not fatigued does not happen. Interestingly, a study in which a single bout of 10 seconds of sprint cycling was assessed following 5 bouts of 6-second sprinting with a 30-second recovery between bouts did show an increase in power (Balsom et al., 1995). So when there is an element of fatigue due to previous activity, creatine may help to improve single bouts of intense exercise.

Creatine and repeated bouts of high-intensity exercise

Since enhanced stores of creatine and phosphocreatine result from creatine loading, there is the significant possibility that during recovery phases of repeated bouts of exercise, the elevated creatine will be more rapidly phosphorylated. Enhanced performance may then result in subsequent bouts of exercise. This has already been reported above in the study by Balsom et al. (1993a). Positive ergogenic effects of creatine loading have been exhibited for repeated bouts of high-intensity cycling (Greenhaff et al., 1994; Earnest et al., 1995; Casey et al., 1996), running (Aaserud et al., 1998), swimming

(Peyrebrune *et al.*, 1998) and vertical jumping (Bosco *et al.*, 1997). In most cases, the significant effects are noted in the later bouts of exercise and not usually in the first bout. Furthermore, the significant effects are normally associated with mean power or total work done rather than peak power values. All in all, these findings support the notion of greater rephosphorylation in the recovery period when creatine stores have been enhanced.

It should be noted, however, that not all studies have reported significant effects. Some studies on repeated sprint cycling have shown no significant effect of creatine ingestion (Barnett *et al.*, 1996; Burke *et al.*, 1996; Cooke *et al.*, 1995; Stone *et al.*, 1999). Similar non-responses were obtained for investigations using repeated running (Smart *et al.*, 1998) and swimming (Grindstaff *et al.*, 1997; Leenders *et al.*, 1999).

It is difficult to fathom the reasons why the majority of studies highlight positive ergogenic effects whereas a significant smaller proportion find no such differences. Examination of the dose of creatine ingested and whether carbohydrates were ingested in addition, together with the types of subjects used (i.e. level of training), the sex of the subjects, the dietary habits of the subjects, the number of subjects employed and variations in the mode of testing are all possible confounding variables. On balance, creatine supplementation results in an approximate 4–10 per cent improvement in repeated high-intensity activities. Even some of the studies which reported no significant findings did find 2–4 per cent improvements in performance, but due to the low power of the experimental design produced non-significant results.

Creatine and strength

Phosphocreatine and ATP are likely to be the major energy sources during strength-based activities which are isometric, isotonic or isokinetic. In the cases of isotonic or isokinetic exercise, the activity is repeated in either fast or slow modes, whereas isometric activity involves either an all-out fast action or a hold of the tension for a period of time. The majority of studies in which some form of strength has been assessed have shown positive ergogenic effects. Such studies include the use of isometric (Andrews *et al.*, 1998; Maganaris and Maughan, 1998), isotonic (Earnest *et al.*, 1995; Noonan *et al.*, 1998; Stone *et al.*, 1999) or isokinetic (Greenhaff *et al.*, 1993; Vandenberghe *et al.*, 1996) modes of testing. Improvements of between 6 and 28 per cent in strength were reported in the above studies.

However, as with the studies on repeated bouts of high-intensity exercise, there are a number of studies which reported no significant benefits of creatine on isometric strength (Rawson *et al.*, 1998), isotonic strength (Goldberg and Bechtel, 1997; Stout *et al.*, 1999) and isokinetic strength (Kreider *et al.*, 1996).

The reasons for discrepancies in these findings may be those expressed above, but in addition could include the level of resistance or weight training experienced by the subjects. The latter seems unlikely since studies showing positive effects have included experienced and novice subjects, as have those showing no significant effect. Again, on balance the evidence for a positive effect is greater than no effect.

Creatine and endurance performance

In spite of the fact that creatine and phosphocreatine are involved in high-intensity and anaerobic energy-requiring activities, there has been some speculation that creatine supplementation may help more prolonged, aerobic events owing to an enhanced interval training effect which may lead to an increase in TCA cycle enzyme activity, i.e. citrate synthase (Viru et al., 1994, Greenhaff et al., 1997; Volek et al., 1999). Of course, a potential 'down side' for running events would be the potential increase in body mass.

Smith et al. (1998a) used 15 subjects in a study which employed cycling to exhaustion at 3.0, 3.3 and 3.7 watts/kg. Following creatine supplementation of 20 g/day for 5 days, the subjects only improved time to exhaustion at 3.7 watts/kg. No significant effect was noted for the other two exercise intensities. Since the time to exhaustion for the trial using the highest work load improved from 236 s to 253 s, the event may be considered aerobic. The greater the aerobic contribution the less likely creatine is to have an effect.

In spite of the above findings, Bosco et al. (1995) found that their subjects improved their Cooper 12 minute run/walk test following creatine supplementation of 5 g/day for 42 days. Furthermore, Viru et al. (1994) found that middle distance runners improved their total time for four 1000 m interval runs.

In studies which have examined longer duration activities, no significant effects of creatine have been found (Balsom et al., 1993b; Stroud et al., 1994; Myburgh et al., 1996; Godly and Yates, 1997). Indeed, the study by Balsom et al. (1993b) actually found impaired performance by those on creatine supplementation.

It would appear that creatine supplementation may have positive effects on intense activities for up to 4 or even 12 minutes where there is a clear involvement in aerobic energy processes. The case for beneficial effects on longer duration events is not proven. Clearly there is a need to examine the effects of interval training, with and without creatine supplementation, to note if there are any ergogenic effects with the combination of more intense training possibly brought about by creatine loading.

Creatine and body composition

One of the proposed ergogenic effects of creatine supplementation is the increase in lean body mass. As previously stated, this may result from the fact that creatine is osmotically active and hence increases the muscle water stores, thereby leading to enhanced protein synthesis. Of course, the increase in muscle mass could also result from an increase in training intensity brought about by enhanced muscle stores of phosphocreatine and creatine. Williams *et al.* (1999) reported that out of 58 studies which assessed body mass changes with creatine supplementation, 43 reported significant increases in body mass whereas 15 reported no significant changes. Those studies which reported the increase in body mass showed that a 5- or 6-day loading regimen resulted in an increase of around 1.0 kg (range from 0.6 to 2.8 kg). The more long-term studies reported increases in body mass of up to 5 kg in 12 weeks. In the first instance, the changes may be attributed to fluid retention, although subsequent increases were due to enhanced lean body mass.

There is clear evidence in studies which have used resistance training and creatine supplementation, that significant increases in muscle mass have resulted. This is obviously desirable in sports where an increase in muscle mass is important, but not of benefit in sports such as distance running.

10.6   Health-related aspects

The first reported health problems attributed to creatine loading were published in late 1997 and early 1998. In the first instance, the deaths of three US collegiate wrestlers from renal failure were reported to be linked to creatine supplementation. In fact, only one of the wrestlers had used creatine. The probable cause of renal failure was the extreme weight loss measures undertaken by these athletes in order to make weight for competition. None the less, these tragic deaths brought to light the potential for renal problems if athletes engage in loading with creatine over prolonged time periods without adequate hydration. If athletes are to engage in creatine loading, they should follow appropriate use by not taking more than 5 g/day in the maintenance phase and ensuring plenty of fluid is ingested. Juhn *et al.* (1999) reported that many male collegiate athletes ingested greater than 10 g/day of creatine. This is ill-advised, and if taken in conjunction with diuretics or other dehydration strategies, could conceivably place a strain on the renal system. The evidence of athletes consuming 10 g/day (or more) over 9 weeks failed to show impairment of renal function as measured by creatinine clearance, serum concentration of creatinine and urine analysis (Poortmans and Francaux, 1999).

Another case, which was reported in the *Lancet* in 1998 (Pritchard and Kalra, 1998), concerned the effects of creatine loading and maintenance over a 7-week period in an amateur football player who suffered from focal segmental glomerulosclerosis. Creatine supplementation resulted in a fall in creatinine clearance, and so gave concern to the physicians. It appears that in this instance, when an athlete has a recognized kidney dysfunction, they should be wary of supplementing with creatine.

More recently, a serious case of an apparently healthy 20-year-old male who suffered acute focal interstitial nephritis and focal tubular injury after creatine supplementation of 20 g/day for 4 weeks was reported (Koshy *et al.*, 1999). Taking such a high dose for such a prolonged period is clearly not advisable.

In spite of the anecdotal report on the three wrestlers, and the two case studies reporting renal problems, Poortmans *et al.* (1997) and Poortmans and Francaux (1999) have shown no significant effects on kidney function when creatine is taken over a short or long period. Indeed, Schilling *et al.* (2001) published a retrospective study on 26 collegiate athletes who supplemented their diets with creatine. They concluded that all the subjects' kidney function tests fell within the normal range.

Some clinical studies have added to the debate on safety of creatine supplementation over prolonged periods of time. In one study, the continuous use of lower doses (1.5 g/day) of creatine over a 5-year period for patients suffering from gyrate atrophy of the choroid and retina have shown no adverse effects on kidney or liver (Vannas-Sulonen *et al.*, 1985). Furthermore, studies show that children who are born with an inability to synthesize creatine, and so have diminished muscle and brain creatine stores, suffer impaired motor and mental function. Treatment with oral creatine supplementation of between 4 and 8 g/day over 2 years resulted in normal muscle and brain stores, which in turn led to normal physical and mental development. In these cases no reports of renal or liver damage was found (Stockler *et al.*, 1994, 1996).

Anecdotal reports of creatine supplementation causing muscle cramps, gastrointestinal problems and muscle injuries have appeared in various newspaper and leisure articles without strong scientific back-up. Kreider *et al.* (1998b) found, in a retrospective analysis of five of their published studies, that reports of gastrointesinal distress were isolated and fewer than for subjects taking the placebo supplement. This finding is supported by the retrospective study by Schilling *et al.* (2001).

The results from several studies have refuted the anecdotal reports of creatine supplementation leading to dehydration and thereby causing muscle cramps (Hultman *et al.*, 1996; Kreider *et al.*, 1996, 1998a; Hunt *et al.*, 1999; Rasmussen *et al.*, 1999). Indeed, some of these authors report the potential beneficial influences on body water retention rather than enhanced dehydration and muscle cramps.

The majority of studies in which creatine supplementation has been employed have not reported significant problems either in the form of renal function or in matters relating to muscle cramps or gastrointestinal disturbance. When an athlete with normal kidney function uses creatine in a sensible manner there does not appear to be a problem. Ensuring that a dose of 3–5 g/day for the maintenance phase is taken with sufficient volume of fluid is a minimum safety requirement. Seeking medical advice on renal function is a useful adjunct.

10.7   Creatine and clinical use

As mentioned above, creatine supplementation is used in a clinical setting for conditions such as gyrate atrophy of the choroids and retina, and also for inborn errors of metabolism such as creatine deficiency. In addition, creatine supplementation has been examined in relation to heart disease, neuromuscular disease and recovery from orthopaedic injury and surgery. Conway and Clark (1996) have edited a treatise detailing the clinical applications of creatine and phosphocreatine.

An extensive amount of research has been conducted on the potential medical benefits of both oral creatine and intravenous phosphocreatine supplementation in patients with heart disease. Intravenous administration of phosphocreatine has been reported to improve myocardial metabolism and reduce incidences of ventricular fibrillation in ischaemic heart patients (Andrews et al., 1998; Horn et al., 1998). It appears that phosphocreatine enhances the viability of the cell membrane and so reduces the chance of cell injury during ischaemia. Furthermore, intravenous administration of phosphocreatine may have a cytoprotective effect for cardiac muscle in patients with heart disease (Saks et al., 1996). If interested in further studies relating to the effectiveness of creatine or phosphocreatine administration on skeletal muscle and cardiac function in patients with heart failure, the reader may wish to consult Gordon (2000).

The use of creatine supplementation to reduce lipid profiles has been reported for middle-aged hypertriglyceraemic patients (Earnest et al., 1996). In this study, 56 days of creatine supplementation resulted in a 6 per cent decrease in total cholesterol and a 22 per cent decrease in triglycerides. Creatine ingestion may therefore offer some health benefits by altering blood lipid profiles in a positive manner, although more evidence is needed to confirm this preliminary finding.

Creatine supplementation promotes muscle hypertrophy following resistance training. Consequently, there has been interest in the effectiveness of such supplementation on recovery from injury or surgery. Satolli and Marchesi (1989) found a greater increase in muscle girth of the thigh after knee surgery when supplemented with phosphocreatine, and Pirola et al. (1991) showed a twofold increase in thigh and leg muscle mass when elderly subjects were given 500 mg/day of phosphocreatine intravenously.

Further areas of clinical application include the potential for creatine supplementation on mitochondrial cytopathies (Bourgeois and Tarnopolsky, 2000), neurodegenerative diseases (Kaddurah-Daouk et al., 2000) and improving the quality of life for geriatric patients (Enzi, 2000). In these respects, the simplistic common denominator is that creatine and phosphocreatine increase the 'energy potential' of the various cells and hence can overcome or alleviate the degenerative conditions.

10.8   Should creatine be banned for use in sport?

Creatine is a natural food supplement made up from amino acids. The fact that there is a significant enhancement of power, strength, speed and lean body mass as a consequence of creatine supplementation, particularly when training, means that it is a positive ergogenic aid. Similar statements could be made about the value of carbohydrate loading and amino acid supplementation after exercise to promote both muscle glycogen stores and protein synthesis. So, why ban a natural product? The IOC and World Anti-Doping Agency have not made a position statement concerning creatine, probably because it does occur naturally in food, and it could also prove difficult to determine the level of muscle creatine and phosphocreatine without resorting to invasive biopsies or expensive MRS imaging. Indeed, above what levels of muscle creatine and phosphocreatine would an athlete be banned? Those athletes who eat large amounts of fish could have elevated levels normally. My own view is that creatine supplementation cannot be banned, although careful advice and monitoring of athletes should be undertaken. Further examinations of the effects of creatine on kidney function should be explored.

10.9   Conclusion

The role of creatine in the human body is now largely understood. Its main function is to transfer energy from the mitochondria to the myofibrils. The daily turnover rate of approximately 2 g is only 50 per cent covered by endogenous synthesis, the rest coming from exogenous dietary sources. Supplementation of creatine can lead to an increase in total muscle creatine and also in phosphocreatine, although an upper limit of 160 mmol/kg has been proposed. The increase in muscle creatine stores has generally led to significant improvements in repetitive high-intensity exercise, strength and lean body mass. Equivocal findings have been reported for more prolonged, aerobic-based activities. In the clinical setting, creatine supplementation shows promising therapeutic effects in relation to cardiac failure, some mitochondrial cytopathies and to some neurodegenerative disorders. Adverse effects of prolonged creatine supplementation on renal function have been reported in one or two case studies, although the majority of studies show no detrimental effects. If taken in recommended doses and with adequate hydration, creatine supplementation should be safe.

10.10   References

Aaserud, R., Gramvik, P., Olsen, S.R. and Jensen, J. (1998) Creatine supplementation delays onset of fatigue during repeated bouts of sprint running. *Scand. J. Med. Sci. Sports*, **8**, 247–251.

Andrews, R., Greenhaff, P.L., Curtis, S., Perry, A. and Cowley, A.J. (1998) The effect of dietary creatine supplementation on skeletal muscle metabolism in congestive heart failure. *Eur. Heart J.*, **19**, 617–622.

Balsom, P.D., Ekblom, B. and Soderlund, K. (1993a) Creatine supplementation and dynamic high intensity intermittent exercise. *Scand. J. Med. Sci. Sports*, **3**, 143–149.

Balsom, P.D., Harridge, S.D.R., Soderlund, K., Sjodin, B. and Ekblom, B. (1993b) Creatine supplementation *per se* does not enhance endurance exercise performance. *Acta Physiol. Scand.*, **149**, 521–523.

Balsom, P., Soderlund, K. and Ekblom, B. (1994) Creatine in humans with special reference to creatine supplementation. *Sports Med.*, **18**, 268–280.

Balsom, P.D., Soderlund, K., Sjodin, B. and Ekblom, B. (1995) Skeletal muscle metabolism during short duration high-intensity exercise. *Acta Physiol. Scand.*, **154**, 303–310.

Barnett, C., Hinds, M. and Jenkins, D.G. (1996) Effects of oral creatine supplementation on multiple sprint cycle performance. *Aust. J. Sci. Med. Sports*, **28**, 35–39.

Bernus, G., Gonzale de Suso, J.M., Alonso, J., Martin, P.A., Prat, J.A. and Arus, C. (1993) ^{31}P-MRS of quadriceps reveals quantitative differences between sprinters and long-distance runners. *Med. Sci. Sports Exerc.*, **25**, 479–484.

Bessman, S. and Geiger, P.J. (1981) Transport of energy in muscle: the phosphorylcreatine shuttle. *Science*, **211**, 448–452.

Bessman, S. and Savabi, F. (1988) The role of phosphocreatine energy shuttle in exercise and muscle hypertrophy. In: *Creatine and creatine phosphate: Scientific and clinical perspectives* (eds M.A. Conway and J.F. Clark) Academic Press, San Diego, pp. 185–198.

Boobis, L.H. (1987) Metabolic aspects of fatigue during sprinting. In: *Exercise: benefits, limits and adaptations* (eds D. Macleod, R. Maughan, M. Nimmo, T. Reilly and C. Williams) E&FN Spon, London, pp. 116–143.

Bosco, C., Tranquilli, C., Tihanyi, J., Colli, R., D'Ottavio, S. and Viru, A. (1995) Influence of oral supplementation with creatine monohydrate on physical activity evaluated in laboratory and field tests. *Medicina dello Sport*, **48**, 391–397.

Bosco, C., Tihanyi, J., Pucspk, J. *et al.* (1997) Effect of oral creatine supplementation on jumping and running performance. *Int. J. Sports Med.*, **18**, 369–372.

Bourgeois, J.M. and Tarnopolsky, M.A. (2000) Creatine supplementation in mitochondrial cytopathies. In: *Creatine: from basic science to clinical application* (eds R. Paoletti, A. Poli and A.S. Jackson), Kluwer Academic Publishers, London, pp. 91–100.

Burke, L.M., Pyne, D.B. and Telford, R.D. (1996) Effects of oral creatine supplementation on single-effort sprint performance in elite swimmers. *Int. J. Sports Nutr.*, **6**, 222–233.

Casey, A., Constantin-Teodosiu, D., Howell, S., Hultman, E. and Greenhaff, P.L. (1996) Creatine ingestion favorably affects performance and muscle metabolism during maximal exercise in humans. *Am. J. Physiol.*, **271**, E31–E37.

Clarke, J.F. (1997) Creatine and phosphocreatine: A review of their use in exercise and sport. *J. Athlet. Train.*, **32**, 45–50.

Conway, M.A. and Clark, J.F. (eds) (1996) *Creatine and creatine phosphate: scientific and clinical perspectives*. Academic Press, San Diego.

Cooke, W.H., Grandjean, P.W. and Barnes, W.S. (1995) Effect of oral creatine supplementation on power output and fatigue during bicycle ergometry. *J. Appl. Physiol.*, **78**, 670–673.

Delanghe, J., De Slypere, J.P., De Buyzere, M., Robbrecht, J., Wieme, R. and Vermeulen, A. (1989) Normal reference values for creatine, creatinine, and carnitine are lower in vegetarians. *Clin. Chem.*, **35**, 1802–1803.

Earnest, C.P., Snell, P.G., Rodriguez, R., Almada, A.L. and Mitchell, T.L. (1995) The effect of creatine monohydrate ingestion on anaerobic power indices, muscular strength and body composition. *Acta Physiol. Scand.*, **153**, 207–209.

Earnest, C.P., Almada, A.L. and Mitchell, T.L. (1996) High-performance capillary electrophoresis-pure creatine monohydrate reduced blood lipids in men and women. *Clin. Sci.*, **91**, 113–118.

Edstrom, I., Hultman, E., Sahlin, K. and Sjoholm, H. (1982) The content of high energy phosphates in different fibre types in skeletal muscles from rat, guinea pig and man. *J. Physiol.*, **332**, 47–58.

Enzi, G. (2000) New areas for creatine supplementation: chronic obstructive pulmonary disease and geriatric condition. In: *Creatine: from basic science to clinical application* (eds R. Paoletti, A. Poli and A.S. Jackson), Kluwer Academic Publishers, London, pp. 83–90.

Fitch, C.D. (1977) Significance of abnormalities of creatine metabolism. In: *Pathogenesis of human muscular dystrophies* (ed. L.P. Rowland), Excerpta Medica, Amsterdam, pp. 328–340.

Forsberg, A.M., Nilsson, E., Werneman, J., Bergstrom, J. and Hultman, E. (1991) Muscle composition in relation to age and sex. *Clin. Sci.*, **81**, 249–256.

Godly, A. and Yates, J.W. (1997) Effects of creatine supplementation on endurance cycling combined with short, high-intensity bouts. *Med. Sci. Sports Exerc.*, **29**, S251.

Goldberg, P.G. and Bechtel, P.J. (1997) Effects of low dose creatine supplementation on strength, speed and power events by male athletes. *Med. Sci. Sports Exerc.*, **29**, S251.

Gordon, A. (2000) Creatine supplementation in patients with chronic heart failure. In: *Creatine: from basic science to clinical application* (eds R. Paoletti, A. Poli and A.S. Jackson), Kluwer Academic Publishers, London, pp. 41–50.

Green, A.L., Simpson, E.J., Littlewood, J.J., MacDonald, I.A. and Greenhaff, P.L. (1996a) Carbohydrate ingestion augments creatine retention during creatine feeding in man. *Acta Physiol. Scand.*, **158**, 195–202.

Green, A.L., Hultman, E., MacDonald, I.A., Sewell, D.A. and Greenhaff, P.L. (1996b) Carbohydrate ingestion augments skeletal muscle creatine accumulation during creatine supplementation in man. *Am. J. Physiol.*, **271**, E821–E826.

Greenhaff, P.L. (1997) The nutritional biochemistry of creatine. *Nutr. Biochem.*, **8**, 610–618.

Greenhaff, P.L., Casey, A., Short, A.H., Harris, R., Soderlund, K. and Hultman, E. (1993) Influence of oral creatine supplementation of muscle torque during repeated bouts of maximal voluntary exercise in man. *Clin. Sci.*, **84**, 565–571.

Greenhaff, P.L., Constantin-Teodosiu, D., Casey, A. and Hultman, E. (1994) The effect of oral creatine supplementation on skeletal muscle ATP degradation during repeated bouts of maximal voluntary exercise in man. *J. Physiol.*, **476**, 84P.

Grindstaff, P.D., Kreider, R., Bishop, R. *et al.* (1997) Effects of creatine supplementation on repetitive sprint performance and body composition in competitive swimmers. *Int. J. Sports Nutr.*, **7**, 330–346.

Harris, R.C., Soderlund, K. and Hultman, E. (1992) Elevation of creatine in resting and exercised muscle of normal subjects by creatine supplementation. *Clin. Sci.*, **83**, 367–374.

Harris, R.C., Edwards, R.H.T., Hultman, E., Nordesjo, L.O., Nylind, B. and Sahlin, K. (1976) The time course of phosphorylcreatine resynthesis during recovery of the quadriceps muscle in man. *Pfluegers Arch.*, **367**, 137–142.

Hochachka, P.W. (1994) *Muscles as molecular and metabolic machines.* CRC Press, Boca Raton, Florida.

Horn, M., Frantz, S., Remkes, H. *et al.* (1998) Effects of chronic dietary creatine feeding on cardiac energy metabolism and on creatine content in heart, skeletal muscle, brain, liver and kidney. *J. Mol. Cell. Cardiol.*, **30**, 277–284.

Hultman, E., Greenhaff, P.L., Rem, J.M. and Soderlund, K. (1991) Energy metabolism and fatigue during intense muscle contraction. *Biochem. Soc. Trans.*, **19**, 347–353.

Hultman, E., Soderland, K., Timmons, J.A., Cederblad, G. and Greenhaff, P.L. (1996) Muscle creatine loading in men. *J. Appl. Physiol.*, **81**, 232–237.

Hunt, J., Kreider, R., Melton, C. *et al.* (1999) Creatine does not increase incidence of cramping or injury during pre-season college football training II. *Med. Sci. Sports Exerc.*, **31**, S355.

Ingwall, J.S. (1976) Creatine and the control of muscle-specific protein synthesis in cardiac and skeletal muscle. *Circ. Res.*, **38**, I-115–I-123.

Juhn, M.S., O'Kane, J.W. and Vinci, D.M. (1999) Oral creatine supplementation in male collegiate athletes: a survey of dosing habits and side effects. *J. Am. Diet. Assoc.*, **99**, 593–595.

Kaddurah-Daouk, R., Matthews, R. and Flint Beal, M. (2000) The neuroprotective properties of creatine in animal models of neurodegenerative disease. In: *Creatine: from basic science to clinical application* (eds R. Paoletti, A. Poli and A.S. Jackson) Kluwer Academic Publishers, London, pp. 101–117.

Koshy, K.M., Griswold, E. and Schneeberger, E.E. (1999) Interstitial nephritis in a patient taking creatine. *New Engl. J. Med.*, **340**, 814–815.

Kreider, R., Grindstaff, P., Wood, L. *et al.* (1996) Effects of ingesting a lean body mass promoting supplement during resistance training on isokinetic performance. *Med. Sci. Sports Exerc.*, **28**, S36.

Kreider, R., Ferreira, M., Wilson, M. *et al.* (1998a) Effects of creatine supplementation on body composition, strength, and sprint performance. *Med. Sci. Sports Exerc.*, **30**, 73–82.

Kreider, R., Rasmussen, C., Ransom, J. and Almada, A. (1998b) Effects of creatine supplementation during training on the incidence of muscle cramping, injuries and GI distress. *J. Strength Condition. Res.*, **12**, 275.

Leenders, N., Sherman, W.M., Lamb, D.R. and Nelson, T.E. (1999) Creatine supplementation and swimming performance. *Int. J. Sports Nutr.*, **9**, 251–262.

Maganaris, C.N. and Maughan, R.J. (1998) Creatine supplementation enhances maximum voluntary isometric force and endurance capacity in resistance trained men. *Acta Physiol. Scand.*, **163**, 279–287.

Myburgh, K.H., Bold, A., Bellinger, B., Wilson, G. and Noakes, T.D. (1996) Creatine supplementation and sprint training in cyclists: metabolic and performance effects. *Med. Sci. Sports Exerc.*, **28**, S81.

Nevill, A.M., Jones, D.A., McIntyre, D., Bogdanis, G.C. and Nevill, M.E. (1997) A model for phosphocreatine resynthesis. *J. Appl. Physiol.*, **82**, 329–335.

Nevill, M.E., Boobis, L.H., Brooks, S. and Williams, C. (1989) Effect of training on muscle metabolism during treadmill sprinting. *J. Appl. Physiol.*, **67**, 2376–2382.

Noonan, D., Berg, K., Latin, R.W., Wagner, J.C. and Reimers, K. (1998) Effects of varying dosages of oral creatine relative to fat free mass on strength and body composition. *J. Strength Condition. Res.*, **12**, 104–108.

Peyrebrune, M.C., Nevill, M.E., Donaldson, F.J. and Cosford, D.J. (1998) The effects of oral creatine supplementation in single and repeated swimming. *J. Sports Sci.*, **16**, 271–279.

Pirola, V., Pisani, L. and Teruzzi, P. (1991) Evaluation of the recovery of muscular trophicity in aged patients with femoral fractures treated with creatine phosphate and physiokinesitherapy. *Clin. Ter.*, **139**, 115–119.

Poortmans, J.R., Auquier, H., Renaut, V., Durassel, A., Saugy, M. and Brisson, G.R. (1997) Effect of short-term creatine supplementation on renal responses in men. *Eur. J. Appl. Physiol.*, **76**, 566–577.

Poortmans, J.R. and Francaux, M. (1999) Long-term oral creatine supplementation does not impair renal function in healthy athletes. *Med. Sci. Sports Exerc.*, **31**, 1108–1110.

Pritchard, N.R. and Kalra, P.A. (1998) Renal dysfunction accompanying oral creatine supplementation. *Lancet*, **351**, 1252–1253.

Rasmussen, C., Kreider, R., Ransom, J. *et al.* (1999) Creatine supplementation during pre-season football training does not affect fluid or electrolyte status. *Med. Sci. Sports Exerc.*, **31**, S299.

Rawson, E.S., Clarkson, P.M. and Melanson, E.L. (1998) The effects of oral creatine supplementation on body mass, isometric strength, and isokinetic performance in older individuals. *Med. Sci. Sports Exerc.*, **30**, S140.

Ruggeri, P. (2000) Physiological role of creatine in muscle metabolism during exercise. In: *Creatine: from basic science to clinical application* (eds R. Paoletti, A. Poli and A.S. Jackson), Kluwer Academic Press, London, pp. 59–63.

Sahlin, K. (1998) Anaerobic metabolism, acid–base balance, and muscle fatigue during high intensity exercise. In: *Oxford textbook of sports medicine* (eds M. Harries, C. Williams, W.D. Stanish and L.J. Micheli), Oxford University Press, Oxford, pp. 69–76.

Saks, V.A., Stepanov, V., Jaliashvili, I.V., Konerev, E.A., Kryzkanovsky, S.A. and Strumia, E. (1996) Molecular and cellular mechanisms of action for the cardioprotective and therapeutic role of creatine phosphate. In: *Creatine and creatine phosphate: scientific and clinical perspectives* (eds M.A. Conway and J.F. Clark), Academic Press, San Diego, pp. 91–114.

Satolli, F. and Marchesi, G. (1989) Creatine phosphate in the rehabilitation of patients with muscle hypotrophy of the lower extremity. *Curr. Ther. Res.*, **53**, 67–73.

Schilling, B.K., Stone, M.H., Utter, A. *et al.* (2001) Creatine supplementation and health variables: a retrospective study. *Med. Sci. Sports Exerc.*, **33**, 183–188.

Sharp, R.L., Costill, D.L., Fink, W.J. and King, D.S. (1986) Effects of eight weeks of bicycle ergometer sprint training on human muscle buffer capacity. *Int. J. Sports Med.*, **7**, 7–13.

Smart, N.A., McKenzie, S.G., Nix, L.M. *et al.* (1998) Creatine supplementation does not improve repeat sprint performance in soccer players. *Med. Sci. Sports Exerc.*, **30**, S140.

Smith, J.C., Stephens, D.P., Hall, E.L., Jackson, A.W. and Earnest, C.P. (1998a) Effect of oral creatine ingestion on parameters of the work-time relationship and time to exhaustion in high-intensity cycling. *Eur. J. Appl. Physiol.*, **77**, 360–365.

Smith, S.A., Montain, S.J., Matott, R.P., Zientara, G.P., Jolesz, F.A. and Fielding, R.A. (1998b) Creatine supplementation and age influence muscle metabolism during exercise. *J. Appl. Physiol.*, **85**, 1349–1356.

Soderlund, K., Greenhaff, P.L. and Hultman, E. (1992) Energy metabolism in type I and type II human muscle fibres during short term electrical stimulation at different frequencies. *Acta Physiol. Scand.*, **144**, 15–22.

Steenge, G.R., Lambourne, J., Casey, A., MacDonald, I.A. and Greenhaff, P.L. (1998) Stimulatory effect of insulin on creatine accumulation in human skeletal muscle. *Am. J. Physiol., Endocrinol. Metab.*, **275**, E974–979.

Stockler, S., Holzbach, U., Hanefeld, F., Schmidt, B. and von Figura, K. (1994) Creatine deficiency in the brain: a new, treatable inborn error of metabolism. *Paed. Res.*, **36**, 409–413.

Stockler, S., Hanefeld, F. and Frahm, J. (1996) Creatine replacement therapy in guanidinoacetate methyltransferase deficiency, a novel inborn error of metabolism. *Lancet*, **348**, 789–790.

Stone, M.H., Sanborn, K., Smith, L. *et al.* (1999) Effects of in-season (5 weeks) creatine and pyruvate supplementation on anaerobic performance and body composition in American football players. *Int. J. Sports Nutr.*, **9**, 146–165.

Stout, J.R., Echerson, J., Noonan, D., Moore, G. and Cullen, D. (1999) Effects of creatine supplementation on exercise performance and fat-free weight in football players during training. *Nutr. Res.*, **19**, 217–225.

Stroud, M.A., Holliman, D., Bell, D., Green, A.L., MacDonald, I. and Greenhaff, P.L. (1994) Effect of oral creatine supplementation on respiratory gas exchange and blood lactate accumulation during steady-state incremental treadmill exercise and recovery in man. *Clin. Sci.*, **87**, 707–710.

Vandenberghe, K., Goris, M., Van Hecke, P., Van Leemputte, M., Van Gerven, L. and Hespel, P. (1996) Prolonged creatine intake facilitates the effects of strength training on intermittent exercise capacity. *Insider*, **4**, 1–2.

Vannas-Sulonen, K., Sipila, I., Vannas, A., Simell, O. and Rapola, J. (1985) Gyrate atrophy of the choroids and retina. A five-year follow-up of creatine supplementation. *Ophthalmology*, **92**, 1719–1727.

Viru, M., Oopik, V., Nurmekivi, A., Medijainen, L., Timpmann, S. and Viru, A. (1994) Effect of creatine intake on the performance capacity of middle-distance runners. *Coach. Sports Sci. J.*, **1**, 31–36.

Volek, J.S., Duncan, N.D., Mazzetti, S.A. *et al.* (1999) Performance and muscle fiber adaptations to creatine supplementation and heavy resistance training. *Med. Sci. Sports Exerc.*, **31**, 1147–1156.

Walker, J.B. (1960) Metabolic control of creatine biosynthesis: effect of dietary creatine. *J. Biol. Chem.*, **235**, 2357–2361.

Williams, M.H., Kreider, R.B. and Branch, J.D. (1999) Creatine: the power supplement. Human Kinetics, Leeds.

Wyss, M. and Kaddurah-Daouk, R. (2000) Creatine and creatinine metabolism. *Physiol. Rev.*, **80**, 1107–1213.

Chapter 11

Doping control in sport

Michele Verroken and David R. Mottram

11.1 History of drug testing

The ingestion of substances by athletes with the intention of enhancing or influencing performance in sport is probably as old as sport itself. The widespread use of sophisticated chemical agents in sport and society emerged in the 1950s and 1960s in parallel with the evolution of the modern pharmaceutical industry. As new drugs were being discovered through methods of chemical synthesis rather than from extraction of plant or animal sources, the pharmaceutical industry also developed its processes of chemical analysis in order to test its products for efficacy and safety. It was this evolution of sensitive methods of drug screening that became the basis of the subsequent development of accurate methods of drug testing in sport.

Initially testing programmes were organized by the International Olympic Committee (IOC) and sports federations, mostly at international level; however, testing requirements upon athletes have increased more recently to include national sports federations and national anti-doping organizations, as well as the World Anti-Doping Agency (WADA). The reasons why testing has now become a responsibility of other organizations is explored later in this chapter.

A number of sports federations introduced drug testing in the late 1950s and early 1960s. Tests were targeted at amphetamines, which were at that time the most widely misused performance-enhancing agents. Amphetamines had been implicated in the death of the cyclist Knut Jensen at the 1964 Rome Olympics (Beckett and Cowan, 1979; Voy, 1991) and of the British cyclist Tommy Simpson, who died on the 13th day of the Tour de France in 1967. These most public examples of the misuse of drugs to improve performance pressured some sports organizations into regulating against doping, and testing to detect the misuse of substances, and to sanction the offender.

Early testing methods were relatively unsophisticated. The technology available to analyse an athlete's urine often resulted in inaccurate findings that failed to deter the use of drugs, although exogenous substances like amphetamines would have been relatively easy to detect. With the introduction of testing, athletes soon realized that a clearance time between drug use and testing was all that was needed to avoid traces of banned substances, particularly the metabolites of substances, being detected. At that time athletes were being tested after a competition and had little difficulty in calculating clearance times. Moreover, the detection methods and testing programmes were not capable of unequivocal detection of anabolic steroids, substances known to enhance the effects of training.

Although the IOC were among the first to establish rules about doping and to introduce testing, they were preceded by FIFA (Federation International de Football Association) who introduced testing at the 1966 World Cup in England and by the UCI (Union Cycliste Internationale) who formed their Medical Examination Regulations in 1967. The IOC first set up a Medical Commission in 1961, under the chairmanship of Sir Arthur Porritt. In 1967 the IOC re-established the Medical Commission under the chairmanship of Prince Alexandre de Merode from Belgium, a former cyclist who had been working towards the development of a doping control programme in the 1950s.

The Commission has three main responsibilities:

1. To give guidance and approval to the host country of an Olympic Games on medical and paramedical equipment and facilities at the Olympic Village.
2. To have responsibility for doping controls at the Olympic Games, for classifying the pharmacological substances and methods and for proposing sanctions to the IOC Executive Board when doping rules have been contravened.
3. The Commission is also responsible for femininity control for women's sporting events at the Games and issues certificates of femininity to those who have passed the control.

The IOC instituted its first compulsory doping controls at the Winter Olympic Games in Grenoble, France in 1968 and again at the Summer Olympic Games in Mexico City in the same year. At that time the list of banned substances issued in 1967 included narcotic analgesics and stimulants, which comprised sympathomimetic amines, psychomotor stimulants and miscellaneous central nervous system stimulants. Although it was suspected that androgenic anabolic steroids were being used at this time (Wade, 1972; Beckett, 1981), testing methods were insufficiently developed to warrant the inclusion of anabolic steroids in the list of banned substances.

When testing took place at the Games of 1968 it was of a limited nature. One athlete was disqualified for using alcohol. The IOC itself was clear about the limits of its responsibility on doping control, the IOC Newsletter of August 1968 stated:

The function of the IOC is to alert the National Olympic Committees and the international federations and promote an education campaign. The IOC has its rule and has defined dope and it should see that provisions are made by the Organising Committee for testing but the actual testing is left in the hands of others. This is a responsibility that the IOC is not prepared to take.

The first full-scale testing of Olympic athletes occurred at the 1972 Summer Olympic in Munich, Germany (de Merode, 1979). Again, tests were limited to narcotic analgesics and to the three classes of stimulants; however, testing was much more comprehensive with 2079 samples being analysed. Seven athletes were disqualified; one further athlete had already been disqualified at the Winter Games in Sapporo.

The IOC has overseen testing at subsequent Olympic Games, winter and summer. Olympic Games testing has not been without problems; whilst the organizing committee have to arrange the testing programmes, the international sports federations have the responsibility for guiding the level of testing and for ruling on the substances additional to the basic IOC list that should be controlled. At the Winter Games in Nagano, the identification of marijuana in the urine sample of a snow boarder raised a number of questions about the relevant authority and adequacy of regulations at the Games. Whilst the IOC considered their stance on marijuana was clear, the relevant international federation had vague rules that did not stand up to legal challenge. The Court of Arbitration for Sport Ad Hoc panel that sat during the Nagano Games concluded

> we do not suggest for a moment that the use of marijuana should be condoned, nor do we suggest that sports authorities are not entitled to exclude athletes found to use cannabis. But if sports authorities wish to add their own sanctions to those that are admitted by public authorities, they must do so in an explicit fashion. That has not been done here.
>
> (*NAG OG/98/002, Reeb, 1998*)

Outside of the Olympic Games, some international sports federations (IFs) assumed responsibility for testing. IOC involvement in the control of drug misuse in sport continued through the publication of a list of doping classes and methods adopted by the majority of sports, its guidelines on testing procedures and its accreditation of laboratories. Yet the limitations of the Olympic and IF programmes frustrated some national governments and national sports bodies; lack of confidence soon questioned even the value of testing under the IOC and IF authority.

In this respect the early work of the Council of Europe was significant in bringing governments into the testing arena. The intervention of governments and the development of national sports testing programmes soon increased the volume of testing and the likelihood of being tested.

Competition testing was soon considered of limited value; furthermore there was concern that the testing programmes that were operating in competition were not as accountable as originally suggested. To be effective, testing programmes have had to become more sophisticated and match the regimes of drug misuse. This has evolved in several ways, through the range of substances, the timing of testing and the standards of both programmes and procedures. The fight against doping has been primarily through testing, and it has not been a fight which sport has faced alone; there have been other significant developments that have involved governments, international sports and health organizations. Progress and major landmarks are described more fully in the section on testing programmes in this chapter.

Lack of standardization of testing procedures has emerged as a problem that might undermine the credibility of testing. The Anti-Doping Convention, established by the Council of Europe in 1989, began the move towards standardization of procedures for testing. In 1998 the International Anti-Doping Arrangement (IADA) (the governmental agreement between the countries of Australia, Canada, New Zealand, Norway and the United Kingdom) took the issue of standardization further by drafting an International Standards Organization (ISO 9002) framework for doping control tests and programmes; these standards have become the adopted international principles for sample collection and testing programme organization. More recently, responsibility for world-wide co-ordination of testing standards using the IADA ISO standard has moved under the auspices of the World Anti-Doping Agency as this agency becomes more established. Until the Olympic Games of 2000 in Sydney there was no co-ordinated testing outside the Games; however, the advent of the World Anti-Doping Agency has begun to make a significant impact upon the way doping is controlled in sport. What will be significant for the future credibility of testing is the standards of accountability, independence and transparency that are adopted throughout the world. Proposals for an athlete passport, a mechanism to record the drug tests and be able to track the results as a form of eligibility for athletes, should help to progress the debate about whether athletes should be regarded as national citizens or members of international sports federations, particularly for the purposes of sanctions.

Introduction of tests for anabolic steroids

At St Thomas' Hospital, London Professor Raymond Brooks had been developing methods for detecting anabolic steroids in the early 1970s. Unofficial tests for these substances were undertaken at the 1972 Munich Games. The test for anabolic steroids at that time was based on radioimmunoassay (Brooks *et al.*, 1975). Using this method it was possible to carry out sufficient tests over a short period of time to allow the method to be adopted at a major sporting event. The IOC therefore added anabolic steroids to the list of banned substances in 1975.

The first official tests for anabolic steroids were carried out at the Montreal Olympic Games in Canada in 1976 (Hatton and Catlin, 1987). Of the samples collected, 15 per cent (some 275 samples) were tested for anabolic steroids at these Games, and of the 11 athletes disqualified, eight had been using anabolic steroids. Similar tests were conducted at the Moscow Olympic Games in 1980; however, no incidence of drug taking was reported. The Chairman of the IOC Medical Commission told a press conference that technical difficulties in testing for testosterone cast doubt on the findings. (*Sydney Morning Herald*, 18 August 1980, quoted in *Drugs in Sport: An Interim Report of the Senate Standing Committee on Environment, Recreation and the Arts*, 1989).

Some anabolic steroids were not detectable through radioimmunoassay. A new assay based on gas chromatography/mass spectrometry (GC-MS) was, however, being developed. This method which identified banned substances in the urine in minute quantities (one part per billion) by molecular weight, also permitted the detection of the naturally occurring steroid, testosterone. The adoption of the GC-MS method for testing androgenic anabolic steroids and testosterone at the 1983 Pan American Games in Caracas, Venezuela, led to the disqualification of 19 athletes. However, many athletes withdrew from the Games, presumably to avoid the testing programme. At the 1984 Olympic Games in Los Angeles, of the 1510 samples taken, 12 were found to contain anabolic steroids or testosterone (Catlin *et al.*, 1987). At the Seoul Olympic Games there were 10 positive drug tests, of which four were for anabolic steroids. An additional six cases were reported by the laboratory as containing a substance from a banned pharmacological class, but the IOC Medical Commission decided that these cases should not be considered as positive (IOC Laboratory Statistics, 1991). The Barcelona Games were more indicative of the increased level of testing to disqualify athletes before they compete in the Olympics; although screening programmes are regarded as unethical, the enhanced level of testing that precedes a major event revealed a number of athletes prepared to take the risk and use drugs. At the Games itself, there were only five positive tests reported. Testing at the Winter Olympic Games in Albertville and Lillehammer had revealed no reports of drug abuse. The Sydney Games was preceded by extensive out-of-competition testing programmes that identified a number of doping offences. As these programmes were operated by a range of organizations (from the Australian Government to the World Anti-Doping Agency) it is more difficult to determine precisely the impact of testing. At the Games themselves, 31 findings were reported, of which 20 were not acted upon for justified reasons (control samples or prior medical notification) under the scrutiny of the Independent Observer Team from the World

Anti-Doping Agency. The remaining 11 results (six steroids, four diuretics and one pseudoephedrine) led to a hearing and report to the IOC Executive Board.

Challenges to the detection of anabolic steroids have demonstrated how sophisticated the science of detection has to be if it is to withstand legal argument. Claims that testosterone levels can be increased above the reporting level through use of birth control pills, sex and alcohol consumption have implied the science and the regulations are not as robust as would be required to control drug misuse. Changes in technology have improved the possibilities of detection. In 1998, a working group of directors of IOC accredited laboratories met to harmonize, in a defensible way, the analytical part of reporting low concentrations of anabolic steroids when using the recently implemented techniques of high resolution mass spectrometry (HRMS) and MS/MS. Additional guidance was indicated for analytes of five steroids, clenbuterol, nandrolone, methyltestosterone, methandienone and stanozolol, to harmonize the reporting between laboratories. The IOC were challenged by the Nandrolone Review Committee to clarify the analytical criteria for reporting low concentrations of anabolic steroids (January 2000) and in the case of 19-norandrosterone 'to define the maximum urinary concentration of this steroid above which it is considered that a doping offence may have been committed'. This illustrates how to determine a doping offence has occurred, the reporting of a substance (above a specified level) should be defined in the regulations as the offence. Significantly the 1999 Olympic Movement Anti-Doping Code included reference to a summary of urinary concentrations above which accredited laboratories must report findings for specific substances. This move has heralded greater harmonization across sport, led in part by the laboratories' reporting systems.

Out-of-competition testing

Originally testing was scheduled after a competition had taken place. It was soon evident that testing programmes organized in competitions were not addressing the regime of drug misuse. Athletes taking part in an event knew there was a possibility that they could be selected for testing. To counter this, athletes started to reschedule their drug use to the training period and to calculate clearance times in the body. It was evident that the testing programmes themselves would have to develop. The extension of testing to the out-of-competition period was intended to address the misuse of drugs in training, which could then be stopped a short time before competition and the athlete's drug misuse would not be evident if he/she was tested in competition. In this way the athlete retained most of the effects of the drugs but avoided detection. Such is the sophistication of the drugs in use and the way they are being used, a continuous testing programme has become the only way to control the misuse of drugs.

In the late 1970s testing out of competition was trialled and found to be a useful deterrent as athletes could be tested at any time; moreover, the testing coincided more closely with athletes' drug regimes. Norway was the first country to conduct out-of-competition controls, starting in 1977; the programme was increased to 75 per cent of the total programme by 1988. In the UK, out-of-competition testing was introduced in the early 1980s. In 1985, the Sports Council financed a pilot scheme for out-of-season testing of British track and field athletes eligible for international selection. The (then) British Amateur Athletic Board began a programme of random out-of-competition testing from a register of eligible athletes (Bottomley, 1988).

The experiences of these early testing programmes were significant in shaping the present day systems. Additional measures have been introduced to extend this testing programme abroad, wherever the athlete may be, and to make non-availability for testing (by failure to notify the sport's governing body if the athlete is absent from the notified address for a period of 5 days or longer) a doping offence. The key principle of out-of-competition testing is to give the athlete short or no notice of the test to reduce any opportunity to manipulate the procedure.

At competitions, where testing is expected, athletes are usually selected at random, by place, or by lane. In addition, world, area and national record breakers may be tested. Suspicions that athletes negotiated clearance from competition testing further reduced confidence in the effectiveness of this type of testing. Whilst competition testing will involve the full range of substances, conversely out-of-competition testing focuses on the anabolic agents, peptide hormones and masking agents. This focused analysis reduces the laboratory costs. Out-of-competition testing programmes are also able to concentrate on athletes in representative teams and in the top ranking tables. In team sports, it is possible to organize testing at squad training sessions. For individual activities such as track and field athletics, swimming and weightlifting, testing may take place at any time, at the athlete's home, place of work or training venue. Out-of-competition testing is not appropriate for every sport. Serious consideration of the potential drugs for enhancing or influencing performance helps to target testing towards those sports where drug misuse is a significant danger.

Although other countries and organizations have introduced out-of-competition testing, this type of testing is not carried out world-wide. As Houlihan (1999) points out 'There is little point in the government and domestic governing bodies of sport in one particular country having a clear set of regulations regarding doping, if their elite athletes do not train in their home country nor participate in competition in that country'. The establishment of the World Anti-Doping Agency in 2000 represents a major step forward in the achievement of a world-wide programme of out-of-competition testing. Under the jurisdiction of the relevant international federation, testing of ranked athletes can be organized and delivered through the World Agency. The question is, can this be co-ordinated with the national programmes to provide the most comprehensive and effective coverage. The first weapon in the armoury of the World Agency is the introduction of athlete passports, a mechanism to record tests. These tests might not only include the collection of a urine sample, but following recent advances in the detection of EPO (erythropoietin), the collection of blood samples are now being introduced as part of the out-of-competition testing programme. A key challenge for the World Anti-Doping Agency will be the rationalization of out-of-competition testing among interested organizations, as the athletes may be subject to testing by different organizations at the same time.

11.2   WADA accredited laboratories

Testing of body fluids for the presence of pharmacological substances is routinely carried out in laboratories throughout the world. Until the establishment of the World Anti-Doping Agency, testing was carried out by laboratories accredited by the IOC for major sporting events and for the programmes of doping control in sport. WADA has taken over the accreditation process for laboratories, although it is likely that the IOC will still be involved with the re-accreditation (Table 11.1).

Originally, laboratories received accreditation by complying with written guidelines regarding the equipment to be available, the general analytical procedures to be followed and a code of ethics by which the laboratory must operate. Accreditation of laboratories is dependent upon adequate facilities and expertise being available at the laboratory, both in terms of their range and capability of the analytical equipment and also the capacity of the laboratory for testing the numbers of samples required for a comprehensive control programme.

Accreditation began in 1976, although the proposal to create accredited laboratories was not formally adopted until 1980 (Royal Society of New Zealand, 1990). The first accredited laboratories were those that had already analysed samples from international competitions, namely Cologne, Kriescha, Moscow, Montreal and London. Re-accreditation was introduced in 1985, primarily to avoid legal challenges to the operating standards of these laboratories (Dubin, 1990). Through an increased volume of testing and further development of the laboratory accreditation process, an internationally acknowledged standard has been obtained.

An accredited laboratory must allow itself to be subjected to periodic, 4-monthly testing by WADA and must seek re-accreditation each year. Initial accreditation requires the successful identification of three sets of 10 samples over a period of 6–12 months. Supported by documentation, a similar analytical test on accreditation is carried out in the presence of a delegate of the IOC Sub-Commission on Doping and Biochemistry. Re-accreditation involves analysis of up to 10 control samples within a specified time limit (IOC, 1990).

Table 11.1 WADA accredited laboratories, November 2004

Country	City
Australia	Sydney
Austria	Seibersdorf
Belgium	Ghent
Brazil	Rio de Janeiro
Canada	Montreal
People's Republic of China	Beijing
Colombia	Bogota
Cuba	Havana
Czech Republic	Prague
Finland	Helsinki
France	Paris
Germany	Cologne
Germany	Kreischa
Great Britain	London
Great Britain	Cambridge
Greece	Athens
Italy	Rome
Japan	Tokyo
Malaysia	Penang
Norway	Oslo
Portugal	Lisbon
Poland	Warsaw
Republic of South Africa	Bloemfontein
Russia	Moscow
South Korea	Seoul
Spain	Barcelona
Spain	Madrid
Sweden	Stockholm
Switzerland	Lausanne
Thailand	Bangkok
Tunisia	Tunis
Turkey	Ankara
United States of America	Los Angeles

Source: WADA, 2005.

WADA accredited laboratories currently analyse urine samples, although the use of blood samples as a supplementary form of evidence is presently under investigation. Analysis of blood may provide the evidence of blood doping (or boosting) and may indicate more clearly the levels of endogenous (naturally occurring) substances. For major sporting events the laboratories must be able to report on results within 24–48 hours of receiving the sample.

The 'Requirements for Accreditation and Good Laboratory Practice', version 5 (Dugal and Donike, 1988) were published as an appendix to the International Olympic Charter against Doping in Sport. These requirements were intended to specify the competence levels of laboratories, to standardize the quality of the analytical methods and to identify the essential equipment, such as:

• gas chromatography;
• high-pressure liquid chromatography;
• thin layer chromatography;
• mass spectrometry (MS) in combination with gas chromatography and computer evaluation; and
• access to immunoassay equipment.

The accreditation process came under close scrutiny during the Dubin Inquiry when it became known that the members of the IOC sub-commission who were responsible for accreditation were also heads of IOC laboratories seeking re-accreditation. In correspondence quoted regarding the loss of accreditation of the Calgary laboratory, it was noted 'The structure of the Sub-Commission, which permits your members to be the professionals who act as consultants, then accreditors, subsequently adjudicators, and also the appeal group while maintaining a monopoly commercial interest, defies common standards of public accountability.' (Dubin, 1990). Independent accreditation of laboratory standards was added to the IOC requirements in 1999, although laboratories have been given a lead-in time to achieve this accreditation.

Accreditation of WADA laboratories

In 1994, 24 laboratories were accredited by the IOC, this number had risen to 31 in 2005, reflecting the importance of establishing an accredited laboratory in a country hosting a major event or to serve a geographical area and the tough scrutiny of the accreditation and analytical business. The location of accredited laboratories follows the sites of major events such as the Olympic or Commonwealth Games or world championships.

Accreditation has two levels, full accreditation or Phase I and Phase II restrictions.

Phase I   The laboratory is temporarily suspended from international testing. At the national level (samples originating from the country in which the laboratory is located), the laboratory may perform screening procedures but another accredited laboratory must confirm analytically positive A-samples. The accredited laboratory which has provided confirmation of the A sample will also analyse the corresponding B-sample.

Phase II   The laboratory is temporarily suspended from confirmation of analytically positive A-samples and analysing B-samples. Another WADA accredited laboratory will confirm the A-sample and perform the analysis of the B-sample.

Code of Ethics for WADA accredited laboratories

WADA accredited laboratories are bound by a code of ethics to avoid the misuse of their analytical services.

1. COMPETITION TESTING

The laboratories should only accept and analyse samples originating from known sources within the context of doping control programmes conducted in competitions organized by national and international sports governing bodies. This includes national and international federations, national Olympic committees, national associations, universities and other similar organizations. This rule applies to Olympic and non-Olympic sports. Laboratories should ascertain that the programme calls for specimens collected according to IOC (or similar) guidelines. This includes collection, under observation, of A and B samples, appropriate sealing conditions, athletes' declaration with appropriate signatures, formal chain of custody conditions and adequate sanctions.

2. OUT-OF-COMPETITION TESTING

The laboratories should accept samples taken during training (or out-of-competition) only if the following conditions are simultaneously met:

- That the samples have been collected and sealed under the conditions generally prevailing in competitions themselves as in 1 above.
- Only if the collection is a programme of a national or international sport governing body as defined in 1 above.
- Only if appropriate sanctions will follow a positive case.
- Thus, laboratories should not accept samples from individual athletes on a private basis or from individuals acting on their behalf.
- Laboratories should furthermore not accept samples, for the purposes of either screening or identification, from commercial or other sources when the conditions in the above paragraph are not simultaneously met.
- These rules apply to Olympic and non-Olympic sports.

3. OTHER SITUATIONS

If the laboratory is required to analyse a sample for a banned drug allegedly coming from a hospitalized or ill person in order to assist a physician in the diagnostic process, the laboratory director should explain the pre-testing issue to the requester and agree subsequently to analyse the sample only if a letter accompanies the sample and explicitly certifies that the sample is not from an athlete. The letter should also explain the medical reason for the test.

Finally, the heads of laboratories and/or their delegates will not discuss or comment to the media on individual results. Laboratory directors will not provide counsel to athletes or others regarding the evasion of a positive test.

Where a country is hosting a major international sporting event and does not have a WADA accredited laboratory, that country may apply to have a WADA accredited laboratory temporarily installed to a non-accredited laboratory/facility for the duration of the event. The host city must provide the analytical facilities but the procedures are, partly, staffed and conducted by personnel from the WADA accredited laboratory, with its director being responsible for all results. The accreditation is temporary for the duration of the event.

The WADA laboratory accreditation system lacked a degree of independence in the accreditation and re-accreditation of laboratories. Whilst some laboratories receive considerable support from the government, others rely upon the business they can attract. Laboratories are expected to adhere to ethical standards of laboratories and not to be involved in screening or manipulation of analysis. It was reported that the Italian laboratory had been investigated in respect of problems with tests carried out in football and led to the controlling national body in Italy (CONI) reviewing the operation of the laboratory (Report to the Council of Europe Compliance with Commitments Project). It was not the first time that a WADA accredited laboratory had been implicated in problems with the testing system. There were earlier reports of the involvement of the head of the East German laboratory in Kreischa, Dr Claus Clausnitzer, in the screening of athletes to clear drug tests before taking part in international competitions (Franke and Berendonk, 1997). One significant step forward in making the laboratory accreditation and operations more transparent is the addition of the International Standard ISO 17025 to the accreditation standard for laboratories. Laboratory statistics are reported to the IOC Medical Commission secretary and although this is a useful measure of the amount of testing being carried out, it is difficult to relate the testing programmes with the samples reported upon by laboratories.

11.3   The testing programmes

The control of drug misuse in sport

Most individuals and organizations involved in sport express their condemnation of the misuse of drugs. However, it is not sufficient merely to express condemnation of drug misuse, steps have to be taken to prevent such abuse, to identify abusers and to take sanctions against those who are found to have misused drugs in sport. To this end WADA and sports federations at international and national level, through their rules, have required athletes to undergo testing. Testing programmes help to establish whether an individual has been involved in drug misuse; at the same time, they may also help to establish which athletes have made themselves available for testing and whose tests are analysed as negative.

Testing programmes were originally based at competitions, but as has already been explained, testing organized in this way did not address the regime of drug misuse that athletes began to engage in. The extension of testing out of competition goes some way to counter the use of drugs in training that are then stopped a short time before competition when testing would be almost certain. The athlete retains most of the effects of the drugs but avoids detection. Such is the sophistication of the drugs now in use, a continuous testing programme has become the only way to control the misuse of drugs. At competitions, athletes are usually selected at random, by place, or by lane. In addition, world, area and national record breakers may be tested. Competition testing consists of the full range of substances, conversely out-of-competition testing focuses on the anabolic agents, peptide hormones and masking agents. Out-of-competition testing programmes concentrate on athletes in representative teams and in the top ranking tables. In team sports, it is possible to organize testing at squad training sessions. For individual activities such as track and field athletics, swimming and weight-lifting, testing may take place at any time, at the athlete's home, place of work or training venue. This type of testing is not appropriate for all sports.

In most countries, the responsibility for organizing testing lies with the governing bodies of individual sports. There is, however, a growing trend towards the establishment of a national anti-doping body to deliver a testing service, independent of sports and of a consistent standard.

In the UK, the national organization for doping control is UK Sport. Governing bodies are required to submit details of their competitive and training calendar, and of nationally ranked competitors as a condition of the recognition and funding they receive from the Sports Council. The service is also available to professional sports (i.e. those not in receipt of funding) with adequate regulations. A charge is made to these bodies. Similar organizations exist in Australia, United States, France, Sweden, Finland, Canada, Norway and the Netherlands. Samples were previously collected in accordance with IOC and international federation procedures and analysis takes place at the IOC accredited laboratory. In 1999 the International Standards Organization recognized a specification standard for doping control, the International Standard for Doping Control that had been developed by countries in partnership under a governmental agreement on anti-doping, the International Anti-Doping Arrangement. The standards set out in the International Standard for Doping Control (ISDC) have been endorsed by WADA and are the key standards now operating across the majority of sports and countries. The benefit of the ISDC is the clear specified standard to be followed and the association of this standard with the quality system standard ISO 9002:1994, which involves independent third party audits to retain the quality system certification. For national anti-doping organizations, certification by this standard is a main objective for international recognition.

The emergence of a range of organizations with an interest in the testing of athletes does give rise to possible duplication unless the testing programmes are co-ordinated. The national federation or international federation as well as a national agency or legislative body may test athletes. Regrettably this does mean that athletes themselves are likely to be the victims of rigorous testing programmes as well as the beneficiaries. Unless the testing procedures meet the minimum standards of the ISDC, the overlap of testing programmes might also provide opportunities for loopholes to occur. Testing procedures must be adequate to ensure the validity and integrity of the sample. Some testing procedures require a longitudinal study and if vital information is dispersed between several organizations, it can be some time before steroid profiling or testosterone/epitestosterone ratios can be monitored.

One of the disadvantages of a testing programme to control drug misuse effectively is its focus only on catching athletes who have already used prohibited substances. No further investigation is made into the circumstances that led to the athlete using drugs, and whether responsibility should be attached to any other person or organization.

Currently competitors could be subject to testing at any time, both in and out-of-competition, however it has taken some time to achieve this situation. The heavy reliance by athletes on the testing programmes to protect their reputations and to catch the cheats has never been more evident. For this reason it is imperative that testing programmes are high quality, credible and deliver expectations.

Key individuals in the anti-doping movement levelled criticisms of the sports-led testing programmes in a number of government reports on drug misuse in sport. One of these individuals, Dr Robert Voy, formerly Chief Medical Officer for the United States Olympic Committee observed:

> There is simply too much money involved in international sports today. One needs to understand that the officials in charge of operating sport at the amateur level need world-class performances to keep their businesses rolling forward. The sad truth is that people don't pay to watch losers, and corporations don't sponsor teams that can't bring home the gold. The athletes and officials realise this, so they're willing to do whatever it takes to win. And sometimes that means turning their backs on the drug problem.
>
> (*Voy, 1991*)

The pressure within the sports environment to win at all costs and not to pursue drug testing as rigorously as would be necessary to maintain a deterrent was evident through the emergence of institutionalized drug misuse and cover-ups. The Australian Senate Inquiry (1989) concluded that the drug testing programme of the Australian Institute of Sport 'was worse than having no programme at all. It provided the protection of appearing to do something to prevent the use of drugs, but was conducted in such a manner that it may have been possible for athletes using drugs to claim that the programme showed them how to be drug free'.

In most countries, the responsibility for organizing testing has moved from sport and the governing bodies of individual sports to a government-funded organization. The growing trend towards the establishment of a national anti-doping body, which can deliver a testing service, independent of sports and to a consistent standard is a major step forward to delivering testing of a consistent standard. An independent, accountable national body has the potential to deliver testing on behalf of international federations, the national federations and to work in conjunction with WADA to deliver testing at the international level.

Responsibilities for testing

Regrettably there may be no co-ordination or planning of the testing programmes undertaken so that in some sports a competitor may be subject to testing under several jurisdictions, for example the authority of a country's law, of a competition or championship, of an international federation and a national programme. The emergence of a range of organizations with an interest in the testing of athletes means that duplication is almost inevitable unless the testing programmes are co-ordinated. It was evident around the time of the Olympic Games in Sydney that athletes would be tested by different jurisdictions, including the national federation and international federation as well as a national agency or legislative body. Regrettably this does put pressure upon the athletes and adds to the possible confusion about notification of test results or inconsistencies in the collection procedures. Some testing procedures require a longitudinal study and if vital information is dispersed between several organizations, it can be some time before longitudinal studies like steroid profiling or testosterone/epitestosterone ratios can be monitored effectively and concluded.

On the other hand, in some sports and in some countries testing is not as comprehensive. Intentions to intensify and co-ordinate anti-doping efforts, including testing were announced, in January 1994, following a meeting of the IOC and International Sports Federation. At this meeting, the following principles were agreed:

• To unify their anti-doping rules and procedures for the controls they perform both during and out-of-competition (unannounced tests).
• To adopt, each year, as a basic document the list of banned classes and methods established by the IOC Medical Commission and to undertake the necessary controls for each sport.

- To accelerate unification of the minimum sanctions provided for by the IOC Medical Commission for violations of the anti-doping regulations and to ensure their application at both international and national levels.
- To recognize the sanctions imposed by another International Federation.
- To use the laboratories accredited by the IOC for all international competitions and for out-of-competition tests.
- To develop the co-operation between the IOC, the International Sports Federations, the National Olympic Committees, the National Federations and governmental or other organizations concerned in order to organize and carry out doping controls and to combat the trafficking of doping substances in sport.
- To set up a special financial assistance programme for those International Sports Federations that need it, in order to help them intensify their anti-doping controls.
- To provide that sports included in the Olympic programme must be governed by International Federations that agree to comply with the above-mentioned principles.

This agreement had little impact, in particular the recommendation that the IOC sanctions should be used, as a basis for harmonization, seemed to be a forlorn hope (Vrijman, 2001). Further criticisms arising primarily from the scandal surrounding the Tour de France in 1998 led to the IOC convening a World Conference on Doping 1999 in Lausanne. The Lausanne Declaration produced by this conference (www.nodoping.org/declaration) recommended among other things the establishment of a new independent, international anti-doping agency. Consequently WADA emerged as a partnership between governments and sports organizations. Houlihan (2001) observes that the 'future success of WADA assumes that the mutual suspicion between the IOC and the IFs can be subsumed by their common fear of greater government intervention'. It is also evident that full accountability for testing programmes has yet to be achieved as, despite the high quality of testing programmes and procedures, it is the international federation of the sport that controls the determination of a positive test and the application of a sanction if any.

At national level many countries have a national organization responsible for anti-doping. In Australia, New Zealand, France and South Africa, these organizations have been set up by statute, in other countries the responsibility has been delegated by the government or by the consensus of the sports community. In the UK the organization responsible is the UK Sports Council. Compliance requirements upon governing bodies of sport to submit details of their competitive and training calendar, and of nationally ranked competitors as a condition of recognition, grant and services has formalized the relationship between sports bodies and the government agency. Generally government funding has enabled the national agency to arrange a significant domestic testing programme, usually for the Olympic sports. In addition the testing service is also available to professional sports with adequate regulations and to international federations. Usually a charge is made to these bodies. Similar national anti-doping organizations exist throughout most of Europe, the Nordic Countries, in Ireland and the United States of America. It has been the establishment of an independent anti-doping agency in the USA (www.usantidoping.org) which has demonstrated clearly this country's intent to respond to the problems of managing testing and results and in particular the concerns noted in the Independent International Review Commission on Doping Control – US Track and Field Association.

Significant standardization of sample collection procedures is emerging; originally sample collection would have been in accordance with IOC and international federation procedures, but gaps and differences have encouraged WADA to endorse the IADA International Standard for Doping Control as the accepted standard. An international certification for sampling officers is also being developed. Analysis takes place at the WADA accredited laboratory. Results management should be administered with accountability and transparency.

One of the continual failures of anti-doping programmes generally is the focus upon the athlete as the target of testing and when a test is positive the transgressor who has been found to have cheated by using performance-enhancing drugs. Rarely is there an investigation into the circumstances that led the athlete to use drugs, knowingly or unknowingly, and whether responsibility should be attached to any other person or organization. Calls for athletes to 'blow the whistle' on other competitors are unlikely to be successful unless the international sports federations demonstrate how serious they are about drug-free sport by claiming back medals and prize money and redistributing them to those who have not failed the drugs test. Athlete passports for drug testing are also under consideration; the ability to register the test of an athlete and provide information to the individual about the result would help to demonstrate the athlete's continued participation in the testing programmes. However, this has to be balanced against reducing the fear that some athletes might have about the inadvertent use of a prohibited substance.

Procedures for drug testing

However a competitor is selected, as a winner, randomly or as part of a programme of out-of-competition testing, the sample collection procedure should follow the same principles. If such principles and policies are not sound and adhered to they become the target of lawsuits (Uzych, 1991).

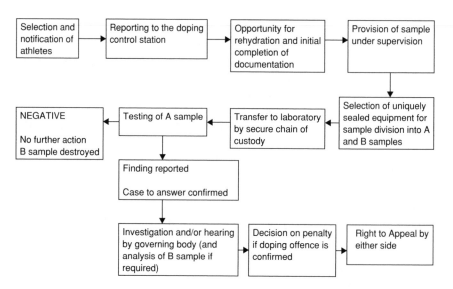

Figure 11.1 The general procedure for drug testing in competition.

The general procedure for drug testing in competition is outlined in Figure 11.1. This process follows the recommended procedure of the Anti-Doping Convention of the Council of Europe and includes the improvements introduced by the International Standard for Doping Control, and is accepted by the majority of countries and sports federations.

Selection of competitors

The policy for selection of competitors at an event where testing is being carried out should clearly define who will be selected. The selection policy is normally specified in the doping regulations that govern the event. This may involve those competitors who are placed in the first three or four of an event, additional randomly selected competitors, all team members or a combination of these. For example, at Olympic competition the usual format is to select the first four competitors in each event with one or two other, randomly selected competitors. Sports that have record performances, such as track and field athletics, swimming and weightlifting, can require negative tests to ratify a record.

For out-of-competition testing, the selection and notification procedures vary slightly from those of competition testing. Selection may be from a register of eligible competitors or from a targeted group within the register. Eligibility depends upon the criteria laid down by the authorizing body, such as ranking, membership of the national team or potential selection for a representative team. Selection procedures are documented to provide a record of who was selected and the selection method used.

Notification

An official from the sample collection team will notify the competitor, in writing, that they have been selected for testing. The sampling official is responsible for accompanying the competitor, at all times, until it is practical to escort him/her to the doping control station. There may be considerable delay between the end of the event and attendance at the doping control station because of award ceremonies, press conferences, treatment for injury, etc. It is therefore vital that the chaperoning of competitors is effective, to ensure there has not been an opportunity for urine manipulation or substitution. The competitor may be accompanied to the doping control station by a coach or other team official.

Documentation

At the doping control station the competitor's identity and time of arrival are recorded. At a convenient point during the testing procedure, the competitor is invited to declare any medications or other substances taken recently (usually in the previous week). Such a declaration is not obligatory but it is in the competitor's interest. Where possible, the name of the substance, its dose and when it was last taken should be recorded. Competitors are reminded that they should declare not only prescription medications but also preparations, which may have been obtained from a pharmacy, health food shop or other outlet.

Providing the sample

At the end of most events, the competitor may be dehydrated. A significant period of time may elapse before a urine sample is produced. The competitor is invited to consume drinks from supplies available at the Doping Control Station; these are individually sealed, non-alcoholic and caffeine free. Such precautions are taken to negate allegations of spiking of drinks. When the competitor is ready to provide a urine sample, he/she is invited to select a collection vessel that should be individually sealed in a plastic wrapping to prevent prior contamination. Collection of the urine takes place under the direct observation of a sampling officer of the same sex. Normally, the competitor must produce a sample of at least 75 ml.

The competitor may then select two, pre-sealed glass bottles labelled A and B, and two bottle containers. The urine sample is divided between these bottles, normally two-thirds of the sample is placed in bottle A and one-third in bottle B. Both bottles are closed and sealed with numbered seals.

Sometimes regulations require that the pH and specific gravity of the urine are measured at the site of collection using a small residue of the sample in the collection vessel. The pH should be between 5 and 7 and the specific gravity should read at least 1.01. If the sample does not meet these specifications, a further sample may be required.

Once the samples have been sealed, the documentation is completed and agreed by the sampling officer, the competitor and any accompanying official. A copy of the form is given to the competitor. Another copy that does not include the name of the competitor but records the sex of the competitor, the volume of urine, the bottle and seal numbers and any medications declared is enclosed with the samples that are sent to the laboratory.

Transfer to the laboratory

The sealed bottles are transported in secure, sealed transit bags to a laboratory along with the laboratory copies of documentation. The chain of custody for the transport of the samples from the Doping Control Station to the laboratory must be documented to ensure integrity of the samples. On arrival at the laboratory the seal numbers are checked and recorded. Any irregularity is noted and the analysis of the sample may be suspended until the integrity can be confirmed. The A sample is prepared for analysis whilst the B sample is stored at low temperatures (the IOC recommend 4°C) pending the result of the analysis of the A sample.

Laboratory testing procedures

There are several analytical techniques that are used alone or in combination, for the detection of drugs in urine. Techniques are selected according to the procedure being adopted. In general, drug-testing procedures are divided into two categories: **screening** and **confirmatory**. Screening procedures provide a sensitive and comprehensive method for identifying whether the sample contains any of the prohibited substances. Confirmatory tests are used to re-analyse the sample and to specifically identify the prohibited substance present and where relevant quantify the substance present.

The additional volume placed in the A bottle enables the full range of screens to be applied and if necessary, further investigations prior to reporting findings. If required the analysis of the B sample will specifically target those substances found in the A sample.

The WADA list of doping substances represents a large and diverse group of chemical substances. Furthermore some sports ban additional substances. Testing procedures must be capable of detecting each of these chemical substances. The problem is compounded by the fact that many of these drugs are metabolized within the body, therefore detection must be capable of identifying these metabolites.

The essential equipment and methods that WADA-accredited laboratories must employ are:

- Gas chromatography (GC)
- High-pressure liquid chromatography (HPLC)
- Mass spectrometry (MS) in combination with gas chromatography
- High-resolution mass spectrometry or tandem MS
- Immunoassay equipment
- Additional or alternative equipment according to new scientific developments

(*WADA Anti-Doping Code, www.wada-ama.org*)

High-pressure liquid chromatography (HPLC)

In HPLC, the matrix on which the drugs are adsorbed is packed in a column and the solvent is forced through the column under high pressure. Mixtures of chemicals will be driven through at different rates and each drug can be identified by the retention time within the column. In addition, many drugs are detected as they leave the column, by ultraviolet light. By selecting appropriate wavelengths, the detector can characterize and quantify the drug present in the urine.

Gas chromatography

In gas chromatography, the matrix on which the drugs are adsorbed is again packed in a column through which a gas such as helium or hydrogen is driven. The column is heated and when the drug reaches the temperature at which it becomes too volatile to remain on the matrix it will be carried by the gas to a detector. The detectors are able to show the presence of certain atoms such as nitrogen or phosphorus. Gas chromatography is therefore a technique which merely indicates the presence of drugs in urine. In order to identify precisely the drug in question, gas chromatography must be accompanied by mass spectrometry.

Mass spectrometry

Mass spectrometry is a technique which enables the tester to identify specifically the drug which is present in the urine. The procedure involves breakdown of the parent drug into its constituent parts by subjecting it to bombardment by a beam of electrons. The machine then measures the levels of the component parts, which are plotted graphically. This mass spectrum is unique for any particular drug.

The combination of GC and MS provides an almost foolproof method for positive identification of drugs in urine. Mass spectrometry can be used as a confirmatory test following any chromatographic or immunoassay screening technique.

Immunoassay

Immunoassay is a technique which is based on the body's allergic response to foreign material within the body. Foreign material is known as an antigen and the immune system produces antibodies to recognize and bind to these antigens. Drugs are a class of antigens. Specific antibodies which selectively bind to particular drugs may be produced in the laboratory. These antibodies normally involve radioactive iodine (radioimmunoassay, RIA) or the enzyme glucose-6-phosphate dehydrogenase (enzyme immunoassay, EIA). Urine samples may be exposed to these antibodies and if the drug which the antibody is designed to recognize is present in the urine, it will be bound to the antibody. This drug/antibody complex can be isolated and identified by one of a number of assay procedures.

Research involving new testing methods and equipment is discussed later in the chapter.

11.4 Reporting test results

A report from a test on an athlete may have several outcomes. If it results from collection of a urine sample that is subsequently analysed, it will be an analytical report that could indicate a finding of a substance prohibited under the relevant doping regulations or a finding of a prohibited substance above the reporting level. If the test result is negative, the governing body should advise the competitor of the result and the laboratory will destroy the B sample.

In the case of a positive result, it is the responsibility of the governing body to act in accordance with their own particular anti-doping policy and regulations. Reports are prepared by the analysing laboratory and relayed in confidence to the relevant governing body. With the evolution of national anti-doping organizations, these bodies usually receive a copy of the report or are the conduit of the report to the relevant sports federation. The competitor should be notified of the results and if the analytical report indicates a finding, further action may follow. The competitor may be invited to explain the finding and will be invited to attend and/or be represented at the analysis of the B sample if they dispute the A sample finding. The B sample analysis usually takes place in the same laboratory as the A sample finding (subject to the accreditation restrictions) and must involve different analysts than those involved in the A sample analysis. A representative of the governing body should also be present at the B sample analysis. This analysis is the opportunity for the chain of custody and sample bottle integrity to be checked and also for any independent scientific expert appointed by the governing body or the athlete to be present to observe the analytical processes. The B sample analysis looks specifically for the substance reported in the A sample. This analysis also involves a chemical standard and a blank sample for comparison. The analytical data are reported to the governing body as before.

If the evidence of the A sample report (and if required the B sample) provides the prima-facie evidence to proceed to the next step, the athlete may be suspended and invited to appear and/or be represented before a disciplinary hearing. In many governing bodies the hearing process is one of investigation to determine the facts and to decide whether these contravene the doping regulations of the sport. Some national governing bodies introduced a hearing at the review stage, which lengthened unnecessarily the disciplinary process. This review hearing stage added further complications to the disciplinary process when the international federation intervened and required the application of strict liability principles in order to proceed to the hearing stage.

A governing body disciplinary hearing is arranged at which the analytical report and possible breach of the doping regulations are considered. The competitor and/or a representative are invited to attend and will be given an opportunity to present their case. Following the hearing, decisions are made about the disciplinary action to be taken and the penalties that will apply. The competitor has the right to appeal, with recourse to law if it is deemed appropriate.

Where a country has a national anti-doping organization, the results of the analysis and subsequent action can be monitored. Reports issued directly to international sports federations may not be subject to the same scrutiny and publication of the information is in the hands of the individual organization.

Irregularities in the sample collection procedure, such as refusal or failure to provide a sample, follow the same investigation and disciplinary procedures. The report originates from the organization responsible for the collection.

Sanctions

The inconsistencies that exist in the sanctions that can be applied in sport for the same offence have been the subject of much criticism. Sanctions are determined by each governing body in accordance with their regulations and those of their international federation. Since sports operate across individual countries that may have to address the need for consistency (either as a consequence of human rights legislation or a concern to achieve uniformity), there are moves towards harmonization of sanctions. The current WADA sanctions are presented in Table 11.2. There are many critics of the sanctions some of whom believe that they are not severe enough, others that they are too severe. Some federations operate their own sanctions appropriate to the career profile of their sport. National rules and legislation can also mean

Table 11.2 The WADA list of sanctions (January 2005)

According to WADA regulations, athletes who test positive may be subject to two forms of sanction, Disqualification and/or Ineligibility.

Disqualification

If an anti-doping rule violation occurs during or in connection with a sports event, the ruling body may disqualify the athlete of all her/his individual results obtained at that event. This includes forfeiture of all medals, points and prizes.

Ineligibility

For all prohibited substances and methods, except those listed as 'Specified substances':

- First violation: 2 years ineligibility
- Second violation: Lifetime ineligibility

For 'Specified substances' where an athlete can establish that the use of such a specified substance was not intended to enhance sport performance, the period of ineligibility is:

- First violation: At a minimum, a warning and reprimand and no period of ineligibility from future events and at a maximum, 1 year's ineligibility
- Second violation: 2 years ineligibility
- Third violation: Lifetime ineligibility

different sanctions: in Greece an anabolic steroid finding can mean 2 years' imprisonment, Canada applies a 4-year ban for a first offence and a life ban for a second offence.

Views concerning the need for testing and the effectiveness of sanctions are varied. Certainly one group of elite, British athletes were in favour of strong action (Radford, 1992). Virtually all (98.3 per cent) of those questioned considered there should be a testing strategy in their particular sport; 79.3 per cent thought that the then current system of doping control in Britain was effective and that out-of-competition testing is a better deterrent than competition testing (82.6 per cent). With regard to penalties, although a more lenient approach to positive results involving OTC drugs was recommended, over half of those questioned considered that the penalty for a positive result involving steroids, amphetamines or blood doping should be a life ban.

A survey carried out by the Australian Sports Drug Agency (ASDA) in 1994 concluded 85 per cent of Australian athletes ($N = 616$) believed the ASDA's drug testing programme would deter Australian athletes from using prohibited drugs; 73 per cent believed the names of athletes testing positive should be made public by their national sporting organization. However, only 11 per cent believed this should be the case if the positive test was the result of inadvertent use (inadvertent use defined as unknowing use of a banned substance contained in a common drug preparation, for example a cough or cold medicine).

Investigation of findings may help to identify the source of supply of the more serious substances, such as steroids, amphetamines and cocaine, and in these cases action can be taken for 'non-use infractions'. In Canada and in many other countries, there are penalties for coaches and administrators who support and encourage the use of drugs.

A survey of United States athletes published prior to the Salt Lake City Winter Olympic Games 2002 (United States Anti-Doping Agency, 2002) indicated that 75 per cent of athletes thought that testing at events was a good idea and that they expected to be tested at least once in the next 12 months. Almost the same percentage of athletes regarded out-of-competition testing as an excellent initiative.

Legal controversy surrounds the possible application of a minimum sanction for a strict liability offence, with no opportunity to plead the circumstances of the case. However, the alternative might lead to a precedent being set that weakens the application of sanctions. The Olympic Movement Anti-Doping Code 1999 sets out a tariff of penalties that now includes financial penalties; it also allows for the possible modification of the 2-year sanction for a first offence 'based upon specific exceptional circumstances to be evaluated in the first instance by the competent IF bodies'.

11.5   Problems in doping control testing

Organizational aspects

Sport is a high profile, internationally recognized activity. Many governments have seen international sporting success as an important propaganda weapon (Waddington, 1996). The exploits of the German Democratic Republic in this context have been documented (Franke and Berendonk, 1997).

Inconsistencies between countries have been found, where short-notice, out-of-competition testing with lifelong bans may apply to one country but not another (Catlin and Hatton, 1991). Similarly, there are inconsistencies between sports federations in terms of the clarity of their rules for drug testing and sanctions (Ng, 1993; Catlin and Murray, 1996). The status of doping agents is constantly changing, particularly with anti-asthma drugs (Frumkin and Price, 1996). Similarly, the application of threshold levels for determining a positive result for certain classes of drugs is constantly under review and subject to change. Even the vagueness of the terminology used in doping control literature may lead to confusion in the athlete's mind (Uzych, 1991).

In recent years, there have been a number of high profile cases of athletes who have tested positive whose cases have highlighted some of the inconsistencies within the organizational framework. Typical defences have included inadvertent use or lack of understanding that over-the-counter (OTC) medicines contain a prohibited drug. A case of this type resulted in a gymnast losing a gold medal at the Sydney 2000 Olympic Games. Other defences have claimed that the positive result was attributable to a mistake in the collection of the sample, a break in the chain of custody, a laboratory error or sabotage (Catlin and Murray, 1996). Although loopholes in the regulations or procedures have been exposed, their exposure has not always led to changes in the regulations, resulting in a lack of trust or respect for the system.

It is clear that the role of the testing bodies is critical. The earlier IOC rules were variably adopted by international sports federation or national governing bodies. It was clear that all governing bodies in sport should operate under the same rules and regulations. This process was begun by the establishment of the World Anti-Doping Agency (WADA) in November 1999 (www.olympic.org, March 2001). WADA was set up as an independent agency, following the Lausanne Declaration at the World Conference on Doping in Sport, held at the IOC headquarters in Lausanne, in February 1999. The mission of WADA is to promote and co-ordinate, at international level, the fight against doping in sport, in all forms.

Harmonization of sanctions between sports continues to be debated. Should equal penalties of disqualification apply between amateur and professional sports? Should periods of ineligibility be the same regardless of whether an athlete's active career is short or long term? These and other questions are difficult to answer, however, the re-introduction of flexibility in sanctions would provide the opportunity for some sporting regulators to take a more lenient approach with offenders and potentially to offer legal loopholes to those sanctioned (Howman, 2003).

WADA at the Sydney 2000 Olympic Games

Under its broad mandate to co-ordinate international anti-doping efforts, WADA nominated a team of independent observers to examine aspects of the testing procedures at the Games. These included sample collection, analysis in the laboratory and review of the test results. From their Executive Summary Report (www.wada-ama.org, 2001), WADA observed that there were changes and improvements in the transparency and process of anti-doping measures at the Games. Furthermore, WADA considered that the principle of independent observers and their involvement in all stages of the process is a key way of ensuring confidence and credibility of the anti-doping process.

WADA at the Salt Lake City 2002 Winter Olympic Games

WADA announced the introduction of the 'Athlete Passport' programme to coincide with the 2002 Winter Olympic Games in Salt Lake City (www.wadapassport.org, 2002). The 'Athlete Passport' programme has three main goals:

EDUCATION

To provide up-to-date and comprehensive information for athletes, including the current rules, regulations and list of banned substances and the adverse effects of doping.

TESTS DATABASE

In which each subscribed athlete's doping control information is held on a secure web-based database.

COMMUNICATION

To provide athletes with a communication link with WADA and thereby enhance their involvement in the anti-doping effort.

Athletes' doping control information can be held on both a paper version of the passport as well as the web-based version. Eventually, the web-based database will enable WADA, International Sports Federations, National Olympic Committees and National Anti-doping Organizations to organize, harmonize and link testing programmes.

An additional benefit of the programme will be that it will improve the ability to maintain longitudinal studies of the natural levels of various chemicals and hormones in elite athletes.

A second WADA initiative at the 2002 Winter Games was the introduction of an e-learning pilot project. This provides an interactive training and education resource. It was intended to have this facility available by July 2002 at www.truegame.org.

WADA at the Athens 2004 Olympic Games

Athens was the first Olympic Games after the publication of the World Anti-Doping Code and the publication of the WADA Prohibited List. Whilst the IOC assumed responsibility for tests, WADA appointed a team of observers for the games. Their report was published in www.wada-ama.org. Testing results revealed 12 cases where prohibited substances were identified, 5 cases of refusal or failure to submit to sample collection and one attempt at tampering with a sample.

Limitations to the testing procedures

In addition to the inherent problems associated with the selection of athletes, the processes in obtaining a urine sample, maintaining accurate documentation and ensuring the accuracy and validity of the testing procedures, Uzych (1991) has identified a number of limitations to the testing procedures.

1. A positive test result merely indicates that the athlete providing the urine specimen was exposed to the drug. Whether this was voluntary or involuntary remains open to question.
2. McBay (1987) has shown that errors may occur in the identification of the specimen or in the analytical procedures. In addition, the presence of a drug or a metabolite in the urine sample provides no scientific basis for determining when, how often or in what dose the drug was taken.
3. In general, a positive test result cannot be used to determine the effects of a drug on an individual and, most critically, the effects on performance.

The limitations identified by Uzych often emerge in a legal challenge to a doping infraction. Rule makers have responded to these limitations by making doping an absolute offence, then allowing for an investigative stage at which any justification, explanation or other information may be considered. At this stage, the legality of the test may be brought into question on the basis of the accuracy and precision of the test. In this context, the issue of false negatives and false positives comes into play. False negatives, where a drug user would not be caught, reflect the accuracy of the testing methods. In the case of false positives, a clean athlete would be falsely accused. The margins for error for these two categories should be zero for false positives and as few as possible for false negatives. In determining whether a test method is acceptable, WADA evaluates both its scientific and legal validity. In other words, its technical accuracy and precision and the likelihood of throwing up false positives.

The question of whether substances do, in fact, improve performance in a particular sport is difficult to establish conclusively. On ethical grounds, it is difficult to justify the use of drugs for research purposes, especially in the quantities detected in some athletes.

Performance improvement is not the only reason why substances are used, there might also be performance or health maintenance. There is a very fine line between treating a minor ailment to 'return health to normal', and the use of substances to improve performance. Some of the benefits that an athlete might derive from the use of a substance (real or placebo) may be psychological. In this context, there has been a significant rise in the use of recreational drugs, particularly marijuana, in society in general and by athletes in particular. This in itself could influence performance measurements.

A major limitation to the testing procedures was the inclusion on the IOC list, in 1989, of the class of drugs known as the peptide hormones, such as erythropoietin (EPO) and human growth hormone (hGH). This created particular limitations due to the fact that validated methods for detection had not been developed. It made a mockery of the doping control system by forbidding athletes from using substances when there was no way of proving their use. By the 2000 Sydney Olympic Games, validated testing procedures for EPO had been approved but not for hGH, a validated test for which was still not available for the January 2005 Prohibited List.

Anabolic steroids and steroid profiling

In the past, the methods for effective testing of anabolic steroids have lagged behind their use in sport. There was a marked increase in published research on drug misuse in sport following the Seoul Olympic Games of 1988, most notably in the area of drug testing for anabolic steroids (Mottram *et al.*, 1997).

Detection of anabolic steroid misuse poses particular problems, particularly since the steroids can be taken prior to competition, allowing a 'washout' period before competing. Clearly, out-of-competition testing provides one means for overcoming this problem. However, this type of testing is not uniformly adopted internationally.

One approach to determine anabolic steroid use involves steroid profiling. In this technique blood samples are taken to determine the amount and endocrine status of endogenous steroids such as androsterone, etiocholanolone, 11-hydroxy-androsterone and 11-hydroxy-etiocholanolone. These endogenous steroids have been shown to be changed when exogenous anabolic steroids are taken, either orally or by injection.

Donike *et al.* (1989) have described the long-term influence of anabolic steroid misuse on the steroid profile and conclude:

1. Taking anabolic steroids decreases the concentrations of endogenous steroids.
2. In steroid users there is a change in the ratios of endogenous isomer steroids like *cis*-androsterone.
3. The decrease in concentration and excretion of endogenous anabolic steroids can be observed even if the exogenous anabolic steroids can no longer be detected in the urine.

Lukas (1993) has suggested that other biochemical markers may be used to determine anabolic steroid use. Such markers could include liver function tests (e.g. lactate dehydrogenase), muscle enzymes (e.g. creatine phosphokinase), blood biochemistry (e.g. high-density/low-density lipoprotein ratios and haematocrit levels) and sperm count and motility. It is suggested that any suspected abnormalities in blood chemistry profiles could be followed with a urine screen for positive identification of the anabolic steroid involved. This could provide a more cost-effective approach. However, these alternative techniques for identifying anabolic steroid misuse require blood samples. This would represent a radical new approach to drug testing for anabolic steroids.

Steroid detection in urine has been difficult. In 1996, it was reported that 40 compounds must be monitored in order to cover the broad range of steroids then available (Schnazer, 1996). The accepted method for detecting anabolic steroids has been gas chromatography coupled with mass spectrometry (GC/MS). This provides a relatively sensitive method of analysis, capable of detecting urine concentrations of as little as 10 ng/ml in a 2–5 ml sample (Cowan, 1997). At the Atlanta 1996 Olympic Games a more sophisticated technology was used for the first time, providing additional selectivity and improving detectability by approximately tenfold to around 1 ng/ml (Bowers, 1997; Cowan, 1997). This was an instrument called a sector mass spectrometer, sometimes referred to as high-resolution mass spectrometry (HRMS). More recently, a technique using tandem mass spectrometry (GC/MS/MS) has been developed which achieves selective detection similar to GC/HRMS (Bowers, 1998). The first mass spectrometer selects an ion originating from a detected banned substance. This ion is then fragmented and one or more fragments is monitored by the second mass spectrometer.

Testosterone

Testosterone and its metabolites are, technically, not difficult to detect in urine and therefore pose no problems for doping control analysis. However, testosterone is an endogenous steroid and, as such, presents difficulties in determining what constitutes 'normal' levels in the population. This, in turn, makes it difficult to determine whether an athlete has taken exogenous testosterone. Possibilities for detection of exogenously administered testosterone include the measurement of the following.

1. Indirect markers, which include the profile of the isomers and metabolites (breakdown products) of testosterone in urine or in blood.
2. Direct markers, such as the presence in blood of testosterone esters which are not produced by the body but which are the product of testosterone production by the pharmaceutical industry.
3. The ratio of carbon isotopes within testosterone, which can be used to distinguish between natural and synthetic testosterone.

These detection methods are reviewed in Segura *et al.* (1999).

A major indirect marker for testosterone is its isomer, epitestosterone. The ratio of unmetabolized testosterone/epitestosterone (T/E) in the urine should be around 1:1. In 1994, the IOC revised its regulations for testosterone. A T/E ratio greater than 6:1 constitutes a doping offence, unless there is evidence that the ratio is due to a physiological or pathological condition, with a mandatory medical investigation being required before a sample is declared positive. In addition, in the absence of previous test data, unannounced testing over a period of 3 months is required.

The threshold value of 6:1 appears to be based on reports that the T/E ratio is unlikely to be above 6 under normal conditions (Chan, 1991). Catlin and Hatton (1991) have reported that the incidence of a T/E ratio above 6 is less than 0.8 per cent and, of those competitors with a ratio between 6 and 9, very few have denied knowingly using testosterone. However, it has been reported that T/E ratios may not exhibit the same urinary profile throughout pubertal development when the ratio may exceed 6 even under normal physiological conditions (Raynaud et al., 1993). These authors recommended caution in applying IOC regulations in such individuals. Similar caution needs to be applied with respect to the fact that the reference range for the T/E ratio, which was established in men, may not be appropriate in women (Honour, 1997). By January 2005 the WADA prohibited list specified that further investigation is obligatory, if the T/E ratio is greater than 4:1 (WADA, 2005).

Clearly, the concomitant use by athletes of epitestosterone and testosterone can confound the testing procedures (Catlin et al., 1997); however, a method of analysis of urinary markers of oral testosterone in the presence of masking epitestosterone has been described (Dehennin and Peres, 1996) and an inter-laboratory collaborative project in this area of research has been described (Catlin et al., 1996). An alternative and, as the authors claim, a more sensitive and specific test involves comparison of levels of testosterone and luteinizing hormone (Perry et al., 1997). This is based on the fact that testosterone administration produces a negative feedback inhibition on the pituitary gonadotrophins, luteinizing hormone and follicle-stimulating hormone.

More recent approaches for testing testosterone have investigated the ratio of the carbon isotopes, ^{12}C: ^{13}C, on the basis that synthetic testosterone has a higher proportion of ^{13}C than endogenous human testosterone (Becchi et al., 1994; Anguilera et al., 1996), and the use of electrospray mass spectrometry for testosterone esters (Shackleton et al., 1997).

Blood doping

Blood doping was added to the IOC list of banned substances and methods after the 1984 Olympic Games, contrary to their policy of not banning anything for which an unequivocal testing procedure was not available.

Blood boosting through legal, altitude training or illegal, blood doping is widely practiced. Blood doping involves transfusion of whole blood or packed red blood cells and may be autologous (the subject's own blood) or homologous (another person's blood). Unfortunately, techniques to detect artificially induced erythrocythaemia are difficult to apply, particularly where autologous transfusion is involved (Catlin and Hatton, 1991). Even if tests were available, their validity would be confounded by altitude acclimatization, hydration status and individual variation in normal haematocrit (Anon, 1987). It is therefore likely that this manipulation is used by athletes, particularly in endurance sports (Ekblom, 1997).

Berglund (1988) describes the development of techniques for the detection of blood doping in sport. Whilst it is possible to demonstrate that an individual has undergone blood doping, there are several factors which must be considered, not least of which is that the method requires a blood rather than urine sample. Furthermore, since the test relies on changes in blood parameters over a period of time, two blood samples must be taken with a minimal interval of 1 to 2 weeks. If these criteria are met, then alteration in the levels of at least two parameters, such as haemoglobin, serum iron, bilirubin and serum erythropoietin, during that period is indicative of blood doping (Birkeland *et al.*, 1997; Birkeland and Hemmersbach, 1999).

Despite the current lack of an unequivocal method for the detection of blood doping, it is likely that the extent of blood doping will remain limited for a number of reasons:

1. Where a subject re-infuses their own blood (autologous transfusion), this requires the help of skilled personnel and storage for 4–5 weeks in a blood bank, which increase the risk of detection.
2. Where a subject uses blood from a matching donor (heterologous transfusion) they run the risk of mismatch of blood, possibly leading to anaphylactic shock or the possibility of contracting blood-borne diseases such as AIDS or hepatitis B.
3. For either technique, the risk of introducing an infection at the site of infusion, leading to a septicaemia, is ever present.

Peptide hormones (human growth hormone and erythropoietin)

The IOC introduced the new doping class of 'Peptide Hormones and Analogues' in 1989, despite the non-existence of unequivocal tests for these agents. Currently, this class includes human growth hormone (hGH), human chorionic gonadotrophin (hCG) and adrenocorticotrophic hormone (ACTH), including all releasing factors for these hormones. The list also includes erythropoietin (EPO).

Evidence for the increasing use of peptide hormones comes from innumerable anecdotes from physicians and others, reports of thefts and forged prescriptions, enquiries to drug hotlines and articles in magazines (Catlin and Hatton, 1991).

Human growth hormone

Abusers believe that hGH can produce desired effects without the risk of the side-effects associated with anabolic steroids and because there is no reliable method available for the detection of hGH through urine testing (Wadler, 1994). From 1988, recombinant hGH has been available. Prior to this date, endogenous hGH was extracted from the pituitary glands of cadavers, with the inherent danger of contamination with viruses and prions, possibly leading to Creutzfeldt–Jakob disease. Recombinant hGH is therefore safer. In addition, its molecular structure is slightly different from naturally occurring hGH. This has provided a valuable marker for the development of a validated test for hGH.

Particular attention is being paid to research into hGH. Kicman and Cowan reviewed the misuse and detection of this class of doping agents, in 1992. The standard methods of chemical analysis for drugs, using gas chromatography and mass spectroscopy, were unsuitable for the detection of the peptide hormones. A review on hGH detection methods has been provided by Rivier and Saugy (1999).

Testing for hGH is made difficult by the fact that metabolism of the hormone is rapid (hGH half-life is around 20 minutes), therefore detection of the parent hormone in blood can only be made for a short time after administration. In addition, the natural levels are low and hGH is released in a pulsatile manner. Secondary markers, such as insulin-like growth factors, have therefore been used.

A multicentred, international research project, entitled GH2000 was established in 1996. This project was financed through joint funding from the European Union, the IOC and pharmaceutical companies. The main objectives of the project were to define the limits of acceptable physiological ranges for hGH in the population as a whole and in elite athletes and to establish an acceptable testing procedure for the 2000 Olympic Games in Sydney. Prior to the GH2000 project, a test to detect hGH in urine, based on an enzyme-linked immunosorbent assay, had been developed (Saugy et al., 1996). This test only applied to out-of-competition situations. Insulin-like growth factors have been used as markers of doping with hGH; however, testing for these markers requires blood samples (Kicman et al., 1997).

The GH2000 project team submitted their final report in January 1999. They described (Sonksen, 1999) detection for hGH by two methods, both of which required blood samples.

1. Detection of the 22 k isomer (the synthetic, recombinant version) of GH in the absence of the naturally occurring 20 k isomer. This method was particularly useful in detecting GH administered within the previous 24 hours.
2. Detection of one or more 'indirect markers' of recombinant GH administration in concentrations higher than is possible within normal physiological variance. This method could detect the use of recombinant GH as long as 14 days before the test.

Both tests were claimed to have very high specificity and adequate sensitivity but before they could be implemented they needed further validation to show, amongst other things, that results applied equally to ethnic groups other than the thousand or so white Europeans who took part in the study.

A future marker for hGH is the turnover of bone and collagen, produced by this hormone. This test has the advantage that these changes persist after hGH withdrawal (Longobardi *et al.*, 2000). A validated test for hGH, acceptable to WADA, was still not available for the January 2005 prohibited list.

Erythropoietin

Erythropoietin (EPO) promotes haematopoietic growth, which stimulates growth and differentiation of erythroids, leading to an increase in red blood cells, thereby increasing the oxygen-carrying capacity of the blood. A validated method for the detection of EPO was not available when it was first banned. Methods of detection, using urine and blood samples, have been investigated (Gareau *et al.*, 1995; Ekblom, 1997). A review on earlier research has been presented by Rivier and Saugy (1999).

The search for a scientifically and legally validated test for EPO was intensified in 1988, following events in that year's Tour de France cycle race. Two research teams, both partially funded by the IOC, have recently been working on the problem. One team, led by Australian scientists, were looking at a method based on blood samples. This study focused on the fact that blood parameters are altered by the administration of recombinant EPO. The other, French-led team, were working on a urine-based method. This study investigated the direct detection of recombinant EPO compared with naturally produced EPO using an electrophoretic technique.

Both research teams subjected their methods to independent, scientific validation, which followed an internationally accepted protocol, consisting of two stages.

1. The test had to be published in an internationally recognized peer-reviewed journal. This allows scrutiny of the methods and results by independently appointed referees for the journal. The Australian study was published in *Haematologica* (Parisotto *et al.*, 2001) and the French study in *Nature* (Lasne and de Ceaurriz, 2000).
2. The original test results, generated by the research team, had to be reproduced in a different laboratory by a different team, following the original protocol.

Following the implementation of these protocols, the IOC Medical Commission, having sought the views of the IOC Juridical Commission, accepted these methods for implementation at the Sydney 2000 Olympic Games. Controversy continues about the necessity of the blood test prior to the urine test; some argue that it helps to control costs by identifying those samples that should be submitted for the more expensive and lengthy EPO test in urine. There is disagreement about whether the blood test is absolutely necessary and also if the blood test could stand alone as an indicator that the athlete should not compete. In cycling this has become part of the medical scrutiny that a cyclist must submit to, to be considered as fit to compete. By 2004, the urine test alone was acceptable to WADA in order to determine misuse of EPO.

Over-the-counter (OTC) medicines

Banned drugs which are available over the counter instil concern in the minds of athletes (Radford, 1992; UK Sports Council, 1995). It is acknowledged that competitors have and will continue to experience problems when purchasing, from a pharmacy, OTC preparations which contain banned substances. The two areas of particular difficulty are with regard to stimulants and narcotic analgesics since members of these groups of drug are available OTC, particularly in cough and cold preparations and as painkillers.

In March 1993, the IOC removed codeine from the list and permitted its use for therapeutic purposes. In September 1994, the IOC allowed two further narcotic analgesics, dihydrocodeine and dextromethorphan, for therapeutic use.

OTC drugs, such as ephedrine, are relatively less potent and non-selective than other stimulants, hence their availability without prescription. This lack of selectivity, with a concomitant likelihood of side-effects, especially if used in supratherapeutic doses, makes them less desirable as potential performance-enhancing drugs, since no improvement in performance has been found in the few research studies on these drugs (Clarkson and Thompson, 1997; Swain *et al.*, 1997; Chester *et al.*, 2003a). In January 2004 a number of OTC medicines (bupropion, caffeine, phenylephrine, phenylpropanolamine, pipradol, pseudoephedrine, synephrine) were removed from the prohibited list. However, they were placed on a monitoring programme in order to continue to detect patterns of their misuse in sport.

Nutritional supplements

In addition to OTC medicines which are known to contain banned substances, there are many other preparations available to athletes, which may possibly contain certain banned drugs (Ayotte, 1999). These include nutritional supplements, where there may be no legal requirement for manufacturers to list the content of the food supplement, therefore making it difficult for an athlete to determine whether taking such a preparation would contravene the doping regulations (Herbert, 1999). Similarly, various 'natural' products such as herbal preparations may, and in some cases frequently do, contain banned substances. These include Ma Huang (Chinese Ephedra) which is a plant that contains ephedrine, and Ginseng, which itself does not contain banned substances in its natural form of ginseng root, but in preparations such as tablets, solutions and teas, other ingredients such as anabolic steroids, ephedrine and other stimulants may be present (Ros *et al.*, 1999).

In 1999, there was a significant number of high-profile cases involving athletes who tested positive for the anabolic steroid, nandrolone and who subsequently claimed that the drug must have been present in nutritional supplements that they had been taking. This issue was reviewed in a series of editorials by Jim Ferstle (Ferstle, 1999a–c).

Since 1996, the US Sport Nutritional Industry has offered a number of natural and, they claim, legal steroids. These include precursors for testosterone such as dehydroepiandrosterone, androstenedione, androstenediol, 19-androstenedione and 19-androstenediol (Ayotte, 1999). These substances may lead to metabolites in the urine, which result in a positive test or alter the testosterone/epitestosterone ratio which again may trigger a positive result. These steroidal supplements are available in a number of other countries and through the Internet. A second study has shown that 14.8 per cent of nutritional supplements contained substances that would have led to a positive dopping test (www.olympic.org; June 2002).

Conflicting conclusions on the acceptance of the claims made by athletes have been reached by the athletes' national sports federation and the international federation. The international federation took the stand of zero tolerance: athletes must take responsibility for what is present in their body, from whatever source. The national federation accepted that there was an element of doubt as to the source of the nandrolone and that the metabolites may have been present in the urine through unwitting ingestion.

Controversy about the natural level of nandrolone in the body led to the publication of a document previously only available to laboratories concerning the urinary concentration of the nandrolone metabolite 19-norandrosterone that should trigger a report. This level was challenged in several hearings in 1999 and 2000. Although early cases accepted arguments for higher levels, later cases confirmed that the IOC reporting guidelines were established. Differences between the reporting level for men and women were also acknowledged. The confusion over the nandrolone issue was exacerbated by claims that low concentrations of metabolites conferred no performance-enhancing effect and were due to the contamination of supplements. This conclusion from a single untimed urine sample could not be substantiated; the possibility that the result arose from the long-term use by injection of nandrolone may seem unlikely in the present climate of testing but evidence to the contrary had to be unequivocal.

It must be remembered that because a product is termed 'natural' or 'herbal' it is not devoid of potential adverse side-effects. Many drugs, whether or not banned by WADA, are derived from plant sources. It is the dose of the product taken which is the principal determinant of whether the drug will be toxic, coupled with the sensitivity of the individual to a particular substance.

Drugs used in the treatment of asthma

β_2-Agonists

Asthma may be triggered by a number of factors, not least of which is exercise. Drug treatment for asthma is complex and may involve a number of drugs which variably act as prophylactic agents to prevent an asthma attack or as bronchodilators to relieve the symptoms of an attack. Two of the main groups of anti-asthma drugs are corticosteroids and β_2-adrenoceptor agonists. Both groups of drugs are subject to WADA doping control regulations. Indeed, the β_2-adrenoceptor agonists are classed as both stimulants and as anabolic agents. It has been reported (Catlin and Murray, 1996) that, in some sports, an inordinately large number of declarations for the use of anti-asthma drugs are submitted compared with the incidence of asthma in the community. This view was substantiated at the Sydney 2000 Olympic Games, where 607 (almost 6%) provided prior notification that they required β_2-agonists for their treatment of asthma. The WADA regulations compound the problem for the athlete in that, in the case of the β_2-adrenoceptor agonists, they are permitted subject to Therapeutic Use Exemption (TUE) approval, whilst certain drugs in this case (salbutamol, terbutaline, formoterol and salmeterol) are permitted for use by inhalation subject to an Abbreviated TUE. Research into methods for testing whether an athlete has taken salbutamol by the prohibited oral route has been reviewed recently by Ventura *et al.* (2000).

In January 2001, the IOC, as part of its annual review of banned substances, changed the list of permitted β_2-agonists by including formoterol as a permitted drug and by banning the previously permitted terbutaline. This led to confusion, as the change was introduced with little prior notice. Soon after, the IOC re-introduced terbutaline as a permitted drug.

Glucocorticosteroids

Glucocorticosteroids are prohibited when administered orally, rectally, intravenously or intramuscularly. Their use requires a TUE. All other routes of administration requires an Abbreviated TUE, except dermatological preparations which are not prohibited. It is not surprising that athletes and their physicians need to be especially vigilant in their selection of an appropriate therapeutic drug regime (Frumkin and Price, 1996).

Recreational drugs

'Recreational' drugs encompass a diverse group of pharmacological agents which are banned under various headings on the IOC list. These include cocaine and amphetamines (stimulants), heroin (narcotic analgesic), and alcohol and marijuana (drugs subject to certain restrictions). It has been suggested that the use of recreational drugs is higher amongst professional athletes than in the general population because athletes can afford them. However, there is little evidence that such substances give unfair advantage to the user, nor is there reason to think that a desire to win motivates abuse.

(Fost, 1986)

The few studies on cocaine and exercise suggest that little or no improvement in performance is produced. Indeed, the sense of euphoria may provide the illusion of a better performance than was actually achieved (Clarkson and Thompson, 1997). The non-performance consequences for the recreational drug taker, as well as for their fellow competitors, could be significant, especially where aggressive instincts are altered (Voy, 1991).

Marijuana use is becoming widespread in society and the impact of this in sport is becoming evident (see Chapter 9). Events surrounding the disqualification and subsequent reinstatement of Ross Rebagliati, following a positive test for marijuana at the Winter Olympic Games at Nagano in February 1998, serve to highlight another problem associated with banning recreational drugs in sport. There appeared to have been no formal agreement between the International Ski Federation and the IOC regarding testing for marijuana at the Games. This highlights the organizational problem discussed earlier in this chapter.

The control of recreational drugs misuse as part of the testing programme for sport is not without controversy. In the UK there is an acceptance by some sports bodies (particularly the professional sports such as association football, cricket and rugby league) that the control of social drug misuse is essential to the well-being of the sport. Hence the delivery through the UK anti-doping organization, UK Sport, of a testing programme where some samples may be submitted to a selective screen involving a social drugs menu only. The players are unaware of the screen the samples will be submitted for. This position is not widely adopted by other countries that have focused their efforts upon the control of substances listed by WADA. Subsequent disciplinary action can involve clinical assessment and rehabilitation during which time the player is suspended from the sport and required to concentrate on responding to treatment. This appreciation of the danger of social drugs in a sporting environment respects the potential for substance misuse related to the sports context but not necessarily directly the sports performance.

Adulteration of urine samples

Adulterants are used by athletes to add to urine samples in order to invalidate assays for banned substances. A review of such adulterants, including a recently developed product entitled 'Urine Luck', is provided by Wu *et al.* (1999). Urine Luck contains pyridinium chlorochromate, which is effective in interfering with tests for carboxy-TCH and opiates. Methods for identifying the presence of pyridinium chlorochromate itself are also described in this chapter.

Adulterants need to be added to urine samples at the time of collection. Vigilance on the part of sampling officers is therefore imperative to prevent their use.

11.6 Alternatives to urine testing in doping control

Blood samples

The detection of blood doping and the use of peptide hormones, such as EPO and growth hormone (GH), is extremely difficult using urine testing alone. Consequently, the use of blood sampling in the doping control system has been contemplated for many years.

Early assessment of drug testing using blood samples was made by Birkeland *et al.* at a series of IAAF meetings in 1993–1994 (Birkeland *et al.*, 1997). The authors investigated a number of potential doping agents and methods. These included EPO, GH, insulin-like growth factor-1, testosterone and blood doping. The authors concluded that, out of the 99 athletes tested, results indicated that blood doping or the use of recombinant EPO or GH was not widespread. However, they acknowledged that the methods adopted may not have been sensitive enough.

Some sport organizations, such as the International Ski Federation (FIS), have conducted routine testing using blood samples. The IOC introduced blood sample tests at the 1994 Winter Olympics in Lillehammer, in line with procedures developed by the FIS. The purpose of blood tests was to detect blood doping and to develop more sophisticated methods to combat other doping methods in sports.

The FIS-approved guidelines for blood sampling included:

1. The doping control notification shall state whether the competitor is required to undergo blood sampling in addition to urine sampling. The procedures for selection and notification are the same as for urine sampling.
2. Blood sampling may be performed before or after the urine sampling procedure. All blood sampling shall be taken by qualified personnel.
3. The same type of equipment will be used to store and transport blood as for urine samples.
4. Only a small amount of blood (4 ml) will be taken. The blood will be taken from a superficial vein in the elbow region; 2 ml will be used for each of Sample A and B.
5. The competitor shall declare to the Doping Control Officer any blood transfusion(s) he or she may have received in the preceding 6 months, with details, including the reason for such transfusions.

6. As soon as possible after arrival at the Doping Control Laboratory, the blood samples shall be tested for the presence of foreign blood cells.
7. Refusal to submit to a blood sample may have the same consequences as failure to submit to a urine sample.

Following events in the 1998 Tour de France, the International Cycling Federation introduced blood sampling for cyclists. However, they were only concerned with measuring haematocrit levels, as an indirect measure of EPO use.

The acceptance of blood sampling for the screening of athletes in all Olympic sports came about at the Sydney 2000 Olympic Games, where competitors were subject to EPO testing, which included a blood test (Parissoto et al., 2001; www.olympic.org). By 2004, the blood test for EPO was not required as the urine test alone was deemed robust enough.

Concerns about the use of blood sampling in doping control have been expressed (Hoppeler et al., 1995; Browne et al., 1999). Apart from issues concerning the validity of the laboratory tests themselves, Browne et al. raised some serious medical and ethical issues:

1. The process is invasive, which leaves the athlete at risk from infection.
2. Sampling requires specially trained personnel.
3. Handling blood samples leaves sampling officers and laboratory staff exposed to infection.
4. Transportation requires refrigeration or other special precautions.
5. There are significant issues concerning blood tests applied to minors, who make up a sizeable proportion of competitors.

The authors concluded that in the, then, present state of development, blood tests should not be implemented.

In a counter argument, Birkeland and Hemmersbach (1999) argued that a major ethical question lay in whether sport itself can continue without proper methods to detect doping agents which can not be satisfactorily evaluated in urine. Furthermore, they raised the point that modern DNA technology could attribute a sample to an individual athlete far more accurately than is possible with urine sampling.

The problems surrounding blood sampling have led to consideration of alternative sampling methods, such as hair samples.

Hair samples

Hair is easily collected and stored, prior to analysis. Hair is not subject to degradation and can reveal a historical record of drug exposure over a period of months (Polettini et al., 1996). These authors reported their research into the detection of the β_2-agonists, clenbuterol and salbutamol in hair samples. They concluded that hair sampling was a suitable alternative to urine sampling, for these drugs.

Kintz (1998) considered that hair samples were suitable for testing all banned substances, except peptide hormones. However, cost was identified as a factor to be borne in mind. Kintz did identify a particular use for hair sampling, in cases concerning false-negative tests, since neither abstaining from using a drug for a few days nor tampering with urine samples would alter the concentration of the drug found in the hair.

Disadvantages to the use of hair samples have been highlighted by Rivier (2000). These include the fact that incorporation rates of drugs into blond and grey hair are poorer than into dark-coloured hair. Additionally, the frequency of hair cutting and head shaving by many athletes is a critical factor. It was concluded that a minority of prohibited substances could be detected in scalp hair with the sensitivity and specificity required, thereby limiting the, then present, usefulness of this technique.

11.7   Is the list of banned substances and methods appropriate?

Do we need a list of prohibited substances for all sports?

The IOC has previously published a list of prohibited substances that has been applied to the majority of sports. The restricted section has enabled those substances to be applied to specific sports. However, a number of sports federations have continued to publish and endorse their own lists. Whilst the general principle for listing certain substances is the same, the slight variations that occur from time to time have caused some difficulty in the management of results. The IOC states that its Medical Code is intended to safeguard the health of athletes, and to ensure respect for the ethical concepts implicit in fair play, the Olympic spirit and medical practice. Adverse reactions to drugs are well documented in the medical literature. The health of athletes is clearly at risk through taking a drug, often in doses far in excess of those recommended for therapeutic use. However, reports of side-effects associated with doping in sport are often anecdotal and circumstantial. The reported incidence of acute life-threatening events associated with anabolic steroid abuse is low, but the actual risk may be underrecognized or underreported (Wu, 1997). The adoption of double-blind control trials would provide a much clearer picture of the effectiveness and toxicity of potential performance-enhancing drugs. The incidence of damaging side-effects due to steroids, resulting from the German Democratic Republic's doping programme, provides strong evidence in support of the IOC objective to safeguard the health of athletes (Franke and Berendonk, 1997).

The ethical basis for testing for performance-enhancing drugs in sport has been questioned on the grounds of infringement of liberty (Fost, 1986; Catlin and Murray, 1996). This argument takes no consideration of the infringement of liberty for fellow competitors subjected to the potential adverse reactions induced by pharmacologically modified behaviour.

The creation of the World Anti-Doping Agency has provided a useful opportunity to consolidate the list of substances prohibited for all sports. The World Anti-Doping Code is intended to bring sports together under one consolidated list and indicate agreed variations, so avoiding confusion among athletes and others about the status of substances for a specific sport.

Should the list be expanded to include nutritional supplements?

In attempting to enhance performance through ergogenic aids, without contravening WADA regulations, many athletes have used nutritional supplements. Unlike drugs, nutritional supplements are not required to have strong scientific and clinical evidence that they are effective before being allowed to be marketed (Clarkson, 1996). This encourages the manufacturers to make claims that their products have ergogenic properties (Beltz and Doering, 1993). There is little if any evidence that nutritional supplements possess ergogenic properties in athletes consuming a balanced diet. Furthermore, some products have the potential for harm (Beltz and Doering, 1993). Indeed, studies in which diet was manipulated to induce metabolic acidosis by reducing carbohydrate intake or increasing fat and protein intake have resulted in impaired performance (MacLaren, 1997).

Creatine has been the subject of many studies, but whether it is capable of producing ergogenic effects is equivocal (Clarkson, 1996; Balsom, 1997). Williams (1994) suggested that cut-off limits could be applied to nutrients or derived byproducts that are shown to be ergogenic.

In the absence of convincing evidence for ergogenic properties for nutritional supplements, coupled with the problems associated with testing substances which occur naturally in the body, their inclusion in the WADA list would seem ill-advised. However, in their Executive Summary Report on the Sydney 2000 Olympic Games (www.wada-ama.org), WADA recommended that the IOC Medical Commission makes an urgent study of the medications and supplements declared by competitors during the Sydney Games, with a view to making proposals, if necessary, for revising the list of prohibited substances and to developing more appropriate and adapted education strategies.

11.8 Conclusions

Doping control, through an agreed set of standards and procedures, must continue as a primary objective for WADA, the sports federations and governments of the world. Constant vigilance and a continued willingness to respond rapidly to change is a prerequisite for the anti-doping system. There are, however, other fundamental issues to be considered. The concept of doping control must be supported by high quality research, effective education and international collaboration.

It is encouraging to note that research into drug misuse in sport has increased significantly since the Seoul Olympic Games and that this research is focused on the problem areas, at least in terms of drug testing (Reilly et al., 1996). What is lacking is research into the factors which induce an athlete to take drugs and into the impact, if any, that education on drugs is having on competitors. The need for good quality education has been identified as a high priority by all sectors in sport, from administrators to elite athletes (Reilly et al., 1996). Educational messages aimed at abstinence alone have not been successful (Littlepage and Perry, 1993) and should therefore be based on motivating athletes not to abuse drugs (Uzych, 1991). Education on drug misuse in sport should extend beyond internationally regulated competitive sports and into public sports, where testing and sanctions do not apply (Hoppeler et al., 1995). There is a continuum between public and internationally regulated sport, with public sport providing the initial training ground for elite competitors who, in turn, become role models for those competing at the recreational level (Hoppeler et al., 1995).

The most important area for change is the overriding need for international collaboration between WADA, governments and sports federations. This applies to uniformity in the rules and regulations, consistency in the application and level of sanctions and co-operation on the dissemination of information and development of education policies. Clearly, such measures require significant funding; however, as Larry Bowers has observed 'Given the amount of financial resources invested in sport, the athletes (and fans) have the right to competition decided by innate ability and hard work not by potentially dangerous pharmacological intervention' (Bowers, 1997). The establishment of the World Anti-Doping Agency offers an exciting future for drug-free sport. Initially funded for its first 2 years by the IOC, the governments of the world have agreed to share the funding from 2002. This will enable a world-wide testing programme to be undertaken, research into problem areas can be commissioned and a standardization of programmes can be promoted. The key test for WADA will be its ability to serve both sport and governments, in particular to require the accountability and independence so desperately needed to regain the confidence of athletes in the anti-doping system.

11.9 References

Anguilera, R., Becchi, M., Casabianca, H. et al. (1996) Improved method of detection of testosterone abuse by gas chromatography/combustion/isotope ratio mass spectrometry analysis of urinary steroids. J. Mass Spectrom., 31, 169–176.

Anon (1987) American College of Sports Medicine position on blood doping as an ergogenic aid. *Med. Sci. Sports Exerc.*, **19**, 540–543.

Australian Sports Drug Agency (1994) *Survey of Athletes' Attitudes to Doping Control*. ASDA publication.

Ayotte, C. (1999) Nutritional supplements and doping controls. *New Studies Athlet.*, **14(1)**, 37–42.

Balsom, P.D. (1997) Creatine supplementation in humans. In: T. Reilly and M. Orme (eds) *Esteve Foundation Symposium. Vol. 7: The clinical pharmacology of sport and exercise.* Amsterdam: Excerpta Medica, 167–177.

Becchi, M., Aguilera, R., Farizon, Y. *et al.* (1994) Gas chromatography/combustion/isotope ratio mass spectrometry analysis of urinary steroids to detect misuse of testosterone in sport. *Rapid Commun. Mass Spectrom.*, **8**, 304–308.

Beckett, A.H. (1981) Use and abuse of drugs in sport. *J. Biosoc. Sci. (Suppl.)*, **7**, 163–170.

Beckett, A.H. and Cowan, D.A. (1979) Misuse of drugs in sport. *Br. J. Sports Med.*, **12**, 185–194.

Beltz, S.D. and Doering, P.L. (1993) Efficacy of nutritional supplements used by athletes. *Clin. Pharm.*, **12**, 900–908.

Berglund, B. (1988) Development of techniques for the detection of blood doping in sport. *Sports Med.*, **5**, 127–135.

Birkeland, K.I., Donike, M., Ljungqist, A. *et al.* (1997) Blood sampling in doping control: first experiences from regular testing in athletes. *Int. J. Sports Med.*, **18**, 8–12.

Birkeland, K.I. and Hemmersbach, P. (1999) The future of doping control in athletes. Issues relating to blood sampling. *Sports Med.*, **28(1)**, 25–33.

Birkett, D.J. and Miners, J.O. (1991) Caffeine renal clearance and urine caffeine concentrations during steady state dosing. Implications for monitoring caffeine intake during sport events. *Br. J. Clin. Pharmacol.*, **31(4)**, 405–408.

Bottomley, M. (1988) Report in P. Bellotti, G. Benzi and A. Ljungqist (eds) *International Athletic Foundation World Symposium on Doping in Sport: Official Proceedings.* International Athletic Foundation, Monte Carlo, pp. 209–211.

Bowers, L.D. (1997) Analytical advances in detection of performance enhancing compounds. *Clin. Chem.*, **43**, 1299–1304.

Bowers, L.D. (1998) Athletic drug testing. *Clin. Sports Med.*, **17(2)**, 299–318.

Brooks, R.V., Firth, R.G. and Sumner, N.A. (1975) Detection of anabolic steroids by radioimmunoassay. *Br. J. Sports Med.*, **9**, 89–92.

Browne, A., Lachance, V. and Pipe, A. (1999) The ethics of blood testing as an element of doping control in sport. *Med. Sci. Sports Exerc.*, **31(4)**, 497–501.

Catlin, D.H. and Hatton, C.K. (1991) Use and abuse of anabolic and other drugs for athletic enhancement. *Adv. Int. Med.*, **36**, 399–424.

Catlin, D.H. and Murray, T.H. (1996) Performance-enhancing drugs, fair competition, and Olympic sport. *JAMA*, **276**, 231–237.

Catlin, D.H., Kammerer, R.C., Hatton, C.K., Sekers, J.H. and Merdink, J.L. (1987) Analytical chemistry at the games of the XXIIIrd Olympiad in Los Angeles, 1984. *Clin. Chem.*, **33**, 319–327.

Catlin, D.H., Cowan, D.A., de laTorre, R. *et al.* (1996) Urinary testosterone (T) to epitestosterone (E) ratios by GC/MS. 1. Initial comparison of uncorrected T/E in 6 international laboratories. *J. Mass Spectrom.*, **31**, 397–402.

Catlin, D.H., Hatton, C.K. and Starcevic, S.H. (1997) Issues in detecting abuse of xenobiotic anabolic steroids and testosterone by analysis of athletes' urine. *Clin. Chem.*, **43**, 1280–1288.

Chan, S.C. (1991) Doping control of anabolic steroids. *J. Forensic Sci. Soc.*, **31**, 217–220.

Chester, N., Reilly, T. and Mottram, D.R. (2003a) Physiological, subjective and performance effects of pseudoephedrine and phenylpropanolamine during endurance running exercise. *Int. J. Sports Med.*, **24**, 3–8.

Chester, N., Mottram, D.R., Reilly, T. and Powell, M. (2003b) Elimination of ephedrines in urine following multiple dosing: the consequencies for athletes, in relation to doping control. *Br. J. Clin. Pharmacol.*, **71**, 62–67.

Clarkson, P. (1996) Nutrition for improved sports performance. Current issues on ergogenic aids. *Sports Med.*, **21**, 393–401.

Clarkson, P.M. and Thompson, H.S. (1997) Drugs and sport. Research findings and limitations. *Sports Med.*, **24**, 366–384.

Cowan, D.A. (1997) Testing for drug abuse. In: T. Reilly and M. Orme (eds) *Esteve Foundation Symposium. Vol. 7: The clinical pharmacology of sport and exercise.* Amsterdam: Excerpta Medica, pp. 13–23.

de Merode, A. (1979) Doping tests at the Olympic Games in 1976. *J. Sports Med.*, **19**, 91–96.

Dehennin, L. and Peres, G. (1996) Plasma and urinary markers of oral testosterone misuse by healthy men in presence of masking epitestosterone administration. *Int. J. Sports Med.*, **17**, 315–319.

Donike, M., Geyer, H., Kraft, M. and Rauth, S. (1989) Long term influence of anabolic steroid misuse on the steroid profile. In: P. Bellotti, G. Benzi and A. Ljungqist (eds) *Official proceedings of the 2nd I.A.F. World Symposium on Doping in Sport.* I.A.F., Monte Carlo, June 1989, pp. 107–116.

Dubin, C.L. (1990) *Commission of inquiry into the use of drugs and banned practices intended to increase athletic performance.* Canadian Government Publishing Center, Ottawa.

Dugal, P. and Donike, M. (1988) *Requirements for accreditation and good laboratory practice.* IOC Medical Commission document, October 1988.

Ekblom, B. (1997) Blood doping, erythropoietin and altitude. In: T. Reilly and M. Orme (eds) *Esteve Foundation Symposium. Vol. 7: The clinical pharmacology of sport and exercise.* Amsterdam: Excerpta Medica, pp. 199–212.

Ferstle, J. (1999a) Explaining nandrolone. *Athletics Weekly*, September 15th, 16.

Ferstle, J. (1999b) Nandrolone, part II. *Athletics Weekly*, September 22nd, 26–27.

Ferstle, J. (1999c) Nandrolone, part III. *Athletics Weekly*, September 29th, 14–15.

Fost, N. (1986) Banning drugs in sports: a skeptical view. *Hastings Centre rEPOrt*, **16**, 5–10.

Franke, W.W. and Berendonk, B. (1997) Hormonal doping and androgenization of athletes: a secret program of the German Democratic Republic government. *Clin. Chem.*, **43**, 1262–1279.

Frumkin, L.R. and Price, J.M. (1996) The IOC and doping status of antiasthma drugs. *Pediatr. Asthma, Allergy Immunol.*, **2**, 41–46.

Gareau, R., Brisson, G.R., Chenard, C. *et al.* (1995) Total fibrin and fibrinogen degradation products in urine: A possible probe to detect illicit users of the physical-performance enhancer erythropoietin? *Horm. Res.*, **44**, 189–192.

Hatton, C.K. and Catlin, D.H. (1987) Detection of androgenic anabolic steroids in urine. *Clin. Lab. Med.*, **7**, 655–668.

Herbert, D.L. (1999) Recommending or selling nutritional supplements enhances potential legal liability for sports medicine practitioners. *Sports Med. Alert*, **5(11)**, 91–92.

Honour, J. (1997) Steroid abuse in female athletes. *Curr. Op. Obstet. Gynecol.*, **9**, 181–186.

Hoppeler, H.H., Kamber, M.F. and Melia, P.S. (1995) Doping and prevention of doping. International co-operation. *Clin. J. Sport Med.*, **5**, 79–81.

Houlihan, B. (1999) *Dying to Win: Doping in Sport and the Development of Anti-Doping Policy*. Strasbourg: Council of Europe.

Houlihan, B. (2001) in O'Leary J. (ed.) *Drugs and Doping in Sport, Socio-legal perspectives*. London: Cavendish Publishing.

Howman, D. (2003) Sanctions under the World Anti-Doping Code. Available at http://www.wada-ama.org (accessed 02/02/05).

IOC (1990) International Olympic Charter against Doping in Sport.

Kicman, A.T. and Cowan, D.A. (1992) Peptide hormones and sport: Misuse and detection. *Br. Med. Bull.*, **48**, 496–517.

Kicman, A.T., Miell, J.P., Teale, J.D. *et al.* (1997) Serum IGF-I and IGF binding proteins 2 and 3 as potential markers of doping with human GH. *Clin. Endocrinol.*, **47**, 43–50.

Kintz, P. (1998) Hair testing and doping control in sport. *Toxicol. Lett.*, **102–103**, 109–113.

Lasne, F. and de Ceaurriz, J. (2000) Recombinant erythropoietin in urine. *Nature*, **405**, 635.

Littlepage, B.N.C. and Perry, H.M. (1993) Misusing anabolic drugs: possibilities for future policies. *Addiction*, **88**, 1469–1471.

Longobardi, S., Keay, N., Ehrnborg, C. *et al.* (2000) Growth hormone (GH) effects on bone and collagen turnover in healthy adults and its potential as a marker of GH abuse in sports: a double blind, placebo controlled study. *J. Clin. Endocrinol. Metab.*, **85(4)**, 1505–1512.

Lukas, S.E. (1993) Current perspectives on anabolic-androgenic steroid abuse. *Trends Pharmacol. Sci.*, **14**, 61–68.

MacLaren, D.P.M. (1997) Alkalinizers: Influence of blood acid–base status on performance. In: T. Reilly and M. Orme (eds) *Esteve Foundation Symposium. Vol. 7: The clinical pharmacology of sport and exercise*. Amsterdam: Excerpta Medica, pp. 157–165.

McBay, A.J. (1987) Drug analysis technology – pitfalls and problems of drug testing. *Clin. Chem.*, **33**, 33B–40B.

Mottram, D.R., Reilly, T. and Chester, N. (1997) Doping in sport: the extent of the problem. In: T. Reilly and M. Orme (eds) *Esteve Foundation Symposium. Vol. 7: The clinical pharmacology of sport and exercise*. Amsterdam: Excerpta Medica, pp. 3–12.

Nandrolone Review – Report to UK Sport, January 2000, UK Sport, London *www.uksport.gov.uk/anti-doping*.

Ng, T.L. (1993) Dope testing in sports: scientific and medico-legal issues. *Ann. Acad. Med. Singapore*, **22**, 48–53.

Olympic Movement Anti-Doping Code 1999. IOC.

Parisotto, R., Wu, M., Ashenden, M.J. *et al.* (2001) Detection of recombinant human erythropoietin abuse in athletes utilizing markers of altered erythropoiesis. *Haematologica*, **86**, 128–137.

Perry, P.J., MacIndoe, J.H., Yates, W.R. *et al.* (1997) Detection of anabolic steroid adminstration: ratio of urinary testosterone to epitestosterone vs the ratio of urinary testosterone to luteinizing hormone. *Clin. Chem.*, **43(5)**, 731–735.

Polettini, A., Montagna, M., Segura, J. *et al.* (1996) Determination of β_2-agonists in hair by gas chromatography/mass spectrometry. *J. Mass Spectrom.*, **31**, 47–54.

Radford, P. (1992) Drug testing and drug education programs. *Sports Med.*, **12**, 1–5.

Raynaud, E., Audrant, M., Pegas, J.Ch. *et al.* (1993) Determination of urinary testosterone and epitestosterone during pubertal development: a cross-sectional study in 141 normal male subjects. *Clin. Endocinol.*, **38**, 353–359.

Reeb, M. (ed.) (1998) *Digest of CAS Awards 1986–1998*. Berne Staemofli Editions SA.

Reilly, T., Mottram, D.R., Chester, N. *et al.* (1996) *Review of Research into Drug Misuse in Sport*. London: UK Sports Council, 1996.

Rivier, L. (2000) Is there a place for hair analysis in doping controls? *Forensic Sci. Int.*, **107**, 309–323.

Rivier, L. and Saugy, M. (1999) Peptide hormones abuse in sport: state of the art in the detection of growth hormone and erythropoietin. *J. Toxicol. Toxin Rev.*, **18(2)**, 145–176.

Ros, J.J.W., Pelders, M.G. and De Smet, P.A.G.M. (1999) A case of positive doping associated with a botanical food supplement. *Pharm. World Sci.*, **21(1)**, 44–46.

Royal Society of New Zealand (1990) *Drugs and Medicines in Sport*. Thomas Publications, Wellington.

Saugy, M., Cardis, C., Schweizer, C. *et al.* (1996) Detection of human growth hormone doping in urine: out of competition tests are necessary. *J. Chromatog. B*, **687**, 201–211.

Schnazer, W. (1996) Metablism of anabolic steroids. *Clin. Chem.*, **42**, 1001.

Segura, J., Peng, S.H. and de la Torre, X. (1999) Recent progress in the detection of the administration of natural hormones: special focus on testosterone. *J. Toxicol. Toxin Rev.*, **18(2)**, 125–144.

Shackleton, C.H.L., Chuang, H., Kim, J. *et al.* (1997) Electrospray mass spectrometry of testosterone esters: Potential for use in doping control. *Steroids*, **62**, 523–529.

Sinclair, C.J.D. and Geiger, J.D. (2000) Caffeine use in sports. A pharmacological review. *J. Sports Med. Phys. Fitness*, **40**, 71–79.

Sonksen, P. (1999) The detection of growth hormone abuse in sport. *5th IOC World Congress on Sport Sciences*, Australia.

Swain, R.A., Harsha, D.M., Baenziger, J. *et al.* (1997) Do pseudoephedrine or phenylpropanolamine improve maximum oxygen uptake and time to exhaustion? *Clin. J. Sports Med.*, **7**, 168–173.

United States Anti-Doping Agency (2002) *Survey of Athletes' Attitudes to Drugs in Sport*, USADA (website).

UK Sports Council (1995) *Doping Control in the UK. Survey of the Experiences and Views of Elite Competitors*. London: UK Sports Council.

Uzych, L. (1991) Drug testing of athletes. *Br. J. Addiction*, **86**, 25–31.

Ventura, R., Segura, J., Berges, R. *et al.* (2000) Distinction of inhaled and oral salbutamol by urine analysis using conventional screening procedures for doping control. *Ther. Drug Monitor.*, **22**, 277–282.

Voy, R. (1991) *Drugs, Sport, and Politics*. Champagne, Illinois, Human Kinetics Inc.

Vrijman, E. (2001) in O'Leary J. (ed.) *Drugs and Doping in Sport, Socio-legal perspectives*. Cavendish Publishing, London.

WADA (2005) The World Anti-Doping Code 2005 Prohibited List. Available at http://www.wada-ama.org (accessed 02/02/05).

Waddington, I. (1996) The development of sports medicine. *Sociol. Sport J.*, **13**, 176–196.

Wade, N. (1972) Anabolic steroids: Doctors denounce them, but athletes aren't listening. *Science*, **176**,1399–1403.

Wadler, G.I. (1994) Drug use update. *Med. Clin. N. Am.*, **78**, 439–455.

Williams, M.H. (1994) The use of nutritional ergogenic aids in sport: Is it an ethical issue? *Int. J. Sports Nutr.*, **4**, 120–131.

Wu, A.H.B., Bristol, B., Sexton, K. *et al.* (1999) Adulteration of urine by 'Urine Luck'. *Clin. Chem.*, **45(7)**, 1051–1057.

Wu, F.C.W. (1997) Endocrine aspects of anabolic steroids. *Clin. Chem.*, **43**, 1289–1292.

Chapter 12

Prevalence of drug misuse in sport

David R. Mottram

12.1 Introduction

Meaningful data on the prevalence of use of performance-enhancing drugs in sport are difficult to obtain. Evidence may be as diverse as statistics on positive dope tests, results of surveys of athletes on their self-reporting or perceptions of drug use through to anecdotal reports and speculation by the media. These sources of evidence are widely inconsistent, leading to speculation of levels of prevalence of drug use ranging from less than 1 per cent to over 90 per cent. A number of studies have been undertaken to evaluate the prevalence of doping within individual countries or sports but these are, in the main, based on analysis of IOC and WADA statistics. The purpose of this chapter is to evaluate the published evidence and, where appropriate, to comment on the validity and accuracy of this evidence.

12.2 Statistics on doping control in sport

Statistics from IOC/WADA accredited laboratories

Statistics on doping control were obtained from the International Olympic Committee's (IOC) Medical Commission and World Anti-Doping Agency. These are based on results from the IOC/WADA accredited laboratories ($n = 32$ in 2005). Overall, the percentage of positive test results from the laboratories has remained consistently low, despite a steady increase in the number of tests conducted annually (Table 12.1). These figures, which themselves may not be a true reflection of the truth, merely tell us how many athletes have tested positive, not how many are using drugs and avoiding detection. The majority of the positive results arise from the misuse of anabolic steroids (Table 12.2), although stimulants and, increasingly, marijuana (the majority of the Other class, see Table 12.7) are frequently detected in urine samples.

In 1993, the IOC changed the class of anabolic steroids to anabolic agents, to include β_2-agonists, such as salbutamol and clenbuterol, which do not possess a steroid structure but which possess anabolic properties (Yang and

Table 12.1 Overview of the results of 'A-Samples' tested by IOC/WADA accredited laboratories from 1993–2003

	No. of A-samples analysed	% of positive results
2003	151 210	1.62
2002	131 373	1.80
2001	125 701	1.65
2000	117 314	1.90
1999	118 259	1.98
1998	105 250	1.83
1997	106 561	1.67
1996	96 454	1.63
1995	93 938	1.61
1994	93 680	1.36
1993	89 166	1.37

Table 12.2 Number of substances identified in the banned classes from IOC/WADA accredited laboratories for 1993–2003

	1993	1994	1995	1996	1997	1998	1999	2000	2001	2002	2003
Stimulants	331	347	310	281	356	412	532	453	352	392	516
Narcotics	46	42	34	37	47	18	9	14	29	13	26
Anabolic agents	940*	891	986	1131	967	856	973	946	914	966	872
β_2-Agonists[†]	–	–	–	–	393	479	536	489	398	382	297
Beta blockers	11	15	14	6	11	12	24	21	20	15	30
Diuretics	65	63	59	54	90	80	118	75	106	144	131
Masking agents	7	8	3	0	13	16	11	5	11	8	11
Peptide hormones	4	3	9	4	5	12	20	12	26	41	79
Others	48	77	224	155	184	295	401	466	423	665	754

* Classed as anabolic steroids prior to the introduction of the class anabolic agents.
[†] Include inhalation preparations which are permitted and clenbuterol (recorded under anabolic agents up to 1996).

McElliott, 1989). However, β_2-agonists are primarily classified as stimulants due to their ability to mimic some of the effects of adrenaline. Four of these β_2-agonists (salbutamol, formoterol, terbutaline and salmeterol) are permitted for use by WADA, provided they are administered by inhalation and an Abbreviated TUE has been granted.

In 1997, the IOC statistics on the number of substances identified in the banned classes were published with β_2-agonists categorized separately from stimulants and anabolic agents. Tables 12.3 to 12.5 show the incidence of positive test results from IOC/WADA statistics, in recent years, for the more commonly misused stimulants, androgenic anabolic steroids and β_2-agonists. It is clear that stimulants, particularly pseudoephedrine and ephedrine, which are found commonly in over-the-counter (OTC) medicines, constitute the majority of these test results.

Table 12.3 Statistics from IOC/WADA accredited laboratories for the number of positive results for substances classed as stimulants (1993–2003)

Stimulants	1993	1994	1995	1996	1997	1998	1999	2000	2001	2002	2003
Pseudoephedrine	103	89	102	69	77	91	185	136	58	77	189
Ephedrine	51	74	78	69	122	141	143	129	123	147	100
Amphetamine	31	48	25	18	30	22	42	21	19	29	43
Phenylpropanolamine	38	28	16	25	14	35	36	17	13	12	0
Caffeine	17	26	15	18	25	25	28	38	43	25	39
Cocaine	8	8	18	16	20	18	21	21	29	36	48
Others	83	74	56	66	68	80	77	91	67	66	97
Totals	331	347	310	281	356	412	532	453	352	392	516

Table 12.4 Statistics from IOC/WADA accredited laboratories for the number of positive results for substances classed as androgenic anabolic steroids (1993–2003)

Anabolic steroids	1993	1994	1995	1996	1997	1998	1999	2000	2001	2002	2003
Testosterone	308	280	293	331	351	299	347	306	328	325	304
Nandrolone	227	207	212	232	262	259	293	325	304	310	256
Metandienone	100	96	132	111	97	78	60	75	63	57	59
Stanozolol	108	93	78	89	131	103	129	116	101	162	159
Methenolone	73	35	39	39	44	36	57	48	36	29	11
Mesterolone	31	9	20	15	19	26	19	17	15	13	16
Methyltestosterone	23	10	9	11	18	22	15	22	10	25	12
Others	70	161[†]	203[†]	303[†]	45	33	53	37	57	45	55
Totals	940	891	986	1131	967	856	973	946	914	966	872

[†] Includes salbutamol and clenbuterol – in 1997, these β_2-agonists were included in the IOC list under their own heading (see Table 12.2).

Table 12.5 Statistics from IOC/WADA accredited laboratories for the number of positive results for substances classed as β_2-agonists (1994–2003)

β_2-Agonists	1994	1995	1996	1997	1998	1999	2000	2001	2002	2003
Salbutamol*	68[†]	132[†]	250[†]	284	366	437	367	256	261	189
Terbutaline*	–	–	–	79	69	68	110	113	97	76
Clenbuterol	30[†]	31[†]	25[†]	30	41	29	10	26	23	31
Others	–	–	–	–	3	2	2	3	1	1
Totals	98	163	275	393	479	536	489	398	382	297

* Results on salbutamol and terbutaline may correspond to administration by inhalation, which is permitted by IOC/WADA regulations.
[†] Recorded under anabolic agents category.

In the late 1990s the IOC introduced urinary cut-off levels for over-the-counter stimulants, such as ephedrine, pseudoephedrine and phenyl-propanolamine. These levels were increased in April 2000. Only when the drugs are present in the urine at levels above 10 or 25 μg/ml, respectively, were the IOC laboratories required to report their findings. In 2004, WADA removed pseudoephedrine, phenylpropanolamine and a number of other OTC stimulants from the prohibited list but continue to monitor their use in sport. Ephedrine remains on the prohibited list but is also included on the WADA list of specified substances that includes substances that are particularly susceptible to unintentional anti-doping rule violations because of their general availability. Doping violations involving specified substances may result in a reduced sanction, provided the athlete can establish the use was not intended to enhance performance.

There is evidence from Table 12.3 that the numbers of positive results for cocaine has increased in recent years, possibly reflecting its increased use as a recreational drug in society.

Testosterone is the most frequently identified anabolic steroid, although the IOC point out that some of the positive results for testosterone are as a result of multiple measurements performed on the same athlete in the case of longitudinal studies on testosterone.

In 2003, there were 14 positive test results for tetrahydrogestrinone, an 'undetectable designer steroid', which was identified after a tip-off to a WADA accredited laboratory. The consequences of this investigation lead to sanctioning of a number of high-profile athletes. In 2005, a second 'designer steroid', desoxymethyltestosterone, was intercepted by Canadian customs officials. Retrospective tests on stored urine samples showed no positive results for this drug, leading some officials to claim that this was a rare case of the testers being one step ahead of the misusers.

It is clear that the annual numbers, and percentages, of positive tests for anabolic steroids are lower than might be expected. These figures are unlikely to reflect the true prevalence of anabolic steroid use for a number of reasons (Mottram, 1999). Anecdotal reports indicate that athletes are adept at tailoring their anabolic steroid regimes to avoid detection. This is fostered by the fact that athletes take their steroids during training, whereas over 50 per cent of drug tests are conducted at the time of competition. The extent of out-of-competition testing is increasing but is not universal (Catlin and Hatton, 1991). This may change with an increase in international co-operation (Hoppeler et al., 1995) and through the offices of the newly established World Anti-Doping Agency (WADA) (www.wada-ama.org).

There has been a dramatic rise in the number of 'positive' test results for salbutamol and terbutaline. The majority of these results were, however, deemed permissible by the IOC as the drugs were administered by inhalation and written notification that the drug was needed had been provided by the athlete, prior to competing. The results from the Sydney 2000 Games

Table 12.6 Statistics from IOC/WADA accredited laboratories for the number of positive results for substances classed as masking agents (1994–2003)

Masking agents	1994	1995	1996	1997	1998	1999	2000	2001	2002	2003
Probenecid	8	3	–	4	3	2	–	4	5	–
Epitestosterone	–	–	–	9	12	9	5	6	3	10
Physical manipulation	–	–	–	–	1	–	–	1	–	2
Totals	8	3	0	13	16	11	5	11	8	12

Table 12.7 Statistics from IOC/WADA accredited laboratories for the number of positive results for substances classed as 'Others' (1994–2003)

Others	1994	1995	1996	1997	1998	1999	2000	2001	2002	2003
Cannabis	75	224	154	164	233	312	295	298	347	378
Corticosteroids	2	–	–	–	–	–	89	46	249	286
Ethanol	–	–	1	20	1	3	4	–	–	–
Local anaesthetics	–	–	–	–	61	85	77	71	63	82
Tetrazepam	–	–	–	–	–	1	1	1	4	–
Totals	77	224	155	184	295	401	466	416	663	746

suggest that athletes are being encouraged to exploit this loophole in the regulations (see Table 12.14). In 2004, WADA introduced the system for Therapeutic Use Exemption (TUE), which applied to this group of drugs.

The low level of detection of masking agents, such as probenecid, compared with figures from the 1980s, suggests that athletes no longer perceive these agents as being effective in the modern environment of highly selective and accurate testing systems (Table 12.6). On the other hand, the rise in the number of positive tests for epitestosterone, a drug without performance-enhancing properties itself but which is used in an attempt to conceal the use of testosterone, indicates that athletes are trying harder to disguise their use of this popular anabolic steroid (see Table 12.4).

The number of positive test results for marijuana (cannabis) has increased dramatically in recent years (Table 12.7). This reflects the increased use of this 'recreational' drug in society. It probably does not indicate an increasing trend in its use as a performance-enhancing drug, since its pharmacological properties are likely to have adverse, rather than positive, effects on performance in most sports.

A few studies have been undertaken into the extent of drug misuse within specific countries. These are listed in Table 12.8. Bahr and Tjornhom (1998) collected data, on Norwegian athletes, from four IOC accredited laboratories in Germany, Norway, Sweden and the UK. The drugs identified were anabolic agents (75 per cent) (almost half of which were testosterone), stimulants (17 per cent), narcotic analgesics (8 per cent), diuretics (5 per cent) and

Table 12.8 Published statistics on doping control in specific countries

Author	Country	Years data collected	No. of samples	% positive test results
Bahr and Tjornhom (1998)	Norway	1977–1995	12 870	1.2
Ueki *et al.* (1998)	Japan	1985–1996	~14 000	~1.0
Mottram *et al.* (1997)	UK	1991–1995	17 193	1.0–1.5
Delbeke (1996)	Belgium	1987–1994	4374	7.8 in cyclists
Benzi (1994)	Italy	1988–1992	N/A	0.29–0.59
Van der Merwe and Kruger (1992)	S. Africa	1986–1991	2066	5.2–5.9 in most years

manipulation attempts (4 per cent). The majority were unannounced tests. A gradual decrease in the percentage of positive samples was recorded among Norwegian athletes as the frequency of testing, in the high prevalence sports, powerlifting, weightlifting and athletics, was increased during the period from 1987 to 1995. The authors commented on the beneficial effects of unannounced out-of-competition testing.

Japan (Ueki *et al.*, 1998) have conducted tests both in and out-of-competition since 1985. In line with international trends, the major abused drugs were stimulants and anabolic steroids. Ephedrine, methylephedrine and phenylpropanolamine, all available over-the-counter, were the main stimulants and nandrolone and testosterone the main steroids. The authors noted the value of testing agencies being independent from sports federations.

A review of data from the UK (Mottram *et al.*, 1997) shows that anabolic steroids and stimulants are the two main drugs of abuse, with narcotic analgesics also frequently detected. The authors commented on the fact that competitors may have been taking drugs which were undetectable at the time.

In the Belgian study (Delbeke, 1996) the percentage of positive results was higher than most other countries. However, this study was confined to cyclists, as this was the most popular sport in that country, and cycling has a long-standing reputation for being associated with drug misuse. The most frequently used drugs were stimulants, including over-the-counter products and amphetamines. There was also a significant number of positive results for nandrolone. The tests were all conducted unannounced, which may also account for the high level of positive results.

In an Italian study, in 1992, stimulants (55 per cent), anabolic agents (32 per cent), beta blockers (10 per cent) and narcotics (3 per cent) were the main drugs identified (Benzi, 1994). Amphetamine was the most frequently identified stimulant, being associated with cyclists. However, the percentage of positive results overall in Italy decreased from 0.59 per cent in 1988 to 0.29 per cent in 1992. The author provides an interesting observation on the small number of IOC laboratories world-wide. This means that few tests can be conducted relative to the number of athletes participating in sport. The author therefore concludes that the data generated from the laboratories are only the 'tip of the iceberg'. He surmises that millions of athletes who take drugs feel safe from the risk of anti-doping control as checks are conducted on very few elite competitors.

In the South African study (Van der Merwe and Kruger, 1992) analysis was undertaken by the University of the Orange Free State, according to IOC regulations. Samples were taken from athletes in a wide range of sports. The percentage of positive results over the study period was very consistent each year, being relatively high (average 5.5 per cent). The main drugs identified were stimulants (50.4 per cent) and anabolic steroids (41.6 per cent).

These national studies, in general, reflect international trends, with anabolic agents and stimulants being the most frequently identified drugs, although the principal class identified varied from country to country. National differences exist where particular sports dominate the scene or where tests are conducted out-of-competition.

Unfortunately, out-of-competition testing is not conducted internationally. The proportion of tests conducted through this route is shown in Table 12.9. By 2000, each of the IOC accredited laboratories was conducting out-of-competition testing, although the percentage of these tests compared with total tests conducted varied from 72.6 per cent (Los Angeles) and 63.5 per cent (Oslo) to 13.7 per cent (Bangkok) and 3.3 per cent (Gent) with a mean of 40 per cent.

The percentage of positive test results arising through out-of-competition testing is consistently lower than the percentage obtained in competition. These figures are, perhaps, surprising since this type of testing is designed to catch athletes unawares, at a time when they are likely to be using drugs which are perceived to have their greatest potential benefit for the athlete. As long as athletes can train in countries where out-of-competition testing does not take place and therefore use androgenic anabolic steroids and peptide hormones during training, with little risk of being tested, the true incidence of drug taking in sport will continue to be underreported.

Statistics from the 2000 Olympic Games in Sydney

The statistics reported in this section are derived from the IOC website (http://www.olympic.org, March 2001).

Table 12.10 provides an overview of the total number of tests performed by the Australian Sport Drug Testing Laboratory, which was accredited by the IOC. In all, some 400 people were involved in doping control tasks over the period leading up to and during the Games. More than 90 people worked at the laboratory around the clock to ensure a turn-around in results of 24–48 hours for in-competition samples and 2 to 3 days for out-of-competition (OOC) tests. The majority of tests (2052) were performed in competition. In

Table 12.9 Statistics from IOC/WADA accredited laboratories – numbers of samples analysed (% positive results) by classification of event (1994–2002)

Classification of event	Numbers of samples analysed								
	1994	1995	1996	1997	1998	1999	2000	2001	2002
National competitors	30 809 (1.68)	31 097 (2.09)	31 388 (1.88)	31 797 (2.09)	34 943 (2.44)	42 073 (2.38)	41 067 (2.60)	38 157 (2.31)	38 331 (2.55)
International competitors	12 447 (1.32)	14 337 (1.71)	13 868 (1.54)	15 993 (1.64)	10 440 (2.07)	14 143 (2.26)	14 831 (2.57)	17 053 (2.42)	19 353 (2.68)
International championships	9 927 (1.59)	9 827 (1.38)	5 826 (3.24)	8 249 (3.29)	10 659 (2.56)	12 566 (3.15)	14 443 (2.13)	14 717 (1.64)	12 530 (1.86)
Not at competition	40 497 (1.08)	38 677 (1.25)	45 372 (1.63)	50 522 (1.15)	49 208 (1.19)	49 477 (1.27)	46 973 (1.01)	55 774 (0.97)	61 159 (1.05)

Table 12.10 Summary of tests performed at Sydney 2000 Olympic Games

Samples in competition	2052
Samples out-of-competition (OOC)	404
Erythropoietin (EPO) tests	307
World record samples	32
National record samples	25
Specific gravity and/or pH extra samples	20
Blind samples	6
Total	2846

Table 12.11 Erythropoietin OOC tests performed at Sydney 2000 Olympic Games

Sport	Number of tests
Cycling – road	39
Cycling – track	33
Cycling – mountain bike	24
Athletics	61
Triathlon	25
Rowing	56
Canoe/kayak – sprint	26
Swimming	35
Modern pentathlon	8
Total	307

most events, the medallists and two athletes selected by drawing lots were tested. This was a protocol agreed between the IOC and the International Sport Federations.

For the first time in Olympic history, OOC tests were performed prior to and during the Games. OOC tests were conducted both within the Village and at other venues. In all, there were 404 OOC tests which began when the Olympic Village opened and continued through to the end of the Games. The selection method for OOC tests was defined by each of the 99 National Olympic Committees who participated in OOC testing.

The IOC Executive Board had taken the decision to introduce testing for erythropoietin (EPO) at the Sydney Games. This was the result of the development of two validated methods for detecting EPO use. One was based on a urine test (Lasne and de Ceaurriz, 2000), using an enzyme-linked immunosorbent assay. The other method required a blood sample, through venepuncture, which was subjected to analysis for characteristic changes in the blood profile, induced by EPO (Parisotto et al., 2001). In all, 307 tests for EPO were conducted, all OOC. The decision was made to focus on endurance sports, a list of which appears in Table 12.11. It is clear that the

Table 12.12 Blind tests performed at Sydney 2000 Olympic Games as part of the quality assurance system for the laboratory

Substance	Number of tests
Nikethamide (stimulant)	1
Clopamide (diuretic) + clostebol (anabolic steroid)	1
Epimetendiol (metabolite of the anabolic steroid, metandienone) (at the detection level)	1
Clenbuterol (β_2-agonist) (at the detection level)	1
EPO	2

Table 12.13 Positive test results from the Sydney 2000 Olympic Games

Drug	Sport					
	Athletics	Gymnastics	Rowing	Weightlifting	Wrestling	Total
Frusemide (diuretic)				3	1	4
Nandrolone (anabolic steroid)	1 (OOC)		1		2	4
Pseudoephedrine (stimulant)		1				1
Stanozolol (anabolic steroid)	1 (OOC)			1		2
Salbutamol (β_2-agonist)						12[†]
Terbutaline (β_2-agonist)						2[†]

[†] All cases for salbutamol and terbutaline were notified by the athlete prior to competition and therefore permitted.

selection of sports coincided, to a large extent, with sports with which EPO has previously been associated.

As all the EPO tests were conducted OOC, and to increase the probability of selecting potential medallists for testing, the method for selection of athletes was based on (i) drawing lots among the athletes entered by each sport and (ii) drawing lots based on the ranking list established by each International Federation concerned.

In order to ensure the quality and accuracy of the systems employed by the laboratory, the IOC introduced six blind tests. These were 'positive' samples, prepared in advance, and introduced to the laboratory along with normal samples, for analysis. The list of blind samples used is shown in Table 12.12. The epimetendiol and clenbuterol samples were just at the detection limits set by the IOC Medical Commission.

Table 12.13 shows the number and nature of the positive results, excluding blind tests, sent to the Chairman of the IOC Medical Commission by the head of the testing laboratory at the Sydney Olympic Games. The 11 true-positive test results at the Sydney 2000 Games represents a 0.39 per cent rate, well below the IOC annual rate of 1.90 per cent in 2000 (see Table 12.1).

The profile of positive test results is characteristic. Frusemide is a diuretic and, as such, is used by competitors in sports (such as weightlifting and wrestling) where weight categories are important. Diuretics are used to promote fluid excretion, and therefore weight, rapidly. Anabolic steroids, such as nandrolone and stanozolol are widely used to increase lean muscle mass in power sports.

Pseudoephedrine is a stimulant, commonly found in over-the-counter cough and cold medicines. In this case, a gymnast claimed that the drug had been prescribed by her physician for this purpose. The IOC had set urinary concentration levels for drugs such as pseudoephedrine, above which the laboratory must report the findings. This was the case for this gymnast and the positive test resulted in her having her medal withdrawn. The argument for reviewing the IOC urinary levels for these drugs, in the light of them being unrealistically low, was made by Chester (2003a).

The positive results for salbutamol and terbutaline were not considered doping as the athlete's physician had notified the IOC, prior to competing, that the drug was required for the treatment of asthma and that the medicine had been administered by inhaler. The IOC stipulates that at Olympic Games athletes who request permission to inhale a permitted β_2-agonist will be assessed by an independent medical panel. However, the IOC also published a table (http://www.olympic.org, March 2001) of the number of athletes from each country who notified the IOC of their use of β_2-agonists for the treatment of asthma. Overall, the figures for the three permitted β_2-agonists are shown in Table 12.14.

A total of 607 athletes at the Sydney 2000 Olympic Games claimed to require treatment for asthma. Considering that around 10 300 athletes were competing in the Games, almost 6 per cent were asthmatics! This compares with a 1999/2000 national asthma audit in the UK, which estimated around 1 in 25 adults (aged 16 and over) (4 per cent) had asthma symptoms currently requiring treatment (www.asthma.org.uk/infofa18.html). This audit reported that the UK has some of the highest rates of asthma in the world.

Table 12.14 Number of competitors giving notification of the use of β_2-agonists at the Sydney 2000 Olympic Games

β_2-Agonist	Number of athletes giving notification
Salbutamol	548
Terbutaline	39
Salmeterol	20
Total	607

In all, 11 positive test results (from Table 12.13) were acted upon at the Games. Of the 2840 samples tested, 0.39 per cent were positive. This figure is lower than the annual percentage rate declared by the IOC from its international accredited laboratories (Table 12.1). This is not surprising, since national organizations screen their competitors prior to departure for the Olympic Games.

Statistics from the 2002 Winter Olympic Games in Salt Lake City

The statistics reported in this section are derived from the IOC website (http://www.olympic.org, March 2002).

The IOC conducted 1960 doping control tests at the 2002 Winter Olympic Games. This figure represents a more than 200 per cent increase over the 621 tests that were conducted at the 1998 Winter Olympic Games in Nagano. A breakdown of the types of test conducted is shown in Table 12.15. Approximately 2500 athletes were subject to these tests. Table 12.16 shows the positive test results for the 2002 Winter Olympic Games.

Darbepoetin was a new drug that had only been introduced in October 2001. As such, it was not named on the IOC list of doping substances. However, it is clearly a related substance to EPO and therefore, by IOC definition, a prohibited substance. It is used, clinically, to treat anaemia in patients with renal failure. Its actions and side-effects are similar to those of erythropoetin (EPO) although it is estimated to be 10 times more potent

Table 12.15 Summary of tests performed at Salt Lake City 2002 Winter Olympic Games

Type of test	Number of samples
In competition urine tests	642
Out-of-competition urine tests	96
Blood screening tests	1222
Total	1960

Table 12.16 Positive test results from the Salt Lake City 2002 Winter Olympic Games

Drug	Number of cases
Darbepoetin	3
Methamphetamine	1
Nandrolone	1

than EPO. The most significant difference from a doping control perspective is that, unlike EPO which is produced naturally in the body, darbepoetin is a synthetic drug and its presence in the body can only have occurred through the athlete having taken the drug. The method used for the detection of darbepoetin at the 2002 Games was the one used for EPO and included both the urine and blood tests.

Of the three athletes who tested positive for darbepoetin, two were stripped of the gold medals that they achieved at the time of testing. However, controversially, all three athletes were allowed to keep the medals that they had achieved earlier in the Games, prior to their positive test results. At the time, the IOC President Jacques Rogge said 'They may technically be champions with those medals, but I question their moral authority, and how they can claim to be Olympic champions in the full sense of the word'.

The positive test results for methamphetamine and nandrolone came to light after the completion of the Games and were subject to formal hearings after the Games. The hearing on the nandrolone case resulted in the athlete being disqualified from the event and a recommendation that the athlete's sports federation, the International Ice Hockey Federation, should consider appropriate further action. In this case, the athlete's team doctor was also implicated and the IOC decided that this doctor would be ineligible to participate in the 2004 Summer Games and the 2006 Winter Games.

The hearing on the methamphetamine case, involving Alain Baxter, concluded that, despite the athlete's claim that he took the drug unknowingly in a nasal decongestant, he should be disqualified, lose his bronze medal and recommended that the International Ski Federation consider further action. Subsequently, Baxter's appeal was upheld. It was accepted that he had not been deliberately seeking to enhance performance. His period of ineligibility from competing was reduced, although the IOC refused to reinstate his bronze medal. This case was contributory to WADA's decision, in January 2004, to introduce a class of Specified Substances to the Prohibited List. This list includes substances that are particularly susceptible to unintentional anti-doping rule violations because of their general availability. Doping violations involving Specified Substances may result in a reduced sanction, provided the athlete is able to establish the use was not intended to enhance performance.

A further controversy came to light at the Games when blood transfusion equipment was found in the accommodation used by the Austrian cross-country ski team. An inquiry was set up to investigate this incident.

Statistics from the 2004 Olympic Games in Athens

Table 12.17 shows the drugs that were identified at the 2004 Athens Games.

Table 12.17 Positive test results from the Athens 2004 Olympic Games

Drug	Boxing	Track and field	Weightlifting	Rowing	Wrestling	Cycling	Total
Cathine	1						1
Methyltestosterone			1				1
Testosterone			1				1
Stanozolol	2				1		3
Oxandrolone			1				1
Clenbuterol	2						2
Ethamivan				1			1
Furosemide			1				1
Heptaminol						1	1
Refusal	4	1					5

12.3 Surveys into drug misuse in sport

There have been many survey-based studies published on the prevalence of drug misuse. Unfortunately, very few are based on surveys conducted with athletes and even fewer with elite athletes. Surveys are broadly divided into those that ask about self-use of drugs and those that seek information on perceived use by others. Results from the former type of study tend to reflect underreporting whilst those on perceived use tend to produce exaggerated claims. This section of the chapter reviews some of the more recently published surveys on drug misuse, in which adolescents and athletes, respectively, have been approached.

Surveys into drug misuse in adolescents

Most surveys in this category have been self-use studies, conducted on adolescents in schools, colleges or universities and who variably participate in sport. There are a number of likely reasons for this choice of subjects:

- researchers have easy access to large numbers of students within the institutions in which they work;
- students are more willing to participate in such surveys;
- access to large numbers of competitive athletes is restricted; and
- competitive athletes are unwilling to discuss their drug use.

A number of review articles have been written (Laure, 1997a; Yesalis and Bahrke, 2000) in which comparisons between previously published research on surveys have been drawn. Table 12.18 lists some of the more recent surveys on self-reporting of anabolic steroid use in adolescents, which have

Table 12.18 Self-reporting surveys on anabolic steroid use in adolescents (%)

Authors	Year	Country	Subjects	Age range	♀	♂	Total
Kindlundh et al.	1999	Sweden	2 717	18–19	0.4	2.7	N/A
Lambert et al.	1998	S. Africa	1 136	16–18	0.0	1.2	0.6
		(2 Provinces)	1 411	16–18	0.1	4.4	2.3
Handelsman and Gupta	1997	Australia	13 355	12–19	1.2	3.2	N/A
Melia et al.	1996	Canada	16 119	11–18	N/A	N/A	2.8
Nilsson	1995	Sweden	1 383	14–19	1.0	5.8	N/A
Du Rant et al.	1995	USA	12 272	14–18	1.2	4.08	N/A
Tanner et al.	1995	USA	6 930	14–18	1.3	4.0	2.7

Table 12.19 Overall conclusions drawn from surveys on anabolic steroid use in adolescents

Around 3–5% of adolescents use anabolic steroids
Prevalence is higher among males
Steroid use may begin at a very young age and prevalence increases with age
Prevalence is higher in those who participate in sport
Anabolic steroids are used for purposes other than potential performance enhancement
Other drugs, in addition to anabolic steroids, are simultaneously misused

been conducted in a number of different countries. The results of these studies and of those reported in the reviews of Laure (1997a) and Yesalis and Bahrke (2000) indicate that there are close similarities in the overall conclusions that have been drawn from these surveys. These are listed in Table 12.19. Most of these conclusions are predictable.

Around 3–5 per cent of adolescents use anabolic steroids

A small proportion of adolescents are likely to indulge in illicit drug taking. Anabolic steroids would be particularly attractive to those who have an interest in body image and/or sport. The phenomenon is international, in line with the promotion of sport within an image-conscious society.

Prevalence is higher among males

The higher incidence of anabolic steroid use in males is consistent in all surveys. In the USA, the prevalence in males is around three times that of females (Du Rant et al., 1995; Tanner et al., 1995). In other countries, such as Sweden, it is even higher (Nilsson, 1995; Kindlundh et al., 1999). In South Africa, use by females was insignificant (Lambert et al., 1998).

Steroid use may begin at a very young age and prevalence increases with age

Tanner *et al.* (1995), reported that anabolic steroid use began in children as young as 8 for boys and 11 for girls. In the Melia *et al.* (1996) study, the survey was conducted with children from the age of 11 to 18. Prevalence increased in this study from 1.5 per cent at the age of 11 to 4.7 per cent at the age of 18. The majority of other studies show a similar trend in the increase in prevalence with age (Laure, 1997a). In one study, however, Du Rant *et al.* (1995) did not show a linear trend in steroid use with age.

Prevalence is higher in those who participate in sport

In general, participation in sport increases the tendency to use anabolic steroids (Laure, 1997a). However, this tendency is not marked. Tanner *et al.* (1995) reported a difference of 2.9 per cent users in the group who participated in sport, compared with 2.2 per cent in non-participants. In the Nilsson (1995) study, fewer students who participated in sport used anabolic steroids. In South Africa (Lambert *et al.*, 1998) male participants in First Team sports were significantly more likely to use androgenic anabolic steroids than players in other teams. Unsurprisingly, high prevalence is associated with weightlifting and bodybuilding and with sports such as American football, baseball, basketball, athletics and swimming.

Anabolic steroids are used for purposes other than potential performance enhancement

Anabolic steroids are used by significant numbers of adolescents for the purpose of bodybuilding, with a view to improving appearance (Kindlundh *et al.*, 1999) which leads to social recognition (Laure, 1997a). Gymnasia were the most common source of androgenic anabolic steroids in South Africa (Lambert *et al.*, 1998), where bodybuilding takes place. However, peer pressure is a small but significant influence on anabolic steroid use (Tanner *et al.*, 1995).

Other drugs, in addition to anabolic steroids, are simultaneously misused

Many studies investigated concomitant use of other drugs with anabolic steroids. The most commonly reported drugs were those which could be categorized as social or recreational, including tobacco, alcohol, cannabis, cocaine, heroin and amphetamine. In the Melia *et al.* (1996) study, reference was made to other performance-enhancing drugs, where respondents reported using caffeine (27 per cent), alcohol (8.6 per cent), painkillers (9 per cent), stimulants (3.1 per cent), 'doping methods' (2.3 per cent) and beta

Table 12.20 Limitations to surveys conducted on drug misuse in sport by adolescents

The number of subjects involved is generally small
Subjects are mainly adolescents
Subjects are mainly non-athletes or non-competitive athletes
Most studies have been confined to North America
Too great an emphasis is placed on anabolic steroids with little information on other drugs
The socio-economic background of subjects is very variable
Underreporting on self-use is common

blockers (1 per cent) in attempts to improve performance. Kanayama *et al.* (2001) studied drug use in gymnasia and reported that, of individuals who used anabolic steroids, 83 per cent also took androstenedione and 78 per cent reported using ephedrine.

While providing some useful data, the scope of these surveys is subject to severe limitations, which must put into question the validity and usefulness of these data in trying to establish the true prevalence of drug misuse in sport. Some of these limitations are listed in Table 12.20.

In the majority of studies, the number of subjects involved is too small to warrant statistical evaluation of the data. Evaluation therefore becomes qualitative and liable to subjective interpretation. The profile of subjects used in these studies is too narrow and not representative enough to draw conclusions with regard to drug misuse in sport. Whilst students are an easy target for investigation, the motives for adolescents to participate in such studies may have a significant and detrimental influence on the outcome. Many students may participate in sport but few will have achieved significant rank in their chosen field. Extrapolation of results into conclusions about the extent of drug misuse in sport is flawed.

Too much emphasis has been placed on investigation into the use of anabolic steroids. It is tempting to assume that the reason for this is that anabolic steroids are the most widely misused of the banned drugs and therefore this group is most likely to throw up sufficient data to warrant embarking on such studies. Attempts have been made to include other drugs in surveys, but usually as an addendum to the principal drug, anabolic steroids.

Surveys into drug misuse in athletes

Data which are the most difficult to obtain concern the use of anabolic steroids in elite athletes. Evidence, such as that presented by Franke and Berendonk (1997), relating to the systematic approach to the misuse of drugs in sport by the government of the German Democratic Republic, is

Table 12.21 Surveys on drug misuse in sport by athletes

Author	Year	Country	Subjects
Scarpino *et al.*	1990	Italy	1015
Anshel	1991	USA	126
Laure and Reinsberger	1995	France	53
Spence and Gauvin	1996	Canada	754
Chester *et al.*	2003b	UK	112
La Torre *et al.*	2001	Italy	1056

rare. Part of their evidence reported that special emphasis was placed on administering androgens to women and adolescent girls, where, it was reported, performance enhancement was particularly effective. Elsewhere, it has been concluded that the level of anabolic steroid use in women has been significantly less than that in men (Yesalis *et al.*, 1989).

What is clearly needed are studies into the prevalence of self-use of all types of potential performance-enhancing drug by competitive athletes in various sports. The logistical, social and ethical problems associated with this approach are immense, hence the scarcity of such studies in the literature. A few of the studies which have been published appear in Table 12.21.

In the Scarpino *et al.* (1990) study, the subjects were male and female athletes from various sports, 71 per cent of whom competed at national level or higher. The prevalence of drug misuse was estimated by respondents as androgenic anabolic steroids (16 per cent), amphetamines (11 per cent), blood doping (7 per cent) and beta blockers (2 per cent).

Male and female athletes, representing nine sports, were surveyed in the Anshel (1991) study. Of these, 64 per cent of the respondents felt certain that at least one team-mate was using a drug for the purpose of performance enhancement. However, this figure does not indicate the level of misuse, since several respondents could have been referring to a single team-mate.

Laure and Reinsberger (1995) were interviewing high-level endurance walkers at a national competition. Respondents were predominantly male. Results indicated that 41 per cent of respondents had heard of other endurance walkers using ergogenic drugs.

University athletes, participating in intercollegiate athletics were the subjects in the Spence and Gauvin (1996) study. Painkillers (17.7 per cent), alcohol (94.1 per cent), androgenic anabolic steroids (0.9 per cent), amphetamines (0.7 per cent), marijuana (19.8 per cent) and cocaine (0.8 per cent) were the main drugs from the IOC list which were cited as being used by respondents.

The Chester *et al.* (2003b) study looked specifically at over-the-counter stimulants and surveyed regional, national and international track and field athletes. Results showed that 3.4 per cent of respondents declared that they had used OTC stimulants for the specific purpose of performance enhancement.

La Torre *et al.* (2001) conducted a study using amateur athletes from a number of sports. Doping was considered to be widespread at high-level sport (27.8 per cent of participants); 16.5 per cent of athletes declared using amino acids and/or creatine, while 28.6 per cent of respondents considered it acceptable to use drugs in order to improve performance.

As previously stated, published work on drug use by athletes is scarce. The few studies reported above indicate that results are highly variable. They are based on surveys with widely differing aims and protocols, in some cases seeking information on self-use, in others on predicted use by fellow athletes. Other variables included the type of sport undertaken by respondents and the specificity, or otherwise, of drugs under investigation.

12.4   A perspective on the prevalence of drug misuse in sport through medical practitioners

In this section of the chapter, the role and views of those who currently or who are likely to prescribe performance-enhancing drugs to athletes are considered.

In general, medical practitioners lack knowledge on the issue of drug misuse in sport (Greenway and Greenway, 1997). Consequently, some doctors may be prescribing banned substances to athletes unwittingly (Laure, 1997b). On the other hand, drugs may be prescribed in the full knowledge of the purpose for which they may be used (Laure, 1997b). Either way, this study reported that 61 per cent of performance-enhancing drug supplies for amateur athletes were obtained from medical practitioners.

Dawson (2001) observed that patients who should concern the physician most are not the high-profile, elite athletes but the youth and members of society who are being increasingly drawn to the use of performance-enhancing drugs.

A study by Gupta and Towler (1997) indicated that 53 per cent of medical practitioners had reported that they had seen at least one patient in the previous year who told them that they had used androgenic anabolic steroids for non-medical purposes. Of these practitioners, 6 per cent reported that they had seen more than 20 patients who mentioned steroid use. Moreover, a small minority of these doctors were prepared to prescribe anabolic steroids for bodybuilding purposes. Dawson (2001) has identified four general groups of patients that use performance-enhancing drugs. These are:

1.   Those who are seriously involved in sport and see the use of drugs as a tool to achieve their ultimate goal.
2.   Those who have recently become involved in sport or started to attend a gymnasium.

3. Occupational users who take drugs to overcome the feelings of being threatened at work.
4. The 'recreational user' using these drugs in an effort to enhance aspects of personal well-being.

Dean (2000) discusses the professional dilemma faced by medical practitioners with regard to treating athletes who are involved in drug misuse. It is unethical for a doctor to withhold treatment from a patient on the basis of a moral judgement that the patient's activities or lifestyle might have contributed to the condition for which treatment is sought. On the other hand, doctors who prescribe or collude in the provision of drugs or treatment with the intention of improperly enhancing performance in sport are equally acting unethically. As Dean (2000) surmises, when it comes to therapeutic treatment for athletes, involving banned drugs, practitioners are damned if they do and damned if they don't. This argument applies particularly in the case of those drugs required for the treatment of conditions such as asthma, which may account for the exceptionally high proportion of 'asthmatics' competing in the Sydney 2000 Olympic Games (see Table 12.14).

Likewise, drugs subject to certain restrictions, prescribed for sporting injuries, provide a difficult prescribing dilemma in the treatment of sports injuries. The issue is also raised with respect to providing harm minimization advice to known anabolic steroid users, as highlighted in the study by Gupta and Towler (1997) where 40 per cent of medical practitioners surveyed indicated a willingness to provide such advice. Dawson (2001) suggested that the policy of drug prohibition causes an increased pressure on the ethical dilemma of physicians. If advising patients on the use of performance-enhancing drugs, are physicians being complicit in their patient's drug use or simply upholding their oath to do their best to protect their patient's health?

Again, accurate data on the prevalence of drug misuse in sport are not forthcoming from evidence derived from medical practitioners. However, it does highlight an area of concern regarding the ready availability of drugs for performance enhancement through medical practitioners. There is certainly scope for improved education, for medical practitioners, on prohibited substances in sport (Greenway and Greenway, 1997).

12.5   General discussion

The number of tests conducted annually by the IOC/WADA laboratories has steadily increased over the years (Table 12.1). Despite this increase, the percentage of positive results has remained consistently low, at below 2 per cent. In fact, the percentage of positive results is lower than that published, since the published figures include the significant number of 'positive' results for β_2-agonists which were permitted.

Few people would regard the figures for positive test results as being an indication of the true prevalence of drug misuse in sport. These reasons are that:

- too few tests are conducted relative to the number of athletes competing in sport;
- a large proportion of the drugs do not need to be taken at the time of competing and out-of-competition testing is not universal; and
- athletes are becoming more adept at tailoring their drug use around times when they are least likely to be tested.

Effective though the IOC/WADA methods of detection are, too often there seems to be a reluctance on the part of the regulatory authorities to take a stringent approach on sanctioning elite athletes who test positive. This arises from a fear of litigation, particularly where a false-positive result may be in question. This has led the IOC/WADA to introduce cut-off levels for an increasing number of drugs, such as sympathomimetic cough and cold preparations, permitted β_2-agonists and the anabolic steroid, nandrolone. Although these cut-off levels are unlikely to confer any realistic advantage, their introduction must, inevitably, encourage athletes to take these substances up to the permitted maximum.

Another factor which leads one to believe that statistics are misleading with regard to prevalence is the increasing use of drugs which are naturally occurring in the body. It is extremely difficult to determine what is a 'normal' level of such substances in an 'average' athlete. Indeed, in the case of human growth hormone we do not yet have a validated test procedure available. There must, therefore, be innumerable instances of the use of these drugs which are going undetected.

The statistics from the IOC/WADA laboratories merely provide an international overview of the problem. More detailed analysis is required, particularly with regard to what is happening country by country, sport by sport and drug by drug. Few studies have been undertaken in individual countries. Where this has happened, details are sparse and inconsistent. More detailed analysis on the association between positive test results and individual sports can be obtained from limited sources. For example, UK Sport Antidoping Directorate produces an annual report containing such information (UK Sport, 2000). However, such data are not universally available and, again, report only on the few positive test results. Interesting as they are, statistics do not reflect the true prevalence of use of drugs in sport.

The same has to be said about published surveys. Unfortunately, the data obtained from surveys have, in the main, been based on inappropriate subjects and reveal little in the way of information on the prevalence of use of drugs in sport.

What is needed is good quality research on drug use by athletes at all levels of ability from junior to elite. Unfortunately, ethical constraints and the reluctance of athletes to divulge true and accurate information on the subject makes this an unachievable goal. We are therefore left in the position of mere speculation. This encourages the media to publish unsubstantiated conjecture and rumour. In turn, this fuels misconceptions and fears in the minds of competitors which encourages further drug use in sport.

12.6   References

Anshel, M.H. (1991) A survey of elite athletes on the perceived causes of using banned drugs in sport. *J. Sport Behav.*, **14**(4), 283–307.

Bahr, R and Tjornhom, M. (1998) Prevalence of doping in sports: doping control in Norway, 1977–1995. *Clin. J. Sports Med.*, **8**, 32–37.

Benzi, G. (1994) Pharmacoepidemiology of the drugs used in sports as doping agents. *Pharmacol. Res.*, **29**(1),13–26.

Catlin, D.H. and Hatton, C.K. (1991) Use and abuse of anabolic and other drugs for athletic enhancement. *Adv. Int. Med.*, **36**, 399–424.

Chester, N., Mottram, D.R., Reilly, T. and Powell, M. (2003a) Elimination of ephedrines in urine following multiple dosing: the consequences for athletes in relation to doping control. *Br. J. Clin. Pharmacol.*, **57**(1): 62–67.

Chester, N., Reilly, T. and Mottram, D.R. (2003b) Over-the-counter drug use amongst athletes and non-athletes. *J. Sports. Med. Phys. Fitness*, **43**, 111–118.

Dawson, R.T. (2001) Hormones and sport. Drugs in sport – the role of the physician. *J. Endocrinol.*, **170**, 55–61.

Dean, C. (2000) Performance enhancing drugs; damned if you do and damned if you don't. *Br. J. Sports Med.*, **34**, 154.

Delbeke, F.T. (1996) Doping in cyclism: Results of unannounced controls in Flanders (1987–1994). *Int. J. Sports Med.*, **17**(6), 434–438.

Du Rant, R.H., Escobedo, L.G. and Heath, G.W. (1995) Anabolic-steroid use, strength training and multiple drug use among adolescents in the United States. *Pediatrics*, **96**, 23–28.

Franke, W.W. and Berendonk, B. (1997) Hormonal doping and androgenization of athletes: a secret program of the German Democratic Republic government. *Clin. Chem.*, **43**(7),1262–1279.

Greenway, P. and Greenway, M. (1997) General practitioner knowledge of prohibited substances in sport. *Br. J. Sports Med.*, **31**,129–131.

Gupta, L. and Towler, B. (1997) General practitioners' views and knowledge about anabolic steroid use – survey of GPs in a high prevalence area. *Drug Alcohol Rev.*, **16**, 373–379.

Handelsman, D.J. and Gupta, L. (1997) Prevalence and risk factors for anabolic-androgenic steroid abuse in Australian high school students. *Int. J. Androl.*, **20**, 159–164.

Hoppeler, H.H., Matthias, M.F. and Melia, P.S. (1995) Doping and prevention of doping: International cooperation. *Clin. J. Sports Med.*, **5**, 79–81.

Kanayama, G., Gruber, A.J., Pope, H.G. *et al.* (2001) Over-the-counter drug use in gymnasiums: An under-recognised substance abuse problem? *Psychother. Psychosomat.*, **70**, 137–140.

Kindlundh, A.M.S., Isacson, D.G.L., Berglund, L. *et al.* (1999) Factors associated with adolescent use of doping agents: anabolic-androgenic steroids. *Addiction*, **94**(4), 543–553.

Lambert, M.I., Titlestad, S.D. and Schwellnus, M.P. (1998) Prevalence of androgenic-anabolic steroid use in adolescents in two regions of South Africa. *S. Afr. Med. J.*, **88**(7), 876–880.

Lasne, F. and de Ceaurriz, J. (2000) Recombinant erythropoietin in urine. *Nature*, **405**, 635.

La Torre, G., Limongelli, F., Masala, D. *et al.* (2001) Knowledge, attitudes and behaviour towards doping and food supplementation in a sample of athletes of central-southern Italy. *Med. Sport*, **54**(3), 229–233.

Laure, P. (1997a) Epidemiological approach of doping in sport. *J. Sports Med. Phys. Fitness*, **37**, 218–224.

Laure, P. (1997b) Doping in sport: doctors are providing drugs. *Br. J. Sports Med.*, **31**, 258–259.

Laure, P. and Reinsberger, H. (1995) Doping and high level endurance walkers. Knowledge and representation of a prohibited practice. *J. Sports Med. Phys. Fitness*, **35**, 228–231.

Melia, P., Pipe, A. and Greenberg, L. (1996) The use of anabolic-androgenic steroids by Canadian students. *Clin. J. Sports Med.*, **6**, 9–14.

Mottram, D.R. (1999) Banned drugs in sport: Does the International Olympic Committee (IOC) list need updating? *Sports Med.*, **27**(1), 1–10.

Mottram, D.R., Reilly, T. and Chester, N. (1997) Doping in sport: the extent of the problem. In: T. Reilly and M. Orme (eds) *Esteve Foundation Symposium. Vol. 7. The Clinical Pharmacology of Sport and Exercise.* Amsterdam: Excerpta Medica, pp. 3–12.

Nilsson, S. (1995) Androgenic anabolic steroid use among male adolescents in Falkenberg. *Eur. J. Clin. Pharmacol.*, **48**, 9–11.

Parisotto, R., Wu, M., Ashenden, M.J. *et al.* (2001) Detection of recombinant human erythropoietin abuse in athletes utilizing markers of altered erythropoiesis. *Haematologica*, **86**(2), 128–137.

Scarpino, V., Arrigo, A., Benzi, G. *et al.* (1990) Evaluation of prevalence of 'doping' among Italian athletes. *Lancet*, **336**, 1048–1050.

Spence, J.C. and Gauvin, L. (1996) Drug and alcohol use by Canadian university athletes: a national survey. *J. Drug Educ.*, **26**(3), 275–287.

Tanner, S.M., Miller, D.W. and Alongi, C. (1995) Anabolic steroid use by adolescents: prevalence, motives and knowledge of risks. *Clin. J. Sports Med.*, **5**, 108–115.

Ueki, M., Hiruma, T., Ikekita, A. and Okano, M. (1998) Trends in drug abuse in competitive sports, and the international anti-doping movement. *J. Toxicol. Toxin Rev.*, **17**(1), 73–83.

UK Sport (2000) *Anti-doping programme annual report 1999–2000.* UK Sport, London.

Van der Merwe, P.J. and Kruger, H.S.L. (1992) Drugs in sport – results of the past 6 years of dope testing in South Africa. *S. Afr. Med. J.*, **82**, 151–153.

Yang, Y.T. and McElliott, M.A. (1989) Multiple actions of β adrenergic agonists on skeletal muscle and adipose tissue. *Biochem. J.*, **261**, 1–10.

Yesalis, C.E. and Bahrke, M.S. (2000) Doping among adolescent athletes. In: *Clin. Endocrinol. and Metab. Doping in Sport*. London: Ballière's Best Practice and Research, 25–35.

Yesalis, C.E., Wright, J.E. and Lombardo, J.A. (1989) Anabolic-androgenic steroids: a synthesis of existing data and recommendations for future research. *Clin. Sports Med.*, **1**, 109–134.

Synopsis of drugs used in sport

David R. Mottram

Section 1 of this synopsis provides an overview of each of the major classes of drugs and methods banned by WADA and is presented under the headings:

- WADA category
- Use in sport
- Pharmacological action
- Adverse effects

Section 2 of this synopsis presents information on therapeutic drugs used in the management of common illnesses which athletes may experience. The adverse effects of these drugs and the implications for their use in sport are described.

Section I. WADA prohibited drugs and methods

Alcohol

WADA category

III. Substances prohibited in particular sports. A. Alcohol

Use in sport

Alcohol (ethanol) may be used, potentially, as a performance-enhancing drug due to its anti-anxiety effect. In some team sports, where alcohol is part of a social convention, peer pressure may lead to an overindulgence with consequences for the partaker and for fellow competitors.

Pharmacological action

Alcohol affects neural transmission in the CNS by altering the permeability of axonal membranes and thereby slowing nerve conductance. Alcohol also decreases glucose utilization in the brain. Overall, alcohol impairs concentration, reduces anxiety and induces depression and sedation.

Adverse effects

The adverse effects of alcohol have been extensively documented over many centuries.

Amphetamines

WADA category

II. Substances and methods prohibited in competition. S6. Stimulants

Use in sport

Amphetamines are used, during competition, to reduce fatigue and to increase reaction time, alertness, competitiveness and aggression. Amphetamines may be used out of competition to intensify training.

Amphetamines and derivatives such as ecstasy are recreational drugs, therefore, competitors may test positive for amphetamines having not intended to use them for performance enhancement.

Pharmacological action

There are four mechanisms: (i) by releasing neurotransmitters, such as noradrenaline, dopamine and serotonin, from their respective nerve terminals; (ii) inhibition of neurotransmitter uptake; (iii) direct action on neurotransmitter receptors; and (iv) inhibition of monoamine oxidase activity. Of these, neurotransmitter release is the most important.

Adverse effects

The adverse effects of amphetamines include restlessness, irritability, tremor and insomnia with an increase in aggressive behaviour and the potential for addiction. At higher doses, amphetamines may produce sweating, tachycardia, pupillary dilation, increased blood pressure and heat stroke. Effects on the heart may lead to arrhythmias, of which ventricular arrhythmia is potentially fatal.

Anabolic androgenic steroids

WADA category

I. Substances and methods prohibited at all times (in- and out-of-competition). C. Anabolic Agents 1. Anabolic Androgenic Steroids

Use in sport

Anabolic androgenic steroids (AASs) are used to improve strength by increasing lean body mass, decreasing body fat, prolonging training by enhancing recovery time and increasing aggressiveness.

Pharmacological action

AASs have two major effects: (i) an androgenic or mascularizing action and (ii) an anabolic or tissue building effect. They may be taken orally or by deep intramuscular injection. Injectable preparations may be water- or oil-based. In general, oil-based preparations have a longer biological half-life.

AASs produce their effect through an action on endogenous androgen receptors. They increase protein synthesis and possibly have an anticatabolic effect by antagonizing the effect of glucocorticoid hormones such as cortisol, released during intense exercise.

Adverse effects

Acne and water retention are common, reversible side-effects. Prolonged use may lead to male-pattern baldness. Cardiovascular side-effects associated with AAS use include hypertension and alteration of cholesterol levels.

The liver is a target tissue for androgens and it is the principal site for steroid metabolism, especially after oral administration. A number of effects on the liver have been described, including hepatocyte hypertrophy and, at high doses, cholestasis and peliosis hepatis. Androgens also increase the risk of liver tumours. Psychological effects with AASs, such as mania, hypomania and depression, have been reported.

In females, the extent of AAS use is less well known. The risks of steroid misuse in women are greater than in men, with some side-effects irreversible. Females prefer oral steroids, which are shorter acting than the oil-based injectable steroids, such as testosterone, which are more likely to produce side-effects such as acne, unwanted facial hair, cliteromegaly and a change in the shape of the face, with squaring of the jaw line.

In males, AAS misuse is commonly associated with testicular atrophy and reduced sperm production. Gynaecomastia is a common side-effect among male body builders and may be associated with steroid misuse.

β_2-Agonists

WADA category

I. Substances and methods prohibited at all times (in- and out-of-competition). S3. β_2-agonists and S1 Anabolic Agents 2. Other Anabolic Agents

All β_2-agonists are prohibited but athletes may apply for a Therapeutic Use Exemption (TUE). An Abbreviated TUE may be applied for in the case of salbutamol, formoterol, terbutaline or salmeterol use, by inhalation, to prevent and/or treat asthma or exercise-induced asthma.

Other drugs used in the treatment of asthma, including corticosteroids (subject to restriction, see below), anticholinergics, methyl xanthines and cromoglycate, are permitted in sport.

Use in sport

All β_2-agonists are potent bronchodilators and may, therefore, improve performance in aerobic exercise.

β_2-Agonists, particularly clenbuterol, possess anabolic activity and are used as an alternative or in addition to anabolic steroids.

For salbutamol, a positive test result under the anabolic agent category is determined by a concentration in urine greater than 1000 ng/ml and under the stimulant category, greater than 100 ng/ml.

Pharmacological action

Bronchodilation is mediated through stimulation of the β_2-adrenoreceptors in the smooth muscle of the respiratory tract.

β_2-Adrenoreceptors are also found in skeletal muscle, stimulation of which induces muscle growth. β_2-Agonists are also capable of reducing subcutaneous and total body fat.

Adverse effects

At the higher doses likely to be experienced by misusers in sport, these drugs lose their selectivity, leading to stimulation of β_1-adrenoreceptors. This, commonly, produces fine tremor, usually of the hands and may produce tachycardia, arrhythmias, nausea, insomnia and headache.

When clenbuterol is used in doses producing anabolic effects, additional side effects such as generalized myalgia, asthenia, periorbital pain, dizzy spells, nausea, vomiting and fever have been reported.

Beta blockers

WADA category

III. Substances prohibited in particular sports. P2. Beta blockers

Use in sport

Beta blockers have a use in sport where motor skills can be affected by muscle tremor, caused by anxiety. Beta blockers are therefore prohibited in certain sports, such as archery and other shooting events and in high-risk sports, such as ski jumping, bobsleigh and luge.

Pharmacological action

Beta blockers are first-line drugs in the management of angina pectoris, hypertension, some cardiac arrhythmias, hyperthyroidism and glaucoma and are used occasionally for migraine and essential tremor.

Adverse effects

The adverse effects of beta blockers vary according to the properties of the individual drug. Beta blockers may produce bronchoconstriction, fatigue, cold extremities, sleep disturbances and nightmares.

Caffeine

WADA category

Caffeine was removed from the prohibited list by WADA in January 2004. However, WADA continues to monitor for its misuse in sport.

Use in sport

Caffeine may be used, primarily, for its central stimulant effect, to improve alertness, reaction time and attention span. In addition, caffeine may increase the mobilization and utilization of fatty acids, leading to a sparing of muscle glycogen.

Pharmacological action

Caffeine inhibits the phosphodiesterase group of enzymes, which activate second messengers such as cyclic AMP. They act as one of the links between receptor activation and cellular responses. Caffeine also directly antagonizes adenosine receptors.

Adverse effects

Mild side-effects associated with caffeine include irritability, insomnia and gastrointestinal disturbances. More severe effects include peptic ulceration, delirious seizures, coma and superventricular and ventricular arrhythmias.

Cannabinoids

WADA category

II. Substances and methods prohibited in-competition. S8. Cannabinoids

Passive smoking of cannabinoids has been cited as the reason for a positive test result on a number of occasions.

Use in sport

Cannabinoid effects are incompatible with most sports, therefore tests are only conducted in certain sports.

Pharmacological action

The active constituent of marijuana is 1-5-9-tetrahydrocannabinol (THC). When smoked, 60–65 per cent is absorbed and effects are noted within 15 minutes and last for 3 hours or so. It produces a sedating and euphoric feeling of well-being.

Adverse effects

The central depressant effects of THC decrease the motivation for physical effort and motor co-ordination, short-term memory and perception are impaired. In addition to its psychological effects, THC induces tachycardia, bronchodilation and an increased blood flow to the limbs.

Cocaine

WADA category

I. Substances and methods prohibited at all times (in- and out-of-competition). S6. Stimulants

Other local anaesthetics are permitted in sport.

Use in sport

Studies on the ergogenic effects of cocaine are inconclusive. Cocaine is a 'recreational' drug and many instances of positive doping results have arisen from residual levels remaining in the body after recreational use, rather than an attempt by the athlete to enhance performance. Cocaine is notable for distorting the user's perception of reality, therefore the athlete may perceive enhanced performance where, in reality, a decrease in endurance and strength, due to the drug, exists.

Pharmacological action

The pharmacological effects of cocaine on the brain are complex and include inhibition of the uptake of various central neurotransmitters, particularly dopamine.

Adverse effects

The complex pharmacology of cocaine leads to a wide spectrum of adverse effects, including a negative effect on glycogenolysis, paranoid psychosis, seizures, hypertension and myocardial toxicity, which could lead to ischaemia, arrhythmias and sudden death, especially following intense exercise. Smoked 'crack' cocaine is more dangerous as the rate of absorption is greater, leading to a more intense effect on the cardiovascular system.

Diuretics

WADA category

I. Substances and methods prohibited at all times (in- and out-of-competition). S5. Diuretics and other Masking Agents

Use in sport

Diuretics do not have performance-enhancing effects but have been used to increase urine production in an attempt to dilute other doping agents and/or their metabolites. Diuretics are also used to reduce weight in sports where weight classification applies. In this context they are subject to testing at the time of the weigh-in.

Diuretics are used by body builders to counteract the fluid retentive effects of androgenic anabolic steroids.

Pharmacological action

Diuretics variably exert their pharmacological effect on the kidney, to produce an increased loss of fluid. All pharmacological classes of diuretics are banned by WADA.

Adverse effects

The primary adverse effect results from induced hypohydration, although concomitant electrolyte disturbances compromise the heart and muscles. These effects are exacerbated where hyperthermia and dehydration accompany fatigue and glycogen depletion.

Ephedrine and other sympathomimetics available in over-the-counter (OTC) medicines

This group includes drugs such as ephedrine, methylephedrine and l-methylamphetamine.

WADA category

I. Substances and methods prohibited in-competition. S6. Stimulants

WADA regulations define a positive result for these substances if they appear in the urine at concentrations above 5 or 10 µg/ml, depending on the drug. Competitors should be aware of the fact that even using the manufacturers' recommended doses may result in exceeding permitted levels.

Other drugs which are found, commonly, in OTC medicines, such as antihistamines (e.g. triprolidine, astemizole), analgesics (e.g. paracetamol), imidazole decongestants (e.g. xylometazoline), cough suppressants (e.g. pholcodine) and expectorants (e.g. ipecacuanha) are permitted by WADA.

Use in sport

They produce central stimulant effects.

Pharmacological action

These drugs produce decongestion by decreasing mucus secretion. They are structurally related to amphetamine and therefore produce a similar, though weaker, effect as central stimulants.

Adverse effects

OTC sympathomimetics variably produce side-effects such as headache, tachycardia, dizziness, hypertension, irritability and anxiety.

Erythropoietin

WADA category

I. Substances and methods prohibited at all times (in- and out-of-competition). S2. Hormones and related substances. 1. Erythropoietin

Use in sport

The increase in production of erythrocytes by erythropoietin (EPO) improves the oxygen-carrying capacity of the blood. This effect is particularly useful in endurance sports. Misuse normally involves synthetic, recombinant EPO.

Pharmacological action

EPO is a glycoprotein hormone, produced primarily in the kidney. The stimulus for its production is reduced oxygen delivery to the kidney. Its effect is to increase the number of erythrocytes that are produced from the bone marrow and to increase the rate at which they are released into the circulation.

Adverse effects

EPO can, initially, produce flu-like symptoms, such as headaches and joint pain, but these usually resolve spontaneously, even with continued use. Up to 35 per cent of patients on EPO develop hypertension and the risk of thrombosis is increased.

In sport, the misuse of EPO poses a significant potential risk to health since the raised haematocrit increases blood viscosity, which may be further exacerbated through dehydration.

Glucocorticosteroids

WADA category

II. Substances and methods prohibited in-competition, S9. Glucocorticosteroids

Glucocorticosteroids are permitted if the route of administration is dermatological. For oral, rectal, intravenous and intramuscular routes of administration a TUE is required. For all other routes an Abbreviated TUE is required.

Use in sport

Glucocorticosteroids are important in the management of sports injuries, due to their potent anti-inflammatory properties.

Pharmacological action

These drugs are related to the adrenocorticosteroid hormone released from the adrenal cortex. They have a widespread effect on the body including glucocorticoid effects on carbohydrate, protein and fat metabolism and on electrolyte and water balance, as well as their anti-inflammatory effect. As anti-inflammatory agents they reduce the swelling, tenderness and heat associated with injury.

Adverse effects

Local damage may be produced at the site of injection due to dosage volume and subcutaneous atrophy, with associated depigmentation. Corticosteroids produce a catabolic effect on skeletal muscle, leading to muscle weakness soon after treatment has begun, even with modest doses.

Human growth hormone and insulin-like growth factor

WADA category

I. Substances and methods prohibited at all times (in- and out-of-competition). S2. Hormones and related substances. 2. Growth Hormone, Insulin-like Growth Factor, Mechano Growth Factor

Use in sport

Human growth hormone (hGH) is used to increase muscle mass, allow users to train harder, longer and more frequently and to promote faster recovery after training.

Pharmacological action

Human GH is a polypeptide hormone produced by the pituitary gland, to maintain normal growth from birth to adulthood. It has a short (about

20 minutes) half-life, during which time it activates hepatic GH receptors, mediating the production of insulin-like growth factor 1 (IGF-1). It is IGF-1 which is responsible for most of the anabolic action of hGH.

Adverse effects

Overuse of hGH in children can lead to 'gigantism', in adults it can lead to 'acromegaly'. Features of acromegaly include skeletal deformities, arthritis and enlargement of organs such as the heart, lungs, liver, intestines and spleen. Hypertension, diabetes mellitus, peripheral neuropathy and muscle weakness, despite an increase in size, may develop. Increased protein synthesis also produces thickening and coarsening of the skin. Association between the use of hGH and leukaemia has been reported.

Before 1986, hGH was freeze extracted from the pituitaries of human cadavers. This has led to the risk that recipients may contract Creutzfeldt–Jakob disease (CJD), secondary to viral contaminants. Since there is an average 15-year incubation interval, exposed athletes may not yet have undergone the requisite incubation period. Where athletes use IGF-1, adverse effects are the same as for hGH. IGF-1 commonly produces hypoglycaemia, as it promotes the uptake of glucose into cells.

The use of hGH has become more popular among female athletes, since there is no risk of developing the androgenic side-effects associated with AASs.

Local anaesthetics

WADA category

Local anaesthetics were removed from the list in January 2004.

Use in sport

Local anaesthetics may be used to treat minor sporting injuries.

Pharmacological action

Local anaesthetics act by causing a reversible block to conduction along nerve fibres.

Adverse effects

Little information has been published on the adverse effects of local anaesthetics in sport.

Narcotics

WADA category

II. Substances and methods prohibited in-competition. S7. Narcotics

Some less potent narcotics, such as codeine, dihydrocodeine, dextropropoxyphene and dextromethorphan, are permitted by WADA.

Use in sport

Potent narcotic analgesics are misused in sport for their pain-relieving properties.

Pharmacological action

Alkaloids from the opium poppy and their synthetic analogues interact with the receptors in the brain which are normally acted upon by the endogenous endorphin transmitters. They have the capacity to moderate pain but also affect emotions. Frequent use may induce tolerance and dependency, the extent of which is variable depending on the narcotic used.

Adverse effects

In high doses, narcotic analgesics can cause stupor and coma, with the possibility of death due to respiratory depression. Where dependency has occurred, withdrawal symptoms include craving, anxiety, sweating, insomnia, nausea and vomiting, muscle aches and potential cardiovascular collapse.

Other peptide hormones

This category includes human chorionic gonadotrophin (hCG), luteinizing hormone (LH), adrenocorticotrophic hormone (ACTH) and insulin.

WADA category

I. Substances and methods prohibited at all times (in- and out-of-competition). S2. Hormones and related substances

Use in sport

These peptide hormones are used to potentiate the endogenous levels of other hormones with ergogenic or other performance-enhancing properties.

Pharmacological action

Endogenous levels of testosterone may be increased by the use of hCG and LH. ACTH increases adrenal corticosteroid release.

Adverse effects

There is little published research on the effects of these hormones in athletes. Side-effects to hCG include oedema (particularly in males), headache, tiredness, mood changes and gynaecomastia. The production of hCG from pregnant women's urine may lead to viral contamination. Adverse effects to ACTH are related to released glucocorticoid (see below).

Prohibited methods

WADA category

I. Substances and methods prohibited at all times (in- and out-of-competition)

This category comprises M1. Enhancement of oxygen transfer. M2. Chemical and physical manipulation. M3. Gene doping

Use in sport

Blood doping increases the oxygen-carrying capacity of the blood. Manipulation includes the use of drugs (e.g. probenecid, epitestosterone) to mask the use of other doping agents or the use of physical means (e.g. urine substitution) to avoid detection.

Pharmacological action

Probenecid may delay the excretion of other doping agents, such as anabolic steroids. Epitestosterone is used to maintain the ratio of testosterone: epitestosterone in the urine within WADA accepted limits.

Adverse effects

Blood doping may lead to adverse effects associated with hyperviscocity of the blood, as discussed under EPO. Otherwise, autologous blood doping carries no more risk than any other procedure involving invasive techniques. However, risks due to cross-infection and non-matched blood may occur where non-autologous infusion is carried out.

Section 2.   Therapeutic drugs in the management of illness

In this section, consideration is given to the use of therapeutic drugs in the management of illnesses that athletes may experience and for which they may self-medicate or seek medical advice from a general practitioner, pharmacist or other health professional.

Non-steroidal anti-inflammatory drugs (NSAIDs)

Use in sport

NSAIDs, such as aspirin and indomethacin, are widely used as analgesic and anti-inflammatory drugs for the treatment of sports injuries.

Pharmacological action

The analgesic, anti-inflammatory and antipyretic activity of NSAIDs is based on their ability to inhibit prostaglandin synthesis.

Adverse effects

The most common adverse effects associated with NSAIDs are gastrointestinal, including nausea, dyspepsia and ulcers.

Topical administration of NSAIDs may offer an effective and possibly safer alternative route of administration.

Muscle relaxants

Use in sport

There are a number of drugs, such as benzodiazepines and dantrolene sodium, which have muscle relaxant effects. They are not generally recommended for the treatment of athletic injury.

Benzodiazepines and other anxiolytics

Use in sport

A number of classes of drugs have been used as anxiolytics, including alcohol, beta blockers and benzodiazepines. The first two classes have been described above, as they are restricted in certain sports.

Pharmacological action

Benzodiazepines variously reduce the activity of a number of central neurotransmitters, such as acetylcholine, serotonin and noradrenaline. The anti-anxiety effect is primarily through release of gamma-aminobutyric acid, which inhibits the release of serotonin.

Adverse effects

Benzodiazepines are relatively free of adverse effects. However, they are liable to produce dependency if used for extended periods. Benzodiazepines may also be used by athletes for insomnia. Under these circumstances, athletes need to be aware of the 'hangover' effect of these drugs.

Cough and cold preparations

Use in sport

The use of medication for these self-limiting conditions is questionable. The only potential use for drugs is for the control of symptoms such as headache, fever, runny nose and cough. However, some of the drugs found in OTC cough and cold remedies are banned by WADA, although there are cut-off concentrations in the urine for these drugs.

Pharmacological action

Apart from the sympathomimetic decongestants discussed previously, cough and cold medicines may contain analgesics (paracetamol, codeine), antihistamines (e.g. triprolidine, astemizole), imidazole decongestants (e.g. xylometazoline) cough suppressants (e.g. pholcodine) and expectorants (e.g. ipecacuanha), all of which are permitted by WADA.

Adverse effects

In general, cough and cold preparations are taken for short periods of time and therefore side-effects are limited. However, nasal decongestants are liable to produce rebound congestion if used for more than 1 week. Sedating antihistamines may have adverse effects on performance in most sports.

Antidiarrhoeals

Use in sport

First-line treatment for diarrhoea is oral rehydration therapy (ORT). Antimotility drugs may be used for short-term symptomatic relief of acute diarrhoea if it is likely to affect performance.

Pharmacological action

ORT enhances the absorption of water and replaces electrolytes. Antimotility drugs (codeine, diphenoxylate, loperamide) are opioids with a direct relaxant effect on the smooth muscle of the gastrointestinal tract.

Adverse effects

Tolerance and dependence may develop with prolonged use of antimotility drugs. Loperamide may produce abdominal cramps, drowsiness and skin reactions.

Nutritional supplements

Use in sport

In an attempt to enhance performance through ergogenic aids, without contravening WADA regulations, many athletes have used nutritional supplements.

The manufacture and sale of nutritional supplements is not as closely regulated as that for drugs. Nutritional supplements may therefore contain banned substances or their precursors, which produce the same metabolites as banned substances in the urine. The use of nutritional supplements may therefore lead to a positive dope test result.

Pharmacological action

Manufacturers may make exaggerated claims regarding the ergogenic properties of their products. There is little, if any, evidence that nutritional supplements possess ergogenic properties in athletes consuming a balanced diet.

Adverse effects

Some nutritional supplements have the potential for harm. Creatine has been the subject of many studies, but results are equivocal as to whether it produces ergogenic effects. There are few reliable scientific data on possible adverse effects of creatine, but its potential effect on renal dysfunction and electrolyte imbalance, leading to a predisposition to dehydration and heat-related illness, suggests caution in its use.

Glossary

Absorption The process through which a drug passes from its site of administration into the blood.

Addison's disease A disorder caused by degeneration of the adrenal cortex resulting in impairment of sodium reabsorption from the urine.

Adrenal glands The two glands which comprise an outer cortex that produces the mineralocorticoid and glucocorticoid hormones and the inner medulla that produces the hormone adrenaline.

Adrenaline A hormone released from the adrenal medulla under conditions of stress; sometimes referred to as epinephrine.

Adrenoceptors Receptors (subclassified alpha and beta) through which adrenaline, noradrenaline and sympathomimetic drugs exert their effects.

Agonist A drug that interacts with receptors to produce a response in a tissue or organ.

Agranulocytosis The destruction of granulocytes (blood cells) often induced by drugs. The condition responds to treatment by corticosteroids.

Allergy A hypersensitivity reaction in which antibodies are produced in response to food, drugs or environmental antigens (allergens) to which they have previously been exposed.

Anabolic steroid A hormone or drug which produces retention of nitrogen, potassium and phosphate, increases protein synthesis and decreases amino acid breakdown.

Anaerobic metabolism Biochemical reactions which occur when oxygen supply to cells is lacking.

Analgesic drug   A drug which can relieve pain. Generally they are subclassified as narcotic analgesics, e.g. morphine or non-narcotic analgesics, e.g. aspirin.

Anaphylaxis   An immediate hypersensitivity reaction, following administration of a drug or other agent, in an individual who has previously been exposed to the drug and who has produced antibodies to that drug. It is characterized by increased vascular permeability and bronchoconstriction.

Androgen   A steroidal drug which promotes the development of male secondary sexual characteristics.

Anorectic agent   A drug which suppresses appetite through an action in the central nervous system.

Antagonist drug   A drug that occupies receptors without producing a response but prevents the action of an endogenous substance or an agonist drug.

Antihistamine drug   An antagonist drug which stops the action of histamine and therefore is used in the treatment of hay fever.

Antihypertensive drug   A drug which lowers abnormally high blood pressure.

Anti-inflammatory drug   A drug that reduces the symptoms of inflammation and includes glucocorticosteroids and non-steroidal anti-inflammatory drugs, such as aspirin.

Antipyretic drug   A drug which can reduce an elevated body temperature.

Antitussive drug   A drug which suppresses coughing either by a local soothing effect or by depressing the cough centre in the CNS.

Atherosclerosis   The accumulation of lipid deposits such as cholesterol and triacylglycerol on the walls of arteries. These fatty plaques can lead to a narrowing of arteries and therefore ischaemia or can encourage the formation of a thrombus (blood clot).

Atopy   The acquisition of sensitivity to various environmental substances, such as pollen and house dust, thereby rendering the individual allergic to those substances.

Atrophy   A wasting away or decrease in size of a mature tissue.

Axon   A projection of nerve cell bodies which conduct impulses to the target tissue.

Beta blocker An antagonist of the beta group of adrenoceptors with a wide variety of clinical uses, principally in treating angina and hypertension.

Blind or double-blind trial A method for testing the effectiveness of a drug on a group of subjects where the subjects alone (blind) or the subjects and evaluators (double-blind) are prevented from knowing whether the active drug or a placebo has been administered.

Blood–brain barrier The cells of the capillaries in the brain which impede the access of certain substances in the blood from reaching the brain.

Bronchodilator drug A drug which relaxes the smooth muscle in the respiratory tract thereby dilating the airways. Many bronchodilators are agonist on β_2-adrenoceptors.

Capillaries Blood vessels whose walls are a single layer of cells thick, through which water and solutes exchange between the blood and the tissue fluid.

Cardiac output The volume of blood per minute ejected from the left ventricle of the heart.

Cardiac rate The number of times the heart beats each minute. The normal resting heart rate is around 60 beats per minute.

Cardioselective beta blockers Antagonist of beta-adrenoceptors which have a selective action on the β_1-adrenoceptors, a major site of which is the cardiac muscle in the heart.

Cerebrovascular accident An alternative term for a stroke. This occurs when an area of the brain is deprived of oxygen either through a rupture or spasm of an artery.

Chemotaxis Chemical-mediated attraction of leucocytes to a site of injury.

Cholinergic neurones Nerve fibres that release acetylcholine from their nerve terminals.

Claudication Pain caused by temporary constriction of blood vessels supplying the skeletal muscle.

Coronary heart disease Malfunction of the heart caused by occlusion of the artery supplying the heart muscle.

Coronary occlusion   Obstruction of the arteries supplying heart muscle either through vasoconstriction or a mechanical obstruction such as an atheromatous plaque or blood clot.

Cumulation   The process by which the blood levels of a drug build up, thereby increasing its therapeutic and toxic effects.

Diabetes mellitus   A disorder of carbohydrate metabolism, characterized by an increased blood sugar level, caused by decreased insulin activity.

Diuresis   Increased output of urine which may be induced by disease or the action of drugs.

Dose regime   The amount of drug taken, expressed in terms of the quantity of drug and the frequency at which it is taken.

Drug allergy   A reaction to a drug which involves the production of antibodies when first exposed to the drug.

Drug dependence   A compulsion to take a drug on a continuous basis both to experience its psychic effects and to avoid the adverse physical effects experienced when the drug is withdrawn.

Drug idiosyncrasy   A genetically determined abnormal reactivity to a drug.

Drug metabolism   The chemical alteration of drug molecules by the body to aid in the detoxification and excretion of the drug.

Electroencephalogram (EEG)   A recording of the electrical potential changes occurring in the brain.

Electromyography   The measurement of muscular contraction using needle electrodes inserted into the muscle.

Endogenous biochemical   A chemical substance such as a hormone or neurotransmitter which is found naturally in the body.

Epileptogenic effect   An effect likely to lead to the symptoms of epilepsy.

Epinephrine   *see* Adrenaline.

Epiphyses   The articular end structures of long bones.

Erythropoiesis   The process by which bone marrow produces new red blood cells.

European Antidoping Charter for Sport Recommendations adopted by the Committee of Ministers of the Council of Europe in 1984 for the control of drugs in sport.

Generic name The official name of the active drug within a medicine. Different manufacturers of a drug may use their own proprietary or brand name to describe the drug.

Glomeruli The units within the kidney where filtration of the blood takes place.

Glucocorticosteroids Steroid hormones and drugs which affect carbohydrate metabolism more than electrolyte and water balance (cf. mineralocorticoids). They can be used as anti-inflammatory drugs.

Glycogenolysis The breakdown of the storage material, glycogen, into the energy source glucose. Glycogenolysis is a major function of adrenaline.

Hepatic circulation The arteries, capillaries and veins carrying blood to and from the liver.

Hormones Endogenous biochemical messengers that are released from endocrine glands directly into the bloodstream. They interact with specific receptors on their target tissues.

Hyperpnoea An increase in the rate and depth of respiration.

Hyperpyrexia Increase in body temperature.

Hypertrophy An increase in tissue size due to an increase in the size of functional cells without an increase in the number of cells.

Hypokalaemia A condition in which there is a profound lowering of potassium levels in the extracellular fluid.

Iatrogenic disease Originally the term for physician-caused disease. Now it applies to side-effects of drugs caused by inappropriate prescribing or administration of drugs.

Interstitial fluid The water and solute contents of the fluid found between cells of tissues.

Intracellular fluid The water and solute contents of the fluid found within cells.

Ischaemic pain   Pain within a tissue induced by reduced blood flow to that tissue.

Isometric contraction   Contraction of skeletal (striated) muscle in which the muscle develops tension but does not alter in length.

Isotonic contraction   Contraction of skeletal muscle in which the muscle shortens under a constant load, such as occurs during walking, running or lifting.

Kinins   Endogenous polypeptides (e.g. kallidin, bradyknin, angiotensin and substance P) which have a marked pharmacological effect on smooth muscle.

Leucocytes   White blood cells, comprising several different types with differing functions.

Ligand   An atom or molecule (including drugs) that interacts with a larger molecule, at a specific (receptor) site.

Lipolysis   The breakdown of fats into free fatty acid.

Mast cells   Large cells containing histamine and other substances which are released during allergic responses.

Medicine   A preparation containing one or more drugs designed for use as a therapeutic agent.

Metabolite   The chemical produced by the metabolic transformation of a drug or other substance.

Mineralocorticoid   A steroid hormone which has a selective action on electrolyte and water balance.

Monoamine oxidase   A major metabolizing enzyme responsible for the breakdown of monoamines such as adrenaline and noradrenaline.

Mydriasis   Contraction of the iris in the eye leading to an increased pupil size.

Myocardium   The cardiac muscle which makes up the walls of the heart.

Narcolepsy   A disorder characterized by periodic attacks of an overwhelming desire to sleep.

Narcotic analgesic   A drug that induces a state of reversible depression of the CNS (narcosis) as well as producing pain relief (analgesia). Most narcotic analgesics are related to morphine.

Nasal decongestant   A drug (usually a sympathomimetic) which reduces the mucous secretion in the nasal passages normally by vasoconstriction in the nasal mucosa.

Nebulizer therapy   A method of drug administration in which the drug dissolved in a solution is vaporized and the vapour inhaled. This method is primarily used for bronchodilator drugs.

Necrosis   Tissue death.

Neurotransmitter   A biochemical agent released from nerve endings to transmit a response to another cell.

Non-steroidal anti-inflammatory drug   A drug, such as aspirin or indomethacin, the structure of which is not based on a steroid nucleus and which is able to control the inflammatory response within tissues.

Noradrenaline   The neurotransmitter in certain sympathetic and central nerves. Sometimes referred to an norepinephrine.

Oedema   Tissue swelling due to accumulation of fluid in the interstitial spaces.

Osteoporosis   A condition in which bone tissue becomes demineralized.

Over-the-counter medicines   Drugs which can be purchased directly from a pharmacy or drug store without a medical practitioner's prescription.

Paranoia   A mental disorder characterized by persistent delusions, particularly of persecution or power.

Pepsin   A digestive enzyme, secreted in the stomach, that hydrolyses proteins into smaller peptide fractions.

Phagocytosis   The ingestion of bacteria or other foreign particles by cells, usually a type of white blood cell.

Pharmacokinetics   A study of absorption, distribution and excretion of drugs using mathematical parameters to measure time courses.

Pharmacology   The study of the modes of action, uses and side-effects of drugs.

Placebo   A substance which is pharmacologically inactive and which is usually used to compare the effects with an active drug in blind or double-blind trials.

Plasma proteins   Proteins (albumin and globulins) which circulate in the plasma of the blood. Many drugs are capable of binding to these proteins, thereby reducing their availability as therapeutic agents.

Prepubertical male   A male who has not yet reached the age at which he is capable of adult sexual function.

Prescription-only medicine   A therapeutic agent which can only be obtained on the written authority (prescription) of a medical or dental practitioner.

Prostaglandins   A group of chemical agents found in the body and which have a wide variety of actions, some of which are involved in inflammation.

Psychomotor stimulant drug   A drug which can reduce fatigue and elevate mood. They are also referred to as psychostimulants, psychoanaleptics, psychoactivators and psychotonics.

Pulmonary emphysema   A chronic lung disease in which the walls of adjacent alveoli and bronchioles degenerate forming cavities in the lung tissue.

Purulent secretion   A secretion (e.g. nasal) containing a bacterial infection.

Receptor   An area on a macromolecule through which endogenous bio-chemicals or drugs can interact to produce a cellular response.

Respiratory quotient   A parameter used to indicate the nutrient mole-cules being metabolized within the body. It can be determined by dividing the amount of carbon dioxide produced by the amount of oxygen con-sumed. On a balanced diet the respiratory quotient should approximate to 0.85.

Re-uptake   The mechanism by which neurotransmitters, released from nerve terminals, are taken back into the nerve ending for storage and re-release.

Rheumatic fever   Damage to valves of the heart caused by a streptococcal bacterial infection. It is an autoimmune response to the streptococcal toxin.

Rheumatoid arthritis   An autoimmune disease principally affecting joints, characterized by pain, inflammation and stiffness.

Rhinitis   Inflammation of the mucous membrane within the nose resulting in increased mucus secretion. Rhinitis may be caused by infection or an allergic response.

Salicylates   Drugs that are chemically related to salicylic acid. They possess anti-inflammatory, antipyretic and analgesic activity.

Sedative drug   A drug which can calm an anxious person without inducing sleep.

Selectivity   The ability of a drug to exert a greater effect on a particular population of receptors due to its chemical structure. This property reduces the incidence of side-effects.

Serotonin   A neurotransmitter substance, also known as 5-hydroxytryptamine.

Spermatogenesis   The production of sperm cells from spermatogonia or germ cells within the seminiferous tubules of the testes.

Stroke volume   The amount of blood pumped by the ventricles within each beat of the heart.

Sympathomimetic drug   A drug which mimics some or all of the effects produced by stimulation of the sympathetic nervous system. The effects it produces depend upon the adrenoceptors through which it interacts.

Synapse   The narrow gap between the nerve terminal and its target cell into which the neurotransmitter is released.

Tachycardia   A rate of beating of the heart above the normal rate.

Tachyphylaxis   A rapid decrease in the effect of a drug as the dosage is repeated. It is probably caused by desensitization of receptors.

Therapeutic effect   The desired response of a drug taken to treat or cure a disease.

Tolerance   The effect whereby increasing doses of a drug have to be given to maintain the desired effect.

Urticaria   A localized rash on the skin, usually due to an allergic reaction.

Vascular permeability   The passage of fluid and solutes across the membranes of blood vessels.

Vasoconstriction The reduction in the diameter of blood vessels produced by contraction of the smooth muscle in the walls.

Vasodilation Relaxation of vascular smooth muscle leading to an increase in the diameter of blood vessels resulting in a fall in blood pressure.

Withdrawal syndrome The physical response of an individual who is deprived of a drug on which he or she has become physically dependent.

Index